DFG

Essential
BAT Value Documentations

The MAK-Collection

Current Volumes

Part I: MAK Value Documentations, Volume 21
2005. 3-527-31134-3

Part II: BAT Value Documentations, Volume 4
Drexler, H. (ed.)
2005. ISBN 3-527-27049-3

Part III: Air Monitoring Methods, Volume 9
Parlar, H. (ed.)
2005. ISBN 3-527-31138-6

Part IV: Biomonitoring Methods, Volume 10
Angerer, J. (ed.)
2006. ISBN 3-527-31137-8

The MAK-Collection online
www.mak-collection.com

A special selection to start with...

Essential MAK Value Documentations
Greim, H. (ed.)
2006. ISBN 3-527-31394-X

Essential Air Monitoring Methods
Parlar, H. / Greim, H. (eds.)
2006. ISBN 3-527-31476-8

Essential Biomonitoring Methods
Angerer, J. / Greim, H. (eds.)
2006. ISBN 3-527-31478-4

DFG Deutsche Forschungsgemeinschaft

Essential BAT Value Documentations

from the MAK-Collection
for Occupational Health and Safety

Edited by Hans Drexler and Helmut Greim

Working Group
Setting of Threshold Limit Values
in Biological Materials
(Head of the Working Group: Hans Drexler)

Commission for the Investigation
of Health Hazards of Chemical Compounds
in the Work Area
(Chairman: Helmut Greim)
WILEY-VCH Verlag GmbH & Co. KGaA

WILEY-VCH

WILEY-VCH Verlag GmbH & Co. KGaA

Prof. Dr. med. H. Greim
Senatskommission zur Prüfung
gesundheitsschädlicher Arbeitsstoffe
der Deutschen Forschungsgemeinschaft
Technische Universität München
Institut für Toxikologie
Hohenbachernstr. 15–17
85354 Freising-Weihenstephan
Germany

Prof. Dr. med. H. Drexler
Institut und Poliklinik für Arbeits-,
Sozial- und Umweltmedizin
der Universität Erlangen-Nürnberg
Schillerstr. 25 /29
91054 Erlangen
Germany

Important Notice
This volume presents a selection of documentations or methods taken from published volumes of the MAK-Collection. These include occupational exposure values (MAK and BAT values, EKA, BLW) or classifications which may have changed since the publication of the respective volume. Readers are advised to consult the latest edition of the "List of MAK and BAT Values", which is published annually both in print and online (www.mak-collection.com), for current occupational exposure values and classifications.

Library of Congress Card No.: applied for

British Library Cataloging-in-Publication Data: A catalogue record for this book is available from the British Library.

Bibliographic information published by Die Deutsche Bibliothek
Die Deutsche Bibliothek lists this publication in the Deutsche Nationalbibliografie; detailed bibliographic data is available in the Internet at http://dnb.ddb.de.

Printing betz-druck GmbH, Darmstadt
Binding Litges & Dopf Buchbinderei GmbH, Heppenheim

Printed in the Federal Republic of Germany

Printed on acid-free paper

ISBN-13: 978-3-527-31477-5
ISBN-10: 3-527-31477-6

Preface

The year 2005 has marked both the 50th anniversary of the *Commission for the Investigation of Health Hazards of Chemical Compounds in the Work Area* of the Deutsche Forschungsgemeinschaft (DFG, German Research Foundation) as well as the launch of the new international reference series, the *MAK-Collection for Occupational Health and Safety*. Together with the annual *List of MAK and BAT Values*, this series comprises the Commission's English language publications, which are available both in print and online. The series has four parts, each part continuing an established book series:

- MAK Value Documentations (prior title: *Occupational Toxicants*)
- BAT Value Documentations (prior title: *Biological Exposure Values for Occupational Toxicants*)
- Air Monitoring Methods (prior title: *Analyses of Hazardous Substances in Air*)
- Biomonitoring Methods (prior title: *Analyses of Hazardous Substances in Biological Materials*)

For those unfamiliar with these publications and the wealth and quality of information offered through the *MAK-Collection*, we have an additional new design feature on offer: special editions, named *Essentials*, with 20 highlights from each part of the Collection. These *Essentials* are particularly relevant to professionals and researchers in the fields of occupational health and safety. This *Essentials* features a special selection of *BAT Value Documentations* taken from previous volumes of the *MAK-Collection*. The selected documentations are exemplary for the standards maintained by the Commission, which works strictly according to scientific criteria. Also included are general chapters, which outline the concepts of BAT values, BLW and EKA. We hope that this selection will prove useful for fostering occupational health and safety as well as toxicological research around the globe.

We would like to thank the members and guests of the Commission's working group "Setting of Threshold Limit Values in Biological Materials", who have contributed with all their expertise to the respective documentations. Thanks also go to the Commission's scientific secretariat who have thoroughly reviewed the documentations and for the assistance of the translators, all of whom have made them ready for publication with outstanding accuracy. We would also like to thank the publisher Wiley-VCH for editorial guidance, swift production and world-wide distribution. Last, but not least, we are thankful for the continuing support of the Deutsche Forschungsgemeinschaft (DFG).

December 2005

H. Drexler Chairman of the Working Group "Setting of Threshold Limit Values in Biological Materials"	H. Greim Chairman of the Commission for the Investigation of Health Hazards of Chemical Compounds in the Work Area

Essential BAT Value Documentations. DFG, Deutsche Forschungsgemeinschaft

ISBN 3-527-31477-6

Contents

General Aspects

Concepts of Biological Limit Values – The BAT Concept 3

The BLW Concept (Biologischer Leitwert) 8

The EKA Concept – Exposure Equivalent for Carcinogenic Substances
(Expositionsäquivalent für krebserzeugende Arbeitsstoffe) 13

Comparison of the BAT and EKA
Values with the American Biological Exposure Indices (BEIs) 15

Quality Control of Biological
Monitoring in Occupational Medicine 21

Substances

Acetone 35

Alkali chromates (Cr(VI)) 49

Aniline 67

Arsenic and inorganic arsenic compounds 77
(with the exception of arsenic hydride and its salts)

Arsenic trioxide 85

Benzene 99

2-Butanone 115

2-Butoxyethanol 123

Cobalt 137

Cresols (all isomers) 149

Cyclohexane 159

4,4'-Diaminodiphenylmethane 169

Dimethyl sulfate 179

Ethylene oxide 187

Hydrogen fluoride and inorganic fluorine compounds (Fluorides) 195

Essential BAT Value Documentations. DFG, Deutsche Forschungsgemeinschaft

ISBN 3-527-31477-6

Lead and its compounds (except lead arsenate, lead chromate and alkyllead compounds) 205

Lead and its compounds, Addendum (except lead arsenate, lead chromate and alkyllead compounds) 245

Lead and its compounds (except lead arsenate, lead chromate and alkyllead compounds) 253

Methanol 255

Nickel and sparingly soluble nickel compounds 271
(Nickel as nickel metal, nickel sulphide, sulphidic ores, nickel oxide, nickel carbonate)

2-Propanol 283

Styrene 293

Addendum to Styrene 309

Tetrachloroethene 315

Tetrachloroethene, Addendum 329

Vinyl chloride 333

Xylenes 341

Index for Volumes 1–4 355

General Aspects

Essential BAT Value Documentations. DFG, Deutsche Forschungsgemeinschaft

ISBN 3-527-31477-6

Concepts of Biological Limit Values (BAT Values, EKA and BLW)

The BAT Concept – Biological Tolerance Value for Occupational Exposures (Biologischer Arbeitsstoff-Toleranz-Wert)

Definition

The BAT value ("Biologischer Arbeitsstoff-Toleranz-Wert": biological tolerance value for occupational exposures) is defined as the maximum permissible quantity of a chemical substance or its metabolites or the maximum permissible deviation from the norm of biological parameters induced by these substances in exposed humans. The BAT value is established on the basis of currently available scientific data which indicate that these concentrations generally do not affect the health of the employee adversely, even when they are attained regularly under workplace conditions. As with MAK values, BAT values are established on the assumption that persons are exposed at work for at most 8 hours daily and 40 hours weekly. BAT values established on this basis may also be applied without the use of correction factors to other patterns of working hours.

BAT values can be defined as concentrations or rates of formation or excretion (quantity per unit time). BAT values are conceived as ceiling values for healthy individuals. They are generally established for blood and/or urine and take into account the effects of the substances and an appropriate safety margin, being based on occupational medical and toxicological criteria for the prevention of adverse effects on health.

Prerequisites

By definition, BAT values can be established only for such substances which can be taken up by the body in substantial quantities via the lungs and/or other body surfaces

Essential BAT Value Documentations. DFG, Deutsche Forschungsgemeinschaft

ISBN 3-527-31477-6

(skin, gastrointestinal tract) during occupational exposure. Another prerequisite for the establishment of a BAT value is that sufficient occupational-medical and toxicological data are available for the substance and that these data are supported by observations in man. The data must have been obtained with reliable methods. For the establishment of new BAT values and the annual review of the list, the submission of suggestions and reports of experience with such substances in man is requested.

Derivation of BAT Values

The derivation of a BAT value can be based on various constellations of scientific data which reveal a quantitative relationship between exposure concentration and body burden and therefore permit the linking of MAK and BAT values. These include

- studies which reveal a direct relationship between concentrations of a substance, metabolite or adduct in biological material (body burden) and adverse effects on health
- studies which reveal a relationship between a biological indicator (effect parameter) and adverse effects on health.

The following considerations of sex-specific factors apply for the establishment of BAT values:

1. The range of the variation in human anatomical and physiological differences which affect the toxicokinetics of a substance is very wide even for a single sex; the ranges for the two sexes overlap.
2. The resulting sex-specific differences in toxicokinetics vary in a range which is insignificant compared with the uncertainty involved in establishing threshold values.
3. Pregnancy can be associated with certain changes in the toxicokinetics of xenobiotics. In practice, however, the effects of these changes are limited, so that for health protection at the workplace it is the effects on the embryo and foetus which are of particular importance.

Documentation

The reasons why a BAT value was established at a particular level are documented by the Commission for the Investigation of Health Hazards of Chemical Compounds in the Work Area in a loose-leaf collection entitled “Arbeitsmedizinisch-toxikologische Begründungen von BAT-Werten”. Some of these documents are available in English in the present series. They combine a critical review of the available data with comments on the values for the parameters which have been shown in practice to make a useful contribution to occupational hygiene.

Purpose

In the context of specific occupational-medical check-ups, BAT values are intended to protect employees from impairment of health at work. They provide a basis for deciding whether the amount of a chemical substance taken up by the organism is harmful or not. For substances that can be absorbed through the skin, individual exposures can be determined only by biological monitoring. When using BAT values, the medical exclusion criteria defined by the "Berufsgenossenschaft" (Employers' Liability Insurance Association) in the guidelines for occupational medical check-ups must be observed. BAT values are not suitable for the derivation, by means of fixed conversion factors, of biological threshold values for long-term non-occupational exposures such as from air pollution or contaminants in food.

Correlations between BAT and MAK Values

When a substance is inhaled under steady state conditions in controlled laboratory experiments, the relationship between the BAT and MAK values can be expressed in terms of pharmacokinetic functions. Under workplace conditions, however, it is not necessarily possible to deduce the level of a substance to which a particular person was exposed from its specific biological parameter in that person because a series of other factors in addition to the amount of substance in the air can determine the extent of exposure of the organism. These factors include the level of physical activity (respiratory minute volume), absorption through the skin and individual variations in metabolic or excretory patterns.

It is therefore particularly difficult to evaluate field studies which describe the relationships between internal and external exposure to substances which can be absorbed percutaneously. Experience has shown that studies of such substances frequently yield discrepant results. These discrepancies are attributed to different levels of dermal exposure under the different study conditions. When evaluating such results to determine relationships between MAK and BAT values, priority should be given to studies in which the data suggest that skin absorption played a minor role.

In general for substances with low vapour pressure which are readily absorbed through the skin, there is no correlation between exposure concentration and body burden. For these substances a BAT value can often be established only on the basis of a relationship between body burden and effect.

In addition, the concentrations of substances in the workplace air may vary with time and the biological parameters may not vary to the same extent. Therefore observance of BAT values does not make it unnecessary to monitor the concentrations of substances in the workplace air. This applies especially for local irritants and caustic substances. When evaluating macromolecular adducts of foreign substances it should be borne in mind that the persistance of these adducts can lead to discrepancies between the pattern of external exposure and the behaviour of the biological parameters. Similar considerations apply for all highly cumulative substances such as heavy metals and polyhalogenated hydrocarbons.

In spite of all these interfering factors and the consequent differences in the definitions of MAK and BAT values, the two thresholds are generally based on equivalent effects of substances on the organism. However, for substances for which the MAK value is not established on the basis of systemic effects but because of local irritation of skin and mucous membranes, a BAT value can still be based on "critical toxicity" resulting from systemic exposure. In such exceptional cases where the MAK and BAT values are based on different end points, the two values do not necessarily correspond.

Surveillance

The protection of the health of the individual, which is the reason for establishing BAT values, can be monitored by periodic quantitative determination of the chemical compounds or their metabolites or of biological parameters in biological material. The methods used must be diagnostically specific and sensitive enough for the purpose, acceptable to the employee and practicable for the physician. The sampling time, that is, the measurement strategy, must take into account both the exposure conditions at the workplace and the pharmacokinetics of the substance. As a rule, especially for substances which accumulate in the organism, this may be achieved by taking samples at the end of a working day after an extended period of work (working week).

During exposure to gaseous substances which are metabolized rapidly and for which the blood/air distribution coefficient is larger than 10, it must be taken into account that the concentrations of the substances in blood and tissues are positively correlated with the level of physical activity.

The concentrations of inhaled gaseous substances in blood and tissues of persons working under hyperbaric pressure have been shown to be correlated positively with the pressure. In such cases the observance of the BAT value must be monitored more frequently as the BAT value is attained in such workers at lower exposure concentrations than in persons working at normal pressures.

Whole blood, serum and urine samples are used as assay materials, occasionally and under certain conditions, also samples of alveolar air. Saliva and hair samples are not suitable assay materials for occupational medical biomonitoring.

The analytical methods must yield reliable results and meet the requirements of statistical quality control (TRGS 410 of the regulations for hazardous chemicals at the workplace). In the collection "Analysen in biologischem Material" (available in English in the series "Analyses of Hazardous Substances in Biological Materials"), the Commission's "Analytical Chemistry" group has compiled a series of methods which may be considered reliable for this purpose.

Evaluation of Analytical Data

Like any results of laboratory investigations, toxicological analytical data can only be evaluated given knowledge of the whole situation. As well as the other medical findings, especially
- the dynamics of pathophysiological processes
- the short-term effects of exposure-free periods
- the long-term effects of ageing
- the specific workplace conditions
- intensive physical activity and unusual conditions of atmospheric pressure

and any individual background exposures must be taken into account.

Results from analyses in biological material are subject to medical discretion. Only the physician who is responsible may interpret the results.

BAT values are established on the basis of the results of scientific studies and practical medical experience.

Allergenic Substances

Depending on individual disposition, allergic reactions can be induced by various kinds of substance, more or less rapidly and in differing degrees of severity after sensitization of, for example, the skin or respiratory passages. The observance of BAT values cannot provide a guarantee that such reactions will not occur.

Mixtures of Substances

BAT values apply as a rule for exposure to pure substances. They are not necessarily applicable for persons exposed to preparations containing more than one toxic substance (blends, mixtures, solutions). This is especially true for BAT values requiring determination of the substance itself or its metabolites. For mixtures of components with similar effects, a BAT value based on a biological parameter can be helpful in the assessment of health risks, as long as it provides a measure of critical clinical-functional effects of the components. The Commission makes every effort to define and publish such criteria for the biological effects of interfering components of mixtures.

The BLW Concept (Biologischer Leitwert)

Introduction

Biological monitoring is the analysis of a hazardous chemical, its metabolites or other parameters linked to the substance in the blood or urine of man. It allows an assessment of individual exposure to the chemical or even the effects. In addition to ambient air monitoring it provides an instrument of surveillance and health protection at the workplace.

For practical reasons, it is important that this exposure or its effects can be evaluated by comparing the result of the analysis with a limit value. For this purpose the Deutsche Forschungsgemeinschaft (DFG) has established biological tolerance values for occupational exposures (Biologische Arbeitsstoff-Toleranzwerte, BAT). Ideally, the BAT values are based on the quantitative relationship between the internal dose of the chemical and its effects on health. A historical example is the correlation between the concentration of lead in blood or δ-aminolaevulinic acid in the urine and the effects of the metal on the haematopoietic system. However, due to low exposure levels at modern workplaces, the quantitative relationship between the internal dose and the detrimental effects on health can very often not be determined. In these cases, the BAT value is deduced indirectly from the maximum workplace concentration (Maximale Arbeitsplatz-Konzentration, MAK), which is the limit value in ambient air. This is possible because the MAK value generally guarantees the absence of adverse effects on health. A typical example is the BAT value for toluene in blood and for *o*-cresol in urine. In this case, it is assumed that observance of the BAT value implies compliance with the MAK value and that adverse effects on health can therefore be ruled out. For carcinogenic substances the DFG has established exposure equivalents (Expositionsäquivalente für krebserzeugende Arbeitsstoffe, EKA). These are not limit values; they merely show the quantitative relationship between the external and internal dose.

Yet there are numerous hazardous chemicals at the workplace for which neither BAT nor EKA values can be established. This is especially the case if the external and the internal concentrations cannot be correlated, either as a matter of principle or due to lack of data. Examples are

- substances that penetrate the skin
- substances that are taken up orally
- tasks in which respiratory protection is used
- tasks that are performed outdoors.

In addition, it may be important to consider non-genotoxic end points of carcinogenic chemicals. Exposure surveillance should be established for sensitizing agents, even though a level of safety cannot be determined. For substances for which the evaluation of a BAT value or an EKA correlation is problematical, a new threshold limit has been

Essential BAT Value Documentations. DFG, Deutsche Forschungsgemeinschaft

ISBN 3-527-31477-6

created. The working group Setting of Threshold Limit Values in Biological Material has called this the BLW (Biologischer Leitwert) (see Hallier *et al.* 2001).

Definition

The BLW is the amount of a chemical substance or its metabolites or the deviation from the norm of biological parameters induced by the substance in exposed humans which serves as an indicator for necessary protective measures. BLWs are assigned only for hazardous materials for which the establishment of BAT values is not possible (i.e. for carcinogenic substances and suspected carcinogens in the categories 1 to 3 and for non-carcinogens for which the toxicological data are inadequate).

BLW values are generally established on the assumption that persons are exposed at work for at most 8 hours daily and 40 hours weekly during their working lives.

The BLW is based on occupational-medical information as to the effects of handling the hazardous material together with toxicological data. Since observance of the BLW does not exclude a risk of adverse effects on health, it is necessary to extend our knowledge of the relationships between exposure to the substance, the systemic dose and the resulting risks for health. The BLW values are intended to advance this aim by providing a basis for biomonitoring of exposed persons by the physician. By continual improvement of the industrial situation, occupational hygiene and the protective aspects of work planning, concentrations as far as possible below the BLW should be attained.

Requirements

For substances for which there is no BAT value or for which a value cannot be evaluated, a BLW will therefore be established. These are mainly substances

- which are absorbed readily by the skin (e.g. PAHs, glycol ethers)
- for which at present neither relationships between external and internal exposure nor between internal exposure and the effects can be evaluated, but for which there are sufficient data available from biological monitoring at various workplaces. This is the case when, for example, only relatively few analyses of the workplace air were carried out or the results are not representative of the exposure levels. This often occurs with hazardous substances which are difficult to determine, such as dusts, aerosols etc.
- which at the workplace are ingested to a considerable extent (in the form of dust or as substances bound to dust). Occupational-medical practice has shown that the external exposure of the employee is generally underestimated in such cases. This is also because the actual concentration levels at such workplaces are monitored only very inexactly and on the basis of air samples the exposure cannot be reproduced representatively

- with carcinogenic or genotoxic potential (e.g. aromatic amines)
- with allergic effects, if the sensitizing potential cannot be used at present for establishing a BAT value.

The following must be taken into consideration when establishing BLWs:

- toxicological data, in particular for the mechanism of action and toxicokinetics of the substance
- occupational-medical data
- epidemiology
- background exposure
- existing threshold values in air (MAK)
- validated analytical methods must be available for the selected parameters and the requirements for internal and external quality control must be fulfilled.

Below are some examples to illustrate the problem of setting threshold limit values and offer solutions:

Example 1

Studies performed at workplaces with exposure to polycyclic aromatic hydrocarbons (PAHs) have shown that the excretion of hydroxypyrene in the urine differed by two orders of magnitude between individual workers in spite of comparable ambient exposure. This considerable variation is probably caused by uptake of PAHs by the skin. According to the literature, dermal absorption could account for 50 % to 98 % of the total uptake of PAHs at the workplace (Boogaard and van Sittert 1995, Elovaara *et al.* 1995, Quinlan *et al.* 1995, van Rooji *et al.* 1993a, 1993b).

Even if the concentration of the chemical in ambient air is the same, permeation of the skin can lead to very different internal exposures. Peak values of 700 μg hydroxypyrene per litre urine have been measured. Jongeneelen (1992) calculated that a hydroxypyrene excretion of about 6 μg/g creatinine corresponds to an ambient PAH exposure of about 2 μg benzo(a)pyrene per m^3, which according to the author would lead to a relative cancer risk of 1.3. Thus, at some workplaces substantial improvements in occupational hygiene must be made. This illustrates the necessity for a BLW for evaluating the internal PAH dose.

Example 2

Methyl bromide is used as a fumigant for the control of insects, nematodes and fungi. On account of its marked acute neurotoxic properties, which has led to numerous fatal accidents, methyl bromide is applied solely with respiratory protection independent of the surroundings. Yet methyl bromide is also taken up via the skin, leading to exposure of the fumigators. In addition, the masks may not necessarily be impervious. Since the uptake of methyl bromide by inhalation is prevented by respiratory protection, surveillance of the ambient air at the site of fumigation is insufficient. Therefore a biological monitoring procedure was developed on the basis of serum albumin adducts (determination of *S*-methylcysteine) (Müller *et al.* 1994) and tested in an occupational field study (Hallier 1986). (Note: for reasons of analytical practicability, bromide in serum was later chosen as the biomonitoring parameter for methyl bromide). Among the 28 fumigators tested, two individuals with especially high adduct values were conspicuous, whereas the rest of the workers had adduct values which were only slightly (up to 2.5 times) higher than those in unexposed controls. It could be shown that shortcomings in occupational hygiene were responsible for the two high values.

In this example, a conventional limit value such as the BAT is inappropriate, due to the lack of correlation between the external and the internal dose (respiratory protection equipment, skin absorption). Yet a biological monitoring procedure and data on typical blood levels under workplace exposure are available, so that a BLW could be established. Such a value could lead to an improvement in workplace risk prevention and pinpoint shortcomings in occupational hygiene.

Example 3

Another example is arsenic. According to definition, MAK and BAT values cannot be evaluated for the carcinogenic arsenic compounds. In Germany there was a technically based TRK value of 0.1 mg arsenic per m^3 ambient air. According to the EKA, this level in air corresponds to 130 μg/l arsenic in urine at the end of the shift. Arsenic compounds are not only carcinogenic but are also toxic to the skin, the blood vessels and the nervous system. Adverse toxic effects of arsenic have been reported at urinary excretion levels lower than 130 μg/l (Heyman *et al.* 1956, Lagerkvist *et al.* 1986, 1988).
Therefore, a BLW was evaluated to prevent toxic effects.

Example 4

Sensitization and the induction of allergic symptoms are both concentration-dependent phenomena. Therefore exposure to allergens should be limited. As long as threshold values cannot be derived, sensitization and allergic reactions are not suitable end points for MAK or BAT values. A number of occupational allergens can however be surveilled by biological monitoring (e.g. platinum excretion after occupational exposure to platinum salts) in order to identify hazardous workplaces and to implement occupational hygiene (Drexler and Göen 2000, Drexler *et al.* 1999).

References

Boogaard PJ, van Sittert NJ (1995) Urinary 1-hydroxypyrene as biomarker of exposure to polycyclic aromatic hydrocarbons in workers in petrochemical industries: baseline values and dermal uptake. Sci Total Environ 163: 203–209

Drexler H, Göen T (2000) Der Beitrag des biologischen Monitorings zur Risikoerfassung beim Umgang mit sensibilisierenden Arbeitsstoffen am Beispiel der Diacarbonsäureanhydride. Arbeitsmed Sozialmed Umweltmed 35: 136–145

Drexler H, Schaller KH, Nielsen J, Weber A, Weihrauch M, Welinder H, Skerfving S (1999) Efficacy of hygienic measures in workers sensitised to acid anhydrides and the influence of selection bias on the results. Occup Environ Med 56: 145–151

Elovaara E, Heikkilä P, Pyy L, Mutanen P, Riihimäki V (1995): Significance of dermal and respiratory uptake in creosote workers: exposure to polycyclic aromatic hydrocarbons and urinary excretion of 1-hydroxypyrene. Occup Environ Med 52: 196–203

Hallier E (1986) Arbeitsmedizinische Untersuchungen zur Problematik der Durchführung von Begasungen mit Methylbromid. Deutsche Hochschulschriften Nr. 1089, Verlag Hänsel-Hohenhausen, Egelsbach, 1986

Hallier E, Angerer J, Drexler H, Filser JG, Lewalter J, Stork J (2001) Biologische Leitwerte (BLW). Arbeitsmed Sozialmed Umweltmed 36: 6–9

Heyman A, Pfeiffer JB, Willett RW, Taylor HM (1956) Peripheral neuropathy caused by arsenical intoxication: A study of 41 cases with observation on the effect of BAL. N Engl J Med 254: 401–409

Jongeneelen FJ (1992) Biological exposure limit for occupational exposure to coal tar pitch volatiles at cokeovens. Int Arch Occup Environ Health 63: 511–516

Lagerkvist B, Linderholm H, Nordberg GF (1986) Vasospastic tendency and Raynaud's phenomenon in smelter workers exposed to arsenic. Environ Res 39: 465–474

Lagerkvist B, Linderholm H, Nordberg GF (1988) Arsenic and Raynaud's phenomenon. Vasospastic tendency and excretion of arsenic in smelter workers before and after the summer vacation. Int Arch Occup Environ Health 60: 361–364

Müller AMF, Hallier E, Westphal G, Schröder KR, Bolt HM (1994) Determination of methylated globin and albumin for biomonitoring of exposure to methylating agents using HPLC with precolumn fluorescent derivatization. Anal Bioanal Chem 350: 712-7-15

Quinlan R, Kowalczyk G, Gardiner K, Calvert IA, Hale K, Walton ST (1995) Polycyclic aromatic hydrocarbon exposure in coal liquefaction workers: the value of urinary 1-hydroxypyrene excretion in the development of occupational hygiene control strategies. Ann Occup Hyg 39: 329–346

van Rooji JGM, Bodelier-Bade MM, Jongeneelen FJ (1993a) Estimation of individual dermal and respiratory uptake of polycyclic aromatic hydrocarbons in 12 coke oven workers. Br J Ind Med 50: 623–632

van Rooji JGM, van Lieshout EMA, Bodelier-Bade MM, Jongeneelen FJ (1993b) Effect of the reduction of skin contamination on the internal dose of creosote workers, exposed to polycyclic aromatic hydrocarbons. Scan J Work Environ Health 19: 200–207

The EKA Concept – Exposure Equivalent for Carcinogenic Substances (Expositionsäquivalent für krebserzeugende Arbeitsstoffe)

Definition

BAT values are not established for chemical substances which, by their own action or by that of their reactive intermediates or metabolites, are known to cause malignant growths in man or for which there is good evidence of a human cancer risk because at present it is not possible to specify safe levels of such substances in biological materials. Therefore the handling of carcinogens must take place under the conditions described in Section III of the "List of MAK and BAT Values". The determination of carcinogenic substances in biological material is not carried out for the application of a BAT value in the strict sense but rather for the occupational medical detection and quantification of the individual exposure to the substance. Concentrations of the substance or its metabolites in biological material which are higher than those known to correspond to the concentration of the substance in the workplace air are indicative of additional exposure by other routes, usually percutaneous.

For this reason, the Commission investigates the relationships between the concentration of the carcinogen in the workplace air and that of the substance or its metabolites in biological material ("Expositionsäquivalente für krebserzeugende Arbeitsstoffe", EKA: exposure equivalents for carcinogenic substances). From these relationships, the internal exposure which results from uptake of the substance exclusively by inhalation may be determined.

In addition, the considerations expressed in the section "Correlations between MAK and BAT Values" apply to substances which may be absorbed percutaneously.

Essential BAT Value Documentations. DFG, Deutsche Forschungsgemeinschaft

ISBN 3-527-31477-6

Comparison of the BAT and EKA Values with the American Biological Exposure Indices (BEIs)

Scientifically documented occupational-medical threshold values in biological materials are at present drawn up by only two institutions. One of these is the DFG Commission for the Investigation of Health Hazards of Chemical Compounds in the Work Area whose working group "Setting of threshold limit values in biological materials" establishes the BAT and EKA values. The other institution is the BEI Committee of the American Conference of Governmental Industrial Hygienists (ACGIH), who draw up the Biological Exposure Indices (BEIs). Both groups publish annual lists with biological threshold values for monitoring occupationally exposed persons (3, 4). In the following chapter, the definitions of the two threshold values are presented and discussed.

BAT Values

In 1979 the Commission for the Investigation of Health Hazards of Chemical Compounds in the Work Area set up the working group "Setting of threshold limit values in biological materials". This group has drawn up guidelines for the prevention of disease in the individual on the basis of biological indicators and formulated a concept for the meaning and use in practice and documentation of such indicators (9, 10). The occupational-medical threshold value was given the name "Biological tolerance value for occupational exposures (BAT value)".

Unlike the American definition, the German BAT values are conceived as ceiling values for toxic substances in individuals.

The definition is as follows: The BAT value ("Biologischer Arbeitsstoff-Toleranz-Wert": biological tolerance value for occupational exposures) is defined as the maximum permissible quantity of a chemical substance or its metabolites or the maximum permissible deviation from the norm of biological parameters induced by these substances in exposed humans. The BAT value is established on the basis of currently available scientific data which indicate that these concentrations generally do not affect the health of the employee adversely, even when they are attained regularly under workplace conditions. Like for the MAK values, the exposure period is usually a maximum of 8 hours a day and 40 hours a week. BAT values can be defined as concentrations, formation rates or excretion rates (amount/unit of time).

Unlike in the American BEI list, which does not differentiate between carcinogenic and non-carcinogenic substances, in Germany carcinogenic substances are not given BAT values, as at present no safe value can be given. For these substances the working group establishes relationships between the substance concentration in the air at the

Essential BAT Value Documentations. DFG, Deutsche Forschungsgemeinschaft

ISBN 3-527-31477-6

workplace and the concentration of the substance or its metabolites in biological materials (exposure equivalents for carcinogenic substances (EKA)). These show the level of internal exposure resulting from inhalation exposure only.

The occupational-medical documentation of the BAT values and EKAs is published in German and English (6, 7, 8).

BEIs

The BEI Committee was founded in autumn 1982 as a technical committee of the American Conference of Governmental Industrial Hygienists (ACGIH). The aims of the BEI Committee were to consider the concept of biological monitoring and, in addition to workplace monitoring on the basis of the Threshold Limit Values (TLVs), to evaluate biological threshold values. Furthermore, they intended to make known and promote biological monitoring as an instrument for determining potentially toxic substances at the workplace (2).

The BEI Committee started off with five voting members and two non-voting advisors. Importance was laid on both multi-disciplinary and international co-operation in the committee. In the meantime the committee is made up of eleven members. As a result of one member belonging to both the BAT and BEI group, an intensive and successful exchange of experience between the two groups is guaranteed. The procedure of the BEI group is in accordance with that of the TLV Committee. The working group meets twice a year to discuss the BEI documentation which is drawn up by individual members of the committee. This toxicological documentation contains the data necessary to establish a threshold value. The documentation is discussed in detail and revised many times and the suggested BEI then passed by vote. In a second stage the recommended BEIs are submitted to the ACGIH Board and subsequently to the members at the annual business meeting for approval. The BEIs are then published in the annual TLV/BEI list. The values are kept on a provisional list for at least two years (notice of intent to establish or change). During this period all ACGIH members and other interested parties are asked to make their comments. After this period the BEIs are then finally adopted (adopted biological exposure determinants). The TLV list contained BEIs for the first time in 1984/85. The occupational-medical–toxicological documentation for the BEIs are published in a loose-leaf collection (1).

The concept of the BEIs has often been discribed in the literature (5, 11, 12, 13).

BEIs are reference values intended as guidelines for the evaluation of potential health hazards in the practice of industrial hygiene. BEIs represent the levels of determinants which are most likely to be observed in specimens collected from a healthy worker who has been exposed to chemicals to the same extent as a worker with inhalation exposure to the TLV. Exceptions are the BEIs for substances for which the TLVs serve as protection against non-systemic effects (e.g. irritation or respiratory disorders) or for substances which require biological monitoring due to other routes of absorption, in particular the skin. The BEIs for such chemicals can be based on the avoidance of systemic effects and it is therefore possible that the internal exposure exceeds the pulmonary uptake resulting from exposure at the level of the TLV.

BEIs do not indicate a sharp distinction between hazardous and non-hazardous exposures. Due to biological variability, it is possible for an individual's measurements to exceed the BEI without incurring an increased health risk. If, however, measurements in specimens obtained from a worker on different occasions persistently exceed the BEI, or if the majority of measurements in specimens obtained from a group of workers at the same workplace exceed the BEI, the cause of the excessive values must be investigated and proper action taken to reduce the exposure.

BEIs, like BAT values, apply to eight-hour exposures, five days a week. BEIs for other working schedules can be extrapolated on pharmacokinetic and pharmacodynamic bases. BEIs should not be applied either directly or through a conversion factor, in the determination of safe levels for non-occupational exposures. The BEIs are not intended for use as a measure of adverse effects or for diagnosis of occupational illness.

Discussion

For many substances and groups of substances the BAT/EKA values differ from the BEIs, sometimes considerably. Usually the BEIs are lower than the corresponding BAT values. This is already apparent from the definitions the threshold values are based on. The BEI is understood as the average value in human samples of persons exposed at the level of the TLV. Individual measurements may have concentrations above the BEI, but must be compensated for by a comparable number of values below the BEI. The BEI is therefore to be interpreted as an advisory level, which may be exceeded in a group of exposed persons and also by individuals. Only after the BEI has been exceeded over a longer period of time are measures to reduce exposure necessary. A further criteria for such measures is the frequent occurrence of high levels of exposure in a group of persons employed in the same work area. In America, both the works medical centre and also the industrial hygienist carry out biological monitoring in practice.

The BAT values, however, serve to protect the individual and are conceived as ceiling values for healthy individuals, which may not be exceeded. They are used as part of special medical monitoring programmes to protect the health of the workers at the workplace. The BAT values serve as a basis for evaluating the risk represented by certain amounts of hazardous substances taken up by the organism. If the threshold values are exceeded, measures must be taken which can range from improved occupational hygiene at the workplace to imposing temporary or permanent non-exposure. The medical exclusion criteria according to the guidelines issued by the German Employers' Liability Insurance Association (Berufsgenossenschaft) for occupational-medical health surveillance must be taken into consideration when using BAT values. The results of analyses in biological materials are subject to medical discretion in Germany. Generally it is the doctor who interprets them and bears the responsibility.

When comparing BAT/EKAs and BEIs, it must further be borne in mind that, as a result of diverging MAK and TLV-TWA values, the biological threshold values can vary. These differences in the tolerable external exposure are noticeable when the evaluation of the threshold value is based on the relationship between external to internal exposure.

The biological exposure parameters selected can cause further differences between the two lists. In the list of BAT values, parameters of effect are listed more often for biological monitoring than in the American list. Also in Germany, unlike in America, solvent concentrations in blood are used as parameters. Due to the often very short biological half-lives of solvents in biological materials, they can only be used if the sampling times are strictly adhered to. This is obviously possible in Germany, as monitoring is carried out by well-trained occupational physicians. In America monitoring is often carried out by industrial hygienists. With this structure blood sampling causes problems, particularly if they must be received by a certain time. In the American list the solvent metabolites are therefore preferred as monitoring parameters.

The above explains the differences observed when comparing the threshold values of the two lists, but the main reason is the different philosophies on which they are based. In recent years, however, more values have corresponded. The current wish for harmonisation of the threshold values, first expressed at the international workshop of 1996, is to be welcomed. The initiative for harmonisation of occupational-medical threshold values comes from both ACGIH and the DFG Commission for the Investigation of Health Hazards of Chemical Compounds in the Work Area.

References

1. ACGIH: Documentation of the threshold limit values and biological exposure indices, Sixth Edition, American Conference of Governmental Industrial Hygienists, Inc., Cincinnati, Ohio (1991)
2. ACGIH: Topics in Biological Monitoring, American Conference of Governmental Industrial Hygienists, Inc., Cincinnati, Ohio (1995)
3. ACGIH: Threshold Limit Values for Chemical Substances and Physical Agents and Biological Exposure Indices, American Conference of Governmental Industrial Hygienists, Inc., Cincinnati, Ohio (1995–1996)
4. Greim, H. (Ed.): List of MAK and BAT Values 1997, Maximum Concentrations and Biological Tolerance Values at the Workplace, Commission for the Investigation of Health Hazards of Chemical Compounds in the Work Area, Report No. 33, VCH-Verlagsgesellschaft, Weinheim (1997)
5. Fiserova-Bergerova, V.: History and Concept of Biological Exposure Indices, in: Fiserova-Bergerova, V., Ogata, M.: Biological Monitoring of Exposure to Industrial Chemicals, American Conference of Governmental Industrial Hygienists, Inc., Cincinnati, Ohio (1990), pp 19–23
6. Greim, H., Lehnert, G. (Eds.): Biological Exposure Values for Occupational Toxicants and Carcinogens – Critical Data Evaluation for BAT and EKA Values, Vol. 2, VCH-Verlagsgesellschaft, Weinheim (1995)

7. Henschler, D., Lehnert, G. (Eds.): Biologische Arbeitsstoff-Toleranz-Werte (BAT-Werte) und Expositionsäquivalente für krebserzeugende Arbeitsstoffe (EKA), Band 1, VCH-Verlagsgesellschaft, Weinheim (1983–1994)
8. Henschler, D., Lehnert, G. (Eds.): Biological Exposure Values for Occupational Toxicants and Carcinogens – Critical Data Evaluation for BAT and EKA Values, Vol. 1, VCH-Verlagsgesellschaft, Weinheim (1994)
9. Lehnert, G.: Biologischer Arbeitsstoff-Toleranz-Werte: Ein Konzept zur Individualprävention bei Exposition gegenüber gesundheitsschädlichen Arbeitsstoffen. Arbeitsmed. Sozialmed. Präventivmed. *15* (1980), 266–270
10. Lehnert, G., Schaller, K.H.: Strategy of biological monitoring and setting of biological threshold limits (BAT values) in Germany, Isr. J. Med. Sci. *31* (1995), 175–182
11. Lowry, L. K.: The Biological Exposure Index: Its use in assessing chemical exposures in the workplace, Toxicology *47* (1987), 55–69
12. Lowry, L. K.: Biological Limit Values, in: Kneip, J., Grable, J. V. (Eds.): Methods for Biological Monitoring, American Public Health Association, Washington, D.C. (1988), pp 109–119
13. Rosenberg, J., Rempel, D.: Biological Monitoring, Occupational Medicine: State of the Art, Reviews *5* (1990), 491–498

Author: K.H Schaller

(translated from Arbeitsmed. Sozialmed. Umweltmed. *31*, 95–106 (1996))

Quality Control of Biological Monitoring in Occupational Medicine

One of the essential elements of biological monitoring is the analytical determination of parameters in biological materials. Not only the levels of hazardous substances and their metabolites can be considered as parameters, but also effects of the substances on the organism. Measurement of these parameters is mainly carried out in blood and urine samples. The spectrum of parameters used in biological monitoring has been described in the literature (11, 15).

Determination of the parameters includes the pre-analytical phase, i.e. sample collection, storage and transport, through to the analytical determination of the substances and evaluation of the results. The analytical results obtained are evaluated for their occupational-medical and toxicological relevance using the BAT and EKA values and the reference values for the general population. To guarantee that the results obtained in biological monitoring investigations are comparable with these threshold limit values the pre-analytical phase and analytical phase must be carried out in compliance with sampling recommendations, using tested and reliable analytical methods and accompanied by internal and external quality control. This forms the backbone of efficient occupational-medical health care.

1 Pre-analytical Phase (Sample Collection, Transport and Storage)

In all steps before the actual analysis, from the time of sampling the material until removal of a sample from the matrix, confounding influences and interference factors can falsify the results and make interpretation more difficult or even impossible. The main *in vivo* factors that influence the results are the time of sampling and the great variations in the composition of spontaneous urine samples as a result of diuresis. The most important *in vitro* interference factors are:

- exogenous contamination of the material (at the site of sampling)
- contamination of the material from the sampling utensils or the vessels used
- evaporation of volatile components from the material
- absorption of the components to be analysed onto the walls of the vessels used
- changes in the samples during storage and transport (e.g. coagulation of blood samples, sedimentation of urinary components, chemical changes in the parameters).

This means that interference can occur during sampling, transport of the samples—which in the case of occupational-medical toxicology is usually by post or courier—and their subsequent storage in the laboratory. The pre-analytical phase therefore encompasses the time of sampling, correct sampling, the choice of vessel, and transport and

Essential BAT Value Documentations. DFG, Deutsche Forschungsgemeinschaft

ISBN 3-527-31477-6

storage of the samples. Usually the works medical department oversees that these steps in the procedure towards obtaining occupational-medical findings are carried out correctly. Possible confounding influences or interference factors cannot be recognised by quality control. The pre-analytical phase must therefore be co-ordinated with the laboratory before the beginning of an investigation. It is recommended that the services generally offered by the analytical laboratories be taken advantage of and sampling utensils, transport vessels and information on sampling be ordered from them. This is particularly important if specially cleaned vessels or special containers are necessary (5).

1.1 Procedure

Table 1 shows the procedure in the pre-analytical phase for sampling whole blood, plasma/serum, erythrocytes and urine (9, 15).

The materials are usually sampled at the end of the shift, if possible after 3 working days. In some cases the requirements in the current list of BAT/EKA values must be followed (8). The time of sampling is particularly important with substances which are quickly absorbed in relevant amounts and excreted again. This is especially true of many solvents.

The sampling and transport vessels must be adequately labelled for identification. The parameters to be analysed should be listed in an accompanying letter. For analysis of CO-Hb, aromatic hydrocarbons and adducts with chemical agents, data on smoking habits are necessary. For the determination of PCB the age of the person must be given and for blood lead analyses the sex and age. To guarantee optimum sampling, the guidelines on sampling from experienced analytical laboratories should be taken into account (9, 15). If these recommendations regarding the procedure, sampling utensils and vessels are followed, relevant interference factors can be excluded or minimised. Particularly when investigating solvents, the laboratory carrying out the analysis should be consulted. These analytical investigations are usually carried out using head-space gas chromatography. It must be ensured that the head-space vials used for transport and storage are gas-proof and free of contamination and suitable for the head-space sampler used in the laboratory.

In some cases, for example the analysis of adducts or the determination of the chromium(VI) level in erythrocytes, special sample preparation must be carried out. When obtaining blood fractions, the guidelines from the laboratories regarding procedure must be followed. This also applies for the storage and transport of these usually sensitive media.

1.2 Contamination and Losses

In biological monitoring, analytical determination is almost exclusively trace analysis and ultratrace analysis. Preparation of the persons giving the samples and the choice of sampling utensils and vessels must therefore be carried out bearing in mind possible exogenous contamination.

Tab. 1: Recommendations for sampling, storage and transport of biological materials for biological monitoring investigations

Step in the procedure or material	Source of information or aids
1. *Time of sampling*	see List of BAT and MAK Values (8)
2. *Sampling*	
2.1 Blood sampling, venous	
2.1.1 Disinfection of the site of puncture	For analysis of solvents use 3 % hydrogen peroxide solution
2.1.2 Sampling utensils and transport vessels	Disposable syringes and needles e.g. Monovetten®, Vacutainer®
2.1.2.1 Whole blood	5 or 10 ml blood with EDTA-K as anticoagulant
Analytical parameters: inorganic and non-volatile organic substances	Sampling utensils as transport vessel
Analytical parameters: volatile organic substances	Aliquots (1 or 2 ml) in head-space vials
2.1.2.2 Plasma	5–10 ml blood with EDTA-K as anticoagulant
Analytical parameters: metals	Plastic vials, approx. 2–3 ml
Analytical parameters: organo-chlorine compounds	Glassvials , approx. 2–3 ml
2.1.2.3 Serum	5–10 ml blood, Do not use separating gels or coagulation aids Transport vessel see 2.1.2.2.
2.1.2.4 Erythrocytes	5–10 ml blood with EDTA as anticoagulant, separation of the corpuscular components by centrifugation as soon as possible, washing with isotonic saline 3 times, determination of packed cell volume, dispatch in plastic vials
2.2 Urine	
Analytical parameters: inorganic and non-volatile organic substances	Plastic containers or bottles Effective volume 50–100 ml, wide neck
Analytical parameters: volatile organic substances	Aliquots (1 or 2 ml) in head-space vials
2.3 Exhaled air	Special air collection vessels made of glass or plastic or special absorption tubes
3. *Storage and transport of samples*	Dispatch of the samples to the laboratory as soon as possible after sampling; 5 days storage in the refrigerator, longer periods of storage at –18 °C
4. *Dispatch*	By post or courier taking into consideration the conditions for dispatch of infectious materials (protective cover)

For many parameters, for example metals, sampling may only take place after changing into street clothes and always after washing the hands or showering in the works medical department. For the analysis of solvents in blood, wipes containing solvents cannot be used to disinfect the skin before sampling venous blood. Cleansing of the site of puncture with soap and water or 3 % H_2O_2 solution is sufficient.

Due to the great danger of contamination, all materials which come into contact with the body fluids must meet high standards of cleanliness. To prevent carry-over, all sampling utensils and vessels should be discarded after use. Contamination of these disposable articles must be prevented during production, transport and storage. Random checks should be carried out to ensure these vessels are free of contamination. For special purposes these vessels should be swilled out before use with 1M nitric acid followed by distilled water.

Analyte losses occur as a result of evaporation or absorption onto the walls of the vessels and in sediments. For highly volatile substances sealable head-space vials should therefore be used. Absorption losses, in particular of metals, can be counteracted by acidification of the urine samples (1 ml glacial acetic acid/100 ml urine).

2 Analytical Methods

Specific and sensitive analytical methods with defined and tested reliability criteria are indispensable for carrying out the analyses necessary to biological monitoring. They must be reproducible, lead to reliable and comparable results, and also be practicable so that they can be used in routine investigations.

The complex matrix of the biological media and the extremely low concentrations of the parameters usually demand complicated instrumental analysis. The investigations can therefore only be carried out in specialised laboratories. The laboratory is responsible for the analytical reliability of the results (13).

The working group "Analyses of Hazardous Substances in Biological Materials" of the DFG Commission for the Investigation of Health Hazards of Chemical Compounds in the Work Area has published a collection of tested methods and analytical procedures for the requirements of occupational-medical analysis in human biological materials. These methods are recommended by the BAT/EKA working group for the biological monitoring of persons exposed to hazardous substances.

Table 2 shows the analytical procedures contained in this collection of methods, listed according to analytical technique and class of substance. In all, 117 methods are available for determining about 170 parameters (6, 7).

In some cases the evaluation of a threshold limit value is closely connected with the analytical procedure. The EKA values for exposure to arsenic, for example, are coupled with the quantitative determination of arsenic using hydride atomic absorption spectrometry. If the total amount of arsenic in the urine is measured there is a high degree of interference from arsenic taken up with food, for example seafood.

Methodological requirements must also be met in adduct analysis. For all the analytical procedures used in biological monitoring, the analytical reliability criteria, and in particular the precision and detection limit, must be in line with those met in the establishment of the reference values and threshold limit values.

Tab. 2: Methods and spectrum of parameters in the series "Analyses of Hazardous Substances in Biological Materials"

	Inorganic substances	Organic substances (individual components and substance classes)	Parameters of effect
Parameters to be analysed	Metals: Al, As, Ba, Be, Cr, Co, Cu, Hg, In, Mn, Ni, Pb, Pt, Sb, Se, Sn, Sr, Ti, Tl, V, Zn Anions: CN^-, F^-, Br^-	Adducts (e.g. hydroxyethylvaline) Aromatic amino and nitro compounds Solvents Solvent metabolites Organochlorine compounds PAH metabolites (e.g. 1-hydroxypyrene) Pesticides (pyrethroids, carbamates, phenoxy-carbonic acids, organo-phosphoric acid esters) Phenols	Acetylcholinesterase β2-Microglobulin Cholinesterase CO-Hb δ-Aminolevulinic acid δ-Aminolevulinic acid dehydratase Erythrocyte porphyrins Methaemoglobin
Analytical techniques	F-AAS, GF-AAS, Hydride-AAS, Cold vapour AAS, Inverse voltammetry, ICP-OES, ICP-MS	GC-FID, GC-ECD, GC-TID, GC-MS, Head-space gas chromatography, HPLC, Photometry, Fluorimetry	Fluorimetry, Photometry, Gas chromatography, Enzyme linked immunoassay, Radioimmunoassay
Number of methods	36	71	10

3 Internal and External Quality Control

The precision and accuracy of the values determined in the occupational-medical laboratory must be continually checked by adequate internal and external quality control measures. In Germany, quality control in these laboratories is regulated by the Hazardous Substances Ordinance. In the technical regulations for hazardous substances (TRGS 410) statistical quality control is prescribed for carrying out occupational-medical analyses in biological materials to evaluate the level of exposure as defined by the ordinance. These technical regulations were introduced by the German Federal Labour Ministry on 3rd April 1979.

TRGS 410 contains detailed information on procedure. It stipulates that the naming of reference laboratories and the carrying out of intercomparison programmes is the responsibility of the Board of the German Society for Occupational and Environmental Medicine. This society, through its commission for questions of quality control in occupational medicine, has also produced guidelines for the carrying out of statistical quality control during toxicological analyses (12).

For quality control of quantitative laboratory data TRGS 410 prescribes both internal and external quality control. In addition, TRGS 410 §6 contains a note that the collection of methods "Analyses of Hazardous Substances in Biological Materials" of the DFG Commission for the Investigation of Health Hazards of Chemical Compounds in the Work Area should be used in toxicological investigations (standard operational procedures – SOP).

3.1 Internal Quality Control

Internal laboratory quality control serves as systematic monitoring of precision of repeated assays for detecting random errors and determining the accuracy of quantitative laboratory investigations. It includes a check of precision for every series of analyses and of accuracy after every fourth series. In practice it is carried out with a control sample system. The control materials used should be as similar as possible to the material being analysed and commercially available. These are standard reference materials with a certified analyte content and control materials with a constant analyte content for "daily use" during precision and accuracy checks.

Standard reference materials are samples whose quantitative composition of certain components has been determined using various methods and by qualified laboratories. They are accompanied by a certificate stating the concentration of these components. Reference materials with certified values are offered, for example, by the Community Bureau of Reference (CBR) of the Commission of the European Union, by the American National Institute of Standards and Technology (NIST) and by the International Atomic Energy Agency (IAEA). In the programmes of these institutions there are only very few materials with parameters relevant to occupational medicine. In addition this material is very expensive due to the complicated certification procedure. It is therefore not used for routine quality control but during validation of an analytical procedure.

Usually, therefore, commercially available control samples are used for routine internal quality control. Table 3 shows the current commercially available control samples. These control samples are sold freeze-dried and have to be reconstituted.

For occupational-medical parameters not contained in these commercially available control samples, control materials that have been produced by the laboratory itself can be used for internal quality control. Animal or human blood and human serum are spiked with defined concentrations of the analytes. These samples are in liquid form and aliquots are stored deep-frozen until analysis (4).

The results of daily internal quality control are registered on control cards and compared with the standard deviation for this method. The standard deviation of the method is determined in a preliminary phase where control samples are analysed on 20 different working days. A result is correct if it does not differ from the actual value by more than three times this relative standard deviation and if there are no trends towards higher or lower values over a longer period.

The possibilities and results of internal quality control for occupational-medical analyses in biological materials have been described elsewhere (3, 14).

Tab. 3: Commercially available control materials for internal quality control of occupational-medical–toxicological analyses

Trade name	Matrix	Spectrum of parameters N	Parameter	Number of concentration settings
Bio Rad Lab, Munich Lyphocheck®	Urine	22	Al, Sb, As, Pb, Cd, Cr, Co, F^-, Cu, Mn, Ni, Se, Tl, Zn, ALA, HA, MA, PGA, PCP, phenol, TCA	2
Nycomed, Oslo Seronorm®-Trace Elements, Urine	Urine	19	Al, Sb, As, Cd, Co, Cu, Cr, F^-, Pb, Mn, Hg, Ni, Tl, Zn, HA, 1-hydroxypyrene, phenol, TCA, formic acid	1
Recipe, Chemicals and Instruments, Munich Clin Rep®-Controls	Urine	20	Al, Sb, As, Pb, Cd, Cr, Co, Cu, Mn, Ni, Hg, Tl, Zn, HA, MA, MHA, PCP, PGA, TCA, *trans,trans*-muconic acid,	2
Recipe, Chemicals and Instruments, Munich Clin Rep®-Controls	Plasma	11	Organochlorine compounds	2
		9	Metals	2
Nycomed, Oslo Seronorm®-Trace Elements, Serum	Serum	9	Al, Cr, Cu, Co, F^-, Mn, Ni, Se, Zn	1
Nycomed, Oslo Seronorm®-Trace Elements, Whole blood	Blood	8	Cd, Co, Cr, Pb, Mn, Hg, Ni, Se	3
Bio Rad Lab, Munich Lyphocheck®	Blood	1	Pb	3
Recipe, Chemicals and Instruments, Munich Clin Rep®-Control	Blood	7	Pb, Cd, Cr, Co, Ni, Hg, Mn	2

3.2 External Quality Control

External quality control on the basis of intercomparison programmes serves as objective monitoring of the accuracy of the results of quantitative laboratory investigations under comparable conditions. Its aim is to guarantee the comparability of results from laboratory to laboratory and with the valid occupational-medical threshold values for tolerable exposures (e.g. BAT/EKA values or BEIs).

Intercomparison programmes for occupational-medical–toxicological investigations are organised by the following institutions:

- Deutsche Gesellschaft für Arbeitsmedizin und Umweltmedizin e.V.; organised by: Institut und Poliklinik für Arbeits-, Sozial- und Umweltmedizin der Universität Erlangen-Nürnberg, Erlangen, Germany.
- Institute of Occupational Health, Helsinki, Finland.

- Danish National Institute of Occupational Health, AME, Copenhagen, Denmark.
- Centre de Toxicologie du Québec, Toxicology Laboratory, Québec, Canada.
- Deutsche Gesellschaft für Klinische Chemie e.V., Bonn, Germany.
- Instant e.V. Ringversuche, Düsseldorf, Germany.

With the exception of the intercomparison programmes organised by the German Society for Occupational and Environmental Medicine (Deutsche Gesellschaft für Arbeitsmedizin und Umweltmedizin), usually only metals or a limited number of parameters are studied.

The external quality control programme of the German Society for Occupational and Environmental Medicine has been organised since 1982. In the meantime the 19th intercomparison programme has been carried out by this society. These intercomparison programmes are now well accepted nationally and internationally. About 150 laboratories from Germany and abroad take part in these intercomparison programmes. The high degree of acceptance is understandable when one bears in mind that a range of 96 parameters for 47 substances is offered, the most extensive quality control programme in the field of toxicological analysis in biological materials currently offered world-wide (1). Table 4 shows the spectrum of parameters offered in the 19th intercomparison programme. This range covers most of the parameters relevant to occupational and environmental medicine. These intercomparison programmes are held twice a year, in accordance with the recommendations of the German Federal Medical Council. Two concentration settings must be measured per parameter.

Evaluation of the results of analysis of the laboratories which participated in the intercomparison programme is carried out using reference values and tolerance ranges. These values are determined by reference laboratories. At present 19 national and international laboratories, who were selected according to fixed criteria, participate in the evaluation of these reference values. Participants in the intercomparison programme have fulfilled the analytical requirements when both results for one parameter are within the tolerance range, i.e. in the ± 3 SD range determined by the reference laboratories. The participants receive a certificate for this parameter which is valid for one year. There are numerous descriptions of the spectrum, organisation and results of these intercomparison programmes (14, 2).

Evaluation of the intercomparison programmes has shown that the percentage of correct analyses for the laboratories taking part is between 50 % and 60 %. Improvement of this unsatisfactory result must be achieved by critical review of the currently used analytical methods, consistent use of internal quality control and improvement in the performance of these laboratories.

Although quality control is primarily the responsibility of the toxicological laboratories, the occupational physician should find out about the quality of the laboratory which he uses. The laboratory receives a certificate for successful participation in the intercomparison programme of the German Society for Occupational and Environmental Medicine. For reasons of liability, physicians carrying out occupational-medical health checks should also only use laboratories which carry out their toxicological analyses under the conditions of statistical quality control (10). In addition, better monitoring of quality control measures by accident insurance companies (Berufsgenossenschaften) and state occupational physicians is necessary.

Tab. 4: Control samples used in the 19th intercomparison programme of the German Society for Occupational and Environmental Medicine

Control urine		Control blood		Control serum	
Inorganic components	Organic components	Metals	Solvents	Organo-chlorine compounds	Metals
Occupational-medical range					
Aluminium Antimony Arsenic Cadmium Chromium Cobalt Copper Fluoride Lead Manganese Mercury Nickel Thallium Zinc	δ-Aminolevulinic acid Butoxyacetic acid *o*-Cresol Ethoxyacetic acid Hippuric acid 1-Hydroxypyrene Mandelic acid 4,4´-Methylene-bis (2-chloroaniline) Methylhippuric acid *trans,trans*-Muconic acid *N*-Methylformamide Pentachlorophenol Phenol Phenylglyoxylic acid 2-Thio-4-thiazolidine carboxylic acid Trichloroacetic acid	Cadmium Chromium Cobalt Lead Manganese Mercury Nickel	Benzene Toluene Xylenes Ethylbenzene Dichloromethane Trichloromethane Trichloroethene Tetrachoroethene	*p,p*-DDE HCB α-HCH β-HCH γ-HCH PCB (6 congeners) PCP	Aluminium Chromium Cobalt Copper Iron Manganese Nickel Platinum Selenium Zinc
Environmental-medical range					
Arsenic Cadmium Chromium Mercury Nickel Platinum	1-Hydroxypyrene Pentachlorophenol Pyrethroid metabolites (Br_2-CA, *cis*-Cl_2-CA, *trans*-Cl_2-CA, 3-PBA)	Cadmium Lead Mercury		*p,p*-DDE HCB α-HCH β-HCH γ-HCH PCB (6 congeners) PCP	

4 Prospects and Conclusions

Quality control of occupational-medical analyses in biological materials should not be limited to quality control of analytical investigations. The pre-analytical phase (sampling, transport, storage) and selection of the analytical methods must be included in the quality control programme.

The pre-analytical phase, which is the responsibility of the works medical department, does not fall under the measures of quality control according to TRGS 410. It should be optimised through conventions and standards. Recommendations from experienced laboratories and close collaboration with the laboratories entrusted with carrying out the analyses can guarantee that confounding influences and interference factors during the pre-analytical phase can be minimised. The provision by the laboratory of sampling utensils, and vessels for collection, storage and dispatch of the samples, with detailed instructions, can reduce interference due to contamination or losses.

The selection of tested and reliable analytical procedures is an important guarantee for reliable and reproducible analytical results. In Germany reference can be made to the collection of methods "Analyses of Hazardous Substances in Biological Materials" produced by the DFG Commission for the Investigation of Health Hazards of Chemical Compounds in the Work Area. Methods tested with regard to their analytical reliability can be found in this series for about 170 analytical parameters. The methods have usually been tested in several independent laboratories.

Even when using this procedure, internal quality control in toxicological laboratories is necessary. Control materials are available from various companies for routine quality control. The spectrum necessary for internal quality control can be supplemented by the laboratory's own control samples. The requirements for adequate internal quality control are thus fulfilled.

The obligatory participation in external intercomparison programmes for analyses in biological materials prescribed by the German Federal Labour Ministry in TRGS 410 completes the possible programme of quality control. The German Society for Occupational and Environmental Medicine organises two intercomparison programmes a year which include a current range of 96 toxicologically important parameters. The certificates received for successful participation certify the quality of the analytical performance of the participating laboratory, so that occupational physicians using the service of the laboratory can be assured of the quality of this laboratory.

If the recommendations for the pre-analytical phase, the selection of reliable analytical methods by the laboratory and the carrying out of adequate quality control are observed, the prerequisites for reliable findings during biological monitoring are fulfilled.

5 References

1. Aitio, A., Valkonen, S., et al.: External quality assessment in biological monitoring, in: Proceedings of the Sixth FIOH-NIOSH Joint Symposium on Occupational Health and Safety, 8–10 August 1995, Espoo, Finland (Eds.: H. Nordman, J. Starck, A. Tossavainen, E. Viikari-Juntura) People and work – Research reports 3, Finnish Institute of Occupational Health, Helsinki 1995
2. Angerer, J., Schaller, K. H., et al.: Externe Qualitätssicherung arbeits- und umweltmedizinisch-toxikologischer Analysen. Arbeitsmed. Sozialmed. Umweltmed. *30* (1995), 191–203
3. Angerer, J., Schaller, K. H., Weltle, D.: Erfahrungen mit der laborinternen Qualitätssicherung bei arbeitsmedizinisch-toxikologischen Untersuchungen im biologischen Material. Arbeitsmed. Sozialmed. Präventivmed. *25* (1990), 248–252
4. Angerer, J., Schaller, K. H.: Erfahrungen mit der statistischen Qualitätskontrolle im arbeitsmedizinisch-toxikologischen Laboratorium. Arbeitsmed. Sozialmed. Präventivmed. *11* (1976), 311–312 and Arbeitsmed. Sozialmed. Präventivmed. *12* (1977), 33–35
5. Angerer, J., Schaller, K. H., Seiler, H.: The pre-analytical phase of toxicological monitoring examinations in occupational medicine. Trends in Analytical Chemistry, 2 *(11)* (1983) 257–261
6. Angerer, J., Schaller, K. H., (Eds.): Analytische Methoden zur Prüfung gesundheitsschädlicher Arbeitsstoffe, Band 2, Analysen in biologischem Material. VCH-Verlagsgesellschaft, Weinheim 1985–1994
7. Angerer, J., Schaller, K. H., (Eds.): Analyses of Hazardous Substances in Biological Materials, Vol. 1–4. VCH-Verlagsgesellschaft, Weinheim 1991–1994
8. Deutsche Forschungsgemeinschaft (DFG), List of MAK and BAT Values 1998, Report No. 34. VCH-Verlagsgesellschaft, Weinheim 1998
9. Ewers, U., Kramer, H., Körting, H.: Diagnostik der inneren Exposition/Human-Biomonitoring, Kapitel III – 2.1, 1–19, in: Handbuch Umweltmedizin (Wichmann, Schlipköter, Fülgraff (Eds.)) eco-med Verlag, 2. Erg.Lfg. 9/93
10. Kalbreier, U., Szadkowski, D.: Haftungsfragen bei arbeitsmedizinischen Vorsorgeuntersuchungen unter Inanspruchnahme fremder Laboratorien. Arbeitsmed. Sozialmed. Präventivmed. *16* (1981), 270–272
11. Lauwerys, R. R., Hoet, P. (Eds.): Industrial Chemical Exposure: Guidelines for Biological Monitoring. Lewis Pub., Boca Raton, 1993
12. Lehnert, G., Rutenfranz, J., et al.: Richtlinie zur Durchführung der statistischen Qualitätssicherung bei arbeitsmedizinisch-toxikologischen Analysen. Arbeitsmed. Sozialmed. Präventivmed. *16* (1981), 56
13. Schaller, K. H., Angerer, J.: Die apparative Ausstattung des Betriebsarztes (III): Das arbeitsmedizinisch-toxikologische Labor. Arbeitsmed. Sozialmed. Präventivmed. *24* (1989), 287–290
14. Schaller, K. H., Angerer, J., Lehnert, G.: Internal and external quality control in the toxicological analysis of blood and urine samples in the Federal Republic of Germany. Int. Arch. Occup. Environ. Health, *62* (1991), 537–542
15. Schaller, K. H., Angerer, J., Lehnert, G.: Praktische Hinweise zum Biomonitoring in der Arbeits- und Umweltmedizin, arbeitsmedizin aktuell (Eds.: H.J. Florian, F. Stollenz, H. Valentin, A. Zober) G. Fischer Verlag, Stuttgart, Jena 1996

Author: K.H. Schaller

(translated from Arbeitsmed. Sozialmed. Umweltmed. *31*, 317–323 (1996))

Substances

Essential BAT Value Documentations. DFG, Deutsche Forschungsgemeinschaft

ISBN 3-527-31477-6

Acetone

BAT	80 mg acetone/l urine Sampling time: end of exposure or end of shift
Date of evaluation	1995
CAS No.	67-64-1
Synonyms	2-Propanone Dimethyl ketone β-Ketopropane
Formula	C_3H_6O 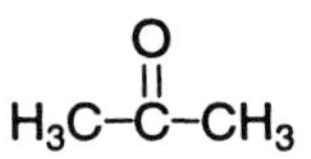
Molecular weight	58.08
Melting point	–95.6 °C
Boiling point	56.3 °C
Vapour pressure at 20 °C	240 mbar
MAK [last established: 1993]	500 ml/m^3 (ppm) (1200 mg/m^3)

In 1993 the working group "Setting of Threshold Values in Biological Materials" of the DFG Commission for the Investigation of Health Hazards of Chemical Compounds in the Work Area set a BAT value of 40 mg/l for the level of acetone excreted in urine. Sampling time was given as the end of exposure or the end of the shift.

The evaluation of the BAT value was based on the relationship between external and internal exposure. The correlations were determined from experimental studies and field studies. These studies were mainly carried out by Italian research groups.

In the meantime new information has become available both in the scientific literature and two unpublished company reports. The complete documentation of these studies was made available to the commission and stored in its archives.

This new data made it necessary to re-evaluate the BAT value for the urinary excretion of acetone.

Essential BAT Value Documentations. DFG, Deutsche Forschungsgemeinschaft

ISBN 3-527-31477-6

1 Metabolism and Kinetics

Acetone can be taken up by inhalation, ingestion and percutaneous absorption. Due to the high volatility of acetone, inhalation of the substance is important from an occupational-medical point of view. Physical activity increases the rate of absorption significantly, the relative amount absorbed, however, remains constant at about 30 %.

Percutaneous absorption of acetone is not detectable after short-term exposure, and over longer periods of contact takes place only slowly and is of no importance in practice (11).

Due to its good water solubility, acetone is readily taken up into the blood stream. The distribution coefficient between blood and air is very large: 218–245. The proportion of inhaled acetone which is absorbed is about 45 % (34). More recent investigations show the percentage of acetone absorbed by the lungs to be 52 % (20). The reason for this relatively low absorption is not saturation of the blood, but the low affinity of acetone for lipids (distribution coefficient 68). This very low affinity influences the passage of acetone through the cell membranes.

After high-level occupational exposure, acetone is eliminated almost unchanged via the lungs and kidneys, and through the skin. After the end of exposure about 20 % is eliminated via the lungs. In the low concentration range, acetone is degraded mainly oxidatively to carbon dioxide and water. In animal experiments and in humans, formic acid was also found to be formed as a degradation product of acetone (3, 24, 25).

Small amounts of acetone are also excreted unchanged in the urine. According to data from Wigaeus *et al.* (34), renal excretion accounts for 1 % of the total uptake, according to Kawai *et al.* (12) about 3 %. The latter authors give an excretion rate of 22 µg acetone/min. According to investigations by Blaszkewicz *et al.* (4), the acetone excreted unchanged in the urine accounts for about 15 % of the amount absorbed. In this study carried out under defined exposure conditions, it was shown that the maximum renal excretion takes place two hours after the end of exposure; according to Wigaeus *et al.* (34) the maximum lies between 3 and 3.5 hours after exposure.

According to Thiess (35) small amounts of acetone are reduced in the organism to 2-propanol. Lewis *et al.* (16) found this metabolite, however, only at very high blood-acetone concentrations, in particular in diabetics.

The elimination of acetone from the human organism follows a linear course. This was demonstrated under experimental conditions in several studies (4, 9, 20, 21).

With external exposure to acetone concentrations below 15 ppm there is no significant increase in the renal excretion of acetone (12). If external exposure to acetone exceeds 300 ppm, the level of acetone excreted is significantly increased, even in the pre-shift urine sample after exposure; after a further exposure-free day the values return to their base level. This means there is no accumulation of acetone in the human organism (31).

There is not much data for the biological half-life of acetone in human blood or for the half-time for renal excretion. Investigations with nine male volunteers yielded a half-life of about three hours for acetone in blood (7). Abshagen and Rietbrock (1) calculated for dogs a considerably longer half-life of 11 hours; for rats the half-life is about five hours. In a more recent study with man the half-life for acetone in venous blood (period of observation 0–4 hours after the end of exposure) was given as 6.1 ± 0.7 hours, for arterial blood (period of observation 0–2 hours after the end of exposure) as 3.9 ± 0.7 (34). For alveolar air the half-life is 4.3 ± 1.1 hours, calculated from measurements obtained between five minutes and nine hours after exposure.

2 Critical Toxicity

(see also MAK documentation and addendum (11))

Acetone, as a liquid or vapour, has a strongly defatting effect on the skin and mucous membranes. The irritative effects are, however, only mild; sensitisation is unknown. In addition, irreversible damage to skin and mucous membranes has not been described to date.

Inhalation of gaseous acetone in high concentrations results at first in a dry mouth and neurotoxic symptoms such as drowsiness, nausea and co-ordination disorders. The potential for causing organ damage seems to be low.

3 Exposure and Effect

3.1 Relationship between External and Internal Exposure

a. Laboratory Experiments with Volunteers

Several research groups have carried out laboratory studies with experimental exposure to acetone, usually under defined conditions of physical activity. These are the studies by Wigaeus *et al.* (34), Pezzagno *et al.* (20,21), Blaszkewicz *et al.* (4) and Satoh *et al.* (26). Some of these studies were already taken into account in the old BAT value documentation (43). The most important is the experimental study by Blaszekewicz *et al.* (4). In this study external exposure to 500 ppm acetone in air corresponded to acetone concentrations of about 40 mg/l in urine. The physiological values for acetone in urine had not yet been completely re-established 15 hours after the end of exposure. In this study investigations were also carried out on discomfort and irritation of the mucous membranes (30, 40). With external exposure to 1000 ppm acetone no significant effects were detected on reaction time, in choice reaction tests and on short term memory. Increases were found in negative estimations of mucous membrane irritation (sum for eyes, mouth, throat, nose). The feeling of ill-health also increased. With exposure to acetone concentrations of 500 ppm this irritation and feeling of discomfort was weak and reversible, and did not occur in all persons. These findings served as a basis for the evaluation of the currently valid MAK value of 500 ppm. A study by Satoh *et al.* (26) with external exposure to acetone of 100 to 400 ppm for only two hours and changing physical activity on a bicycle ergometer (100 watts) revealed after linear extrapolation that 500 ppm acetone in air corresponds to an acetone concentration of about 28 mg/l excreted in urine.

b. Field Studies with Occupationally Exposed Persons

Table 1 summarises the data from the relevant studies for evaluation of the BAT value. Data are given on external and internal exposure. The regression coefficient refers to the simplified regression equation c_u (mg/l) = a × c_{air} (mg/m^3). From this value, the urinary concentrations of acetone corresponding to external exposure to 500 ppm were calculated by linear extrapolation and are given in the last column. It is an average value and can vary considerably in both the high and low concentration ranges.

The first six field studies listed in the table were taken into account in the 1993 BAT value evaluation for excretion of acetone in urine (43). The studies by Wang *et al.* (42) and Mizunuma *et al.* (48) are not of much use for evaluating a BAT value as the average levels of external exposure at 140 and 11 ppm are relatively low. Extrapolation from a low range of exposure to the MAK value of 500 ppm is associated with considerable error. In addition, the values in the study by Wang *et al.* (42) vary greatly.

In the study by Satoh *et al.* (39) 110 workers of a factory producing acetate fibres were investigated. The acetone concentrations in air ranged from below the detection limit to about 1200 ppm, urinary excretion from below the detection limit to 150 mg/l. External exposure was determined using passive personal air samplers. Urine sampling was carried out either on the first day of the week after exposure or on the second day at the end of the shift. The correlation coefficients between external and internal exposure were 0.713 and 0.757. External exposure to 500 ppm corresponded to mean renal elimination of acetone of 50 to 53 mg/l. With acetone concentrations in the air at the level of the MAK value, acetone concentrations in urine varied from about 30 to 70 mg/l. A further finding of this study was that, at the given level of external exposure, the levels of acetone excreted with the urine in pre-shift urine samples after an exposure-free interval of about 16 hours were higher than the base value. These somewhat higher than base levels, however, did not significantly influence urinary excretion at the end of the shift on the next day.

There are two industrial research reports available on the production of acetate fibres (Rhône-Poulenc Rhodia AG, No. FO-C 151/53 and No. FO-C 107/94). During the production of cellulose-2,5-acetate yarns using the dry spinning procedure the spinning solution (collodion: solution of about 30 % cellulose-2,5-acetate in acetone) is intensively filtered in chamber filters. The main exposure to acetone occurs during replacement of the used filter plates, which are still saturated with collodion. Replacement of these sticky filter plates requires a certain amount of physical effort and is carried out by so-called filter changers.

Continual monitoring of the acetone concentration at the workplace was combined in the studies with the measurement of renally excreted acetone. During the investigations the workers were asked not to wear breathing masks. The two series of measurements were carried out in December 1993 and in December 1994.

Tab. 1: Field studies

Authors	Area of production	n	Exposure ppm	Urine sampling	Acetone conc. in urine (mg/l)	Correlation Regression coefficient[1]	Acetone conc. in urine (mg/l) after 500 ppm exp.
Grampella, D. *et al.* (1987)	Production of acetate fibres	30 30	520–640 930–1030	4 hours	62 ± 13 93 ± 15	0.044 0.039	53 47
Ghittori, S. *et al.* (1987)	Various companies producing e.g. acetate fibres	74 30	10–300 600–1400	4 hours	< 35 40–150	0.033 0.027–0.045	40 32–54
Satoh, T. *et al.* (1992)	Production of acetate fibres	11	190–500	8 (10) hours		0.042	50
Fujino A. *et al.* (1992)	Production of acetate fibres	about 20 from 200	0–1200 > 600–1200	8 hours	10 ? –160	0.042 (0.062)[2]	50 75
Blaszkewicz, M. *et al.* (1993)	Production of acetate fibres	68	950 (mean)	8 hours		0.036 (0.026–0.047)[3]	43 (31–56)
Wang, G. *et al.* (1994)	Processing of plastics	44	140 (mean) max. 300	8 hours	22 (mean) up to 90	0.045; ? from 0.015 to 0.075	54
Mizunuma, K. *et al.* (1993	Cleaning	41	11 (mean) max. 165	8 hours	1–50	0.087	104
Rhône-Poulenc Rhodia AG 1995	Production of acetate fibres Filter change	20	Dissolving dept. 1: 250–500 Dissolving dept. 2: 500–750	8 hours	20–200	0.072	86
Satoh *et al.* (1994)	Production of acetate fibres	110	0–1200[5]	8 hours	0–160[5]	0.043	53

[1] simplified regression c_u (mg/l) = a × c_{Air} (mg/m³); [2] when only higher level of exposure considered (> 500 ppm); [3] coefficients from the individual mean values of 6 persons; [4] only the investigation from the processing of plastics is taken into consideration; [5] range taken from figures

In the first study the level of external exposure of 15 persons was determined using passive air samplers, determination of acetone in urine was carried out using head-space gas chromatography. The 8-hour average values for external exposure varied from about 250 to 1500 mg/m^3. In the urine samples, which were collected 5 to 6.5 hours after the beginning of the shift, the amount of acetone excreted ranged between 26 and 120 mg/l. The regression for the relationship between external and internal exposure was calculated using the formula: excretion of acetone in urine (mg/l) = 0.08 × acetone concentration in air (mg/m^3). For exposure to 500 ppm, the calculated urinary acetone concentration was 96 mg/l (Rhône-Poulenc Rhodia AG No. Fo-C 151/53).

In the second study 20 persons were investigated in the same way. For the determination of the external acetone exposure levels, in addition to passive monitoring with personal air samplers, parallel active monitoring was carried out. With the passive air samplers ambient air concentrations were determined which were 10 % lower than those measured with the active samplers. The values from the active personal air samplers were used for the calculations. A regression of 0.072 × acetone concentration in air (mg/m^3) was calculated for the dependence of the urinary concentration on the 8-hour mean value for external exposure. Groups of individual values deviated from this value, however, by more than 20 % in both directions. For exposure to 500 ppm an acetone concentration in the urine samples collected at the end of the shift of 86 mg/l urine can be calculated (Rhône-Poulenc Rhodia AG No. Fo-C 107/94).

After evaluation of the two studies a regression was calculated on the basis of 35 value pairs: acetone excreted in urine (mg/l) = 0.073 × acetone concentration in air (mg/m^3). External exposure to 500 ppm therefore corresponds to urinary excretion of acetone concentrations of 88 mg/l, although individual values can deviate by up to 20 % (Rhône-Poulenc Rhodia AG FE-TA 1/95).

3.2 Relationship between Internal Exposure and Effect

For the evaluation of exposure and effect, there are only a few studies available. Furthermore, it must be noted that the exposure was mainly determined on the basis of the acetone concentration in the ambient air and not through biological monitoring.

The experimental investigation carried out by Dick *et al.* (6) led to acetone concentrations in venous blood of 15.3 ± 2.9 mg/l (range 11.6 ± 19.6 mg/l) and in exhaled air of 25.8 ± 4.0 ppm (range 18.6–34.0 ppm) after the end of a four-hour exposure. The use of a great number of psychometric test procedures and self-rating scales revealed no significant effects at the chosen acetone concentration of 250 ppm, except on two variables. These exceptions were an audiometric discrimination test and the "anxiety scale" of the Profile of Mood Status (well-being questionnaire; only in men). The authors interpret these results as indications that further investigations are necessary. Taking into consideration the overall results of the study, which may be regarded as largely "negative", these findings can have no occupational-medical significance for the evaluation of a threshold limit value.

In an experimental study, 16 men were exposed for 7.5 hours to 1000 ppm acetone, 400 ppm ethyl acetate or a mixture of the two substances (500/200 ppm) (28, 29). The acetone concentrations in the exhaled air averaged about 600 ppm and in the capillary blood about 80 mg/l after exposure to 1000 ppm (4). There was a linear increase in the concentration of acetone in blood during the exposure period. On the following morning, i.e. 15 hours after the end of exposure, no more acetone could be detected in expired air, while in blood the "normal values" had not yet been reached (4). The acetone concentrations in urine showed a linear increase under these exposure conditions up to about 90 mg/l at a concentration of 1000 ppm in air and up to about 40 mg/l at 500 ppm acetone and simultaneous presence of ethyl acetate (4). Also in the urine samples, the physiological values for acetone in urine had not yet been regained 15 hours after the end of exposure. No measurable differences in the psychomotor reaction times could be detected. Mucous membrane irritation and feelings of discomfort were the essential findings. Simultaneous physical activity with ergometry had no effect on the psychic reactions (30).

It can be concluded that at present only a few studies are suitable for evaluating threshold limit values on an exposure/effect basis. The results more or less all show that at acetone concentrations of up to 100 mg/l urine or blood, no neurotoxic effects can be detected. The irritant effects of acetone on the mucous membranes are discussed in Section 2.

4 Selection of the Indicators

For the monitoring of persons exposed to acetone there are only parameters of internal exposure available. Acetone concentrations in the blood and urine samples can be used as indicators. Only the post-shift samples are suitable for analysis. The acetone concentrations in the alveolar air have been measured by some research groups.

Significant correlations between the external and internal exposure (acetone–urine, acetone–blood, acetone–alveolar air) have been found by various research groups (4, 5, 7, 9, 11, 12, 20, 21), both in field studies and also in studies of volunteers exposed to defined concentrations. As a rule, the relationships between the external concentration and internal exposure have been shown to be linear.

In most studies the acetone concentration in urine has proved to be a suitable biological parameter (8). Accordingly, biological threshold limit values are suggested for this parameter by most groups. The suggested American BEI value for occupational exposure to acetone is thus based on the acetone excreted in urine.

Acetone accumulates in blood linearly during the exposure period and the values are still increased even a long time after the end of exposure. These can be differentiated from the background values, however, according to Blaszkewicz *et al.* (4), only when the ambient air concentrations are very high and the periods of exposure are long.

Wigaeus *et al.* (34) carried out parallel investigations on the acetone concentration in arterial and venous blood; no concrete information is given, however, on the sampling of arterial blood. It was probably capillary blood. Both the acetone concentration in venous blood and that in arterial blood increased during exposure to acetone. The venous blood concentrations ran parallel to the arterial levels; they were, however, somewhat lower. The arterio-venous difference was, however, not constant and was influenced by the physical activity during exposure. The results gained with capillary blood are thus not directly transferable to venous blood.

In occupational health surveillance, biological monitoring is generally carried out with venous blood samples and the BAT value should therefore be based on concentrations in venous blood. Venous blood samples were investigated in a study by Dick *et al.* (6) with 137 volunteers after four-hour exposure to 250 ppm acetone. Starting with a background value of 2.0 ± 2.0 mg/l the acetone concentrations after two hours of exposure were 9.0 ± 2.0 mg/l and after four hours 15.3 ± 2.9 mg/l. 90 minutes after the end of exposure the values had decreased to 11.9 ± 2.6 mg/l, 20 hours after exposure to 1.6 ± 1.3 mg/l. The results showed considerable interindividual variation.

Given this situation (different sampling times, investigations using capillary blood, interindividual variation etc.) the database at present does not seem sufficient for the evaluation of a BAT value in venous blood. More recent investigations (8) show that there is a significant correlation between acetone concentrations in the blood and urine so that in future a biological threshold value in blood can possibly be evaluated.

The arterialised capillary blood propagated by Wigaeus *et al.* (34) is for practical reasons not suitable for biological monitoring, as mentioned above.

Alveolar air investigations with persons exposed to acetone show extraordinarily high interindividual and intraindividual variation. Furthermore, the acetone concentration in the alveolar air seems to be constant at 30–40 % of that in the ambient air and is thus independent of the total uptake (34). Under these conditions and given the problems of finding a practicable method of sampling, the acetone concentration in the alveolar air is unsuitable for biological monitoring (4).

Animal experiments have shown that after exposure to acetone there is increased excretion of formic acid. Also in humans slight increases in the formic acid concentration in the urine after exposure to acetone have been observed (3). This was not confirmed, however, in the study by Blaszkewicz *et al.* (4). After exposure to external acetone concentrations up to 2400 mg/m^3 there were no indications of increased excretion of formic acid. Determination of the level of formic acid excreted in the urine is thus not a suitable parameter for the biological monitoring of persons exposed to acetone. The validity of using formic acid excretion as an indicator is furthermore restricted because it is an unspecific parameter. Increased excretion of formic acid is observed after exposure to methanol and formaldehyde and may also be caused by alimentary factors. The normal level of formic acid excreted is subject to considerable interindividual and intraindividual variation (27, 32).

5 Methodology

For the quantitative determination of acetone in blood and urine, only head-space gas chromatography is used today. The DFG Commission for the Investigation of Health

Hazards of Chemical Compounds in the Work Area has published a reliable method in its loose-leaf collection "Analysen in biologischem Material" ("Analyses of Hazardous Substances in Biological Materials") (36). As acetone is a highly volatile substance the materials to be analysed must be transferred to head-space vials with Teflon-coated septa immediately after sampling. These containers are suitable both for the transport and storage of the samples. The analytical determination takes place directly from the head-space in this container.

6 Background Exposure

Table 2 summarises urinary excretion of acetone in samples from not occupationally exposed persons, listed according to country of origin from data in the literature. The amounts excreted physiologically are usually below 3 mg/l. Higher acetone concentrations in urine are, however, observed. Higher background concentrations are found mainly in badly stabilised diabetics or strictly fasting persons (2, 14). Acetone can be excreted in concentrations as high as 30 to 40 mg/l.

Tab. 2: Urinary excretion of acetone in not occupationally exposed persons

n	Mean	Range	Units	References	Country of origin
15	0.76 ± 0.64		mg/l	Pezzagno *et al.* (20)	Italy
994	2.4	< 0.5–19	mg/l	Lewalter (15)	Germany
8	1.4 ± 11.1		mg/l	Wigaeus *et al.* (34)	Sweden
66	1.3 ± 2.4	< detection limit –40.3	mg/l	Satoh *et al.* (39)	Japan
89	0.84 ± 1.5	0.13–9.4	mg/l	Wang *et al.* (42)	Italy

Interference due to exposure to 2-propanol must also be borne in mind. This solvent is metabolised to acetone and excreted with the urine (see BAT documentation for 2-propanol (44)).

Acetone can also be detected as a component of various household products, such as paints, paint remover, nail varnish remover and in felt-tip pens. The same applies for 2-propanol, which can be found in cosmetics and household cleaning agents.

7 Evaluation of a BAT Value

Due to the current lack of data, a BAT value for acetone cannot be evaluated on the basis of relationships between internal exposure and relevant effects. Evaluation must therefore still be carried out using relationships between external and internal exposure. The current MAK value of 500 ppm (1200 mg/m^3) serves as a correlate. Urinary excretion of acetone is used as a biological parameter.

For the re-evaluation of the BAT value experimental investigations with volunteers, field studies and simulation studies are available. These studies are listed in Section 3.1 and the older studies in the documentation of the BAT value from 1993 (43). Field studies (Table 1) and the simulation studies of the BEI group (41) and Kumagai and Matsunaga (37) form the basis for this evaluation. The concentration of renally excreted acetone calculated from correlations and extrapolations for the MAK value of 500 ppm, range between 50 and 100 mg/l urine. This applies in particular for the recent studies. The mean ambient air concentrations measured during the shift and the acetone level measured in urine at the end of the shift are used as parameters for both correlations (Table 1).

The BAT value for the excretion of acetone in urine in post-shift samples was therefore set at

80 mg acetone/l urine.

According to the definition of the BAT value this means that the maximum level of acetone excreted in urine by an individual may only reach this concentration; this is equivalent to average 8-hour inhalation exposure to acetone at the level of the MAK value (500 ppm).

8 Interpretation of the Data

Statements as to the level of internal exposure of the organism to acetone and the adherence to BAT values pre-suppose urine analyses in biological fluids which were sampled at the end of the work shift.

Physical activity leads to an increase in the amount of acetone absorbed and eliminated renally. Light physical work does not have any significant influence on the amount of acetone excreted.

Occupational-medical evaluation must also take into consideration any concurrent exposure to 2-propanol. Endogenous acetone levels in healthy, not occupationally exposed persons are of the order of magnitude of 1 mg/l. In badly controlled diabetics the acetone level can be considerably greater and reach about 30 mg/l (14, 23). Excretion of acetone is also influenced by fasting. According to an investigation by Bales *et al.* (2) in individual cases the acetone concentration in the urine can be of the order of magnitude of the BAT value. There is considerable interindividual variation in the levels of acetone excreted, even in healthy persons.

9 References

1. Abshagen, U., Rietbrock, N.: Kinetik der Elimination von 2-Propanol und seines Metaboliten. Aceton bei Hund und Ratte, Naunyn-Schmiedeberg's Arch. exp. Path. Pharmacol. *264* (1969), 110–118
2. Bales, J. R., Bell, J. D., Nicholson, J. K., Sadler, P. J.: H NMR studies of urine during fasting: Excretion of ketone bodies and acetylcarnitine, Magnetic Resonance in Medicine *3* (1986), 849–856
3. Baumann, K., Angerer, J.: Untersuchungen zur Frage der beruflichen Lösungsmittelbelastung mit Aceton, in: Norpoth (Ed.), 19. Jahrestagung der Deutschen Gesellschaft für Arbeitsmedizin e.V., Gentner Verlag, Stuttgart (1979), 403–408
4. Blaszkewicz, M., Golka, K., Vangala, R. R., Kiesswetter, E. et al.: Biologische Überwachung bei Aceton- und Ethylacetatexposition unter simulierten MAK-Bedingungen, 31. Jahrestagung der Deutschen Gesellschaft für Arbeitsmedizin e.V., in: G. Schäcke, K. Ruppe, C. Vogel-Sührig (Eds.), Gentner Verlag, Stuttgart (1992), 141–144
5. Brugnone, F., Perbellini, L., Grigolini, L., Apostoli, P.: Solvent exposure in a shoe upper factory, Int. Arch. Occup. Environ. Health *42* (1978), 51–62
6. Dick, R. B., Setzer, J. V., Taylor, B. J., Shukla, R.: Neurobehavioral effects of short duration exposures to acetone and methyl ethyl ketone, Br. J. Ind. Med. *46* (1989), 111–121
7. Di Vicenzo, G. D., Yanno, F. J., Astill, B. D.: Exposure of man and dog to two concentrations of acetone vapor, Am. Ind. Hyg. Assoc. J. *34* (1973), 329–336
8. Fujino, A., Satoh, T., Takebayashi, T., Nakashima, H., Sakurai, H., Higashi, T., Matumura, H., Minaguchi, H., Kawai, T.: Biological monitoring of workers exposed to acetone in acetate fibre plants, Br. J. Ind. Med. *49* (1992), 654–657
9. Ghittori, S., Imbriani, M., Pezzagno, G., Capodaglio, E.: The urinary concentration of solvents as a biological indicator of exposure: Proposal for the biological equivalent exposure limit for nine solvents, Am. Ind. Hyg. Assoc. J. *48* (1987), 786–790
10. Grampella, D., Garavaglia, L., Pezzagno, G., Imbriani, M.: Biological Minitoring of workers exposed to acetone, XXII ICOH Congress, Sydney, 27.09–02.10.1987, Occupational Health in the Chemical Industry, WHO-Office Copenhagen (1988)
11. Greim, H. (Eds.): Toxikologische-arbeitsmedizinische Begründungen von MAK-Werten, VCH-Verlagsgesellschaft, Weinheim and in English translation in Occupational Toxicants Volume 7, VCH-Verlagsgesellschaft, Weinheim (1996)
12. Kawai, T., Yasugi, T., Uchida, Y., Iwami, O., Ikeda, M.: Urinary excretion of unmetabolized acetone as an indicator of occupational exposure to acetone, Int. Arch. Occup. Environ. Health *62* (1990), 165–169
13. Kawai, T., Yasugi, T., Mizunuma, K., Horiguchi, S., Iguchi, H., Ikeda, M.: Curvi-linear relation between acetone in breathing zone air and acetone in urine among workers exposed to acetone vapor, Toxicol. Lett. *62* (1992), 85–91
14. Levey, S., Balchum, O. J., Medraxo, V., Jung, R.: Studies of metabolic products in expired air, II. Acetone, J. Lab. Clin. Med. *63* (1964), 574–584
15. Lewalter, J.: personal communication (1990)
16. Lewis, D. G., Laufmann, A., McAnallely, B., Garriott, J.: Metabolism of acetone to isopropyl alcohol in rats and humans, J. Forensic Sci. *29* (1984), 541–549
17. Nelson, K., Ege, J. F., Ross, M., Woodman, L. E., Silverman, L.: Sensory response to certain industrial solvent vapors, J. Ind. Hyg. Tox. *25* (1943), 282–285
18. Oglesby, F. L., Williams, J. E., Fassett, B. W., Sterner, J. H.: cited from Rowe, V. K., Wolf, M. A., in: Patty, Industrial Hygiene and Toxicology, 2nd rev. edition, Vol. II, 1719, Interscience Publishers, New York (1962)
19. Parmeggiani, L., Sassi, C.: Pathologia professionale da acetone. Manifestazioni cliniche indagini negli ambienti di lavoro e ricerche fisiopatologiche, Med. Lav. *45* (1954), 431–468

20. Pezzagno, G., Imbriani, M. Ghittori, S., Capodaglio, E., Huang, J.: Urinary elimination of acetone in experimental and occupational exposure, Scand. J. Work. Environ. Health *12* (1986), 603–608
21. Pezzagno, G., Imbriani, M., Ghittori, S., Capodaglio, E.: Urinary concentration, environmental concentration, and respiratory uptake of some solvents: Effect of the work load, Am. Ind. Hyg. Assoc. J. *49* (1988), 546–552
22. Raleigh, R. L., McGee, M. D., McGee, W. A.: Effects of short, high-concentration exposures to acetone as determined by observation in the work area, J. Occup. Med. *14* (1972), 607–610
23. Ross, D. S.: Acute acetone intoxication involving eight male workers, Ann. Occup. Hyg. *16* (1973), 73
24. Rudney, H.: Propanediol phosphate as a possible intermediate in the metabolism of acetone, J. Biol. Chem. *210* (1954), 361–367
25. Sakami, W.: Formation of formate and labile methyl groups from acetone in the intact rat, J. Biol. Chem. *187* (1950), 369–378
26. Satho, T., Omae, K., Sakurai, H., Nakashima, H., Takebayashi, T., Kawai, T., Higashi, T.: Involvement of pulmonary ventilation in the determination of exposure to acetone: Relationship to urinary excretion of acetone, 23rd International Congress on Occupational Health, Montreal, Canada 22–28.09.1990
27. Schmid, K., Schaller, K. H., Angerer, J., Lehnert, G: Untersuchungen zur diagnostischen Validität der Ameisensäureausscheidung im Urin als Biomonitoring-Parameter, Jahresbericht der Deutschen Gesellschaft für Arbeitsmedizin e.V., in: G. Schäcke (Ed.), Gentner Verlag, Stuttgart (1991)
28. Seeber, A., Kiesswetter, E., Vangala, R. R., Blaszkewicz, M., Golka, K., Bolt, H. M.: Neurobehavioral effects of experimental exposure to acetone and ethyl acetate, 23rd International Congress on Occupational Health, Montreal, Canada 22–29.09.1990
29. Seeber, A., Kiesswetter, E., Giller, D., Vangala, R. R., Blaszkewicz, M., Golka, K., Bolt, H. M.: Wirkungen akuter Exposition gegenüber Aceton und Ethylacetat im MAK-Bereich, in: G. Schäcke, K. Ruppe, C. Vogel-Sührig (Eds.), Verhandlungen der Deutschen Gesellschaft für Arbeitsmedizin e.V. (30. Jahrestagung), Gentner Verlag, Stuttgart (1990), 415–418
30. Seeber, A., Kiesswetter, E., Giller, D., Blaszkewicz, M., Golka, K., Vangala, R. R., Bolt, H. M.: Akute Wirkungen von Aceton und Ethylacetat: Vergleich der Expositionsdauer von 4 gegenüber 8 Stunden, in: G. Schäcke, K. Ruppe, C. Vogel-Sührig (Eds.), Verhandlungen der Deutschen Gesellschaft für Arbeitsmedizin (31. Jahrestagung), Gentner Verlag, Stuttgart (1992), 145–148
31. Takebayashi, T., Kazuyuki, O., Sato, T., Nakajima, H., Omodera, M., Sakurai, H.: Biological Monitoring of Acetone Exposure (2)—Examination on bioaccumulation, 64th Meeting of Japan Soc. Ind. Hyg. (1991) and 50th Meeting of Japan Ass. Ind. Med. (1991)
32. Triebig, G., Schaller, K. H.: A simple and reliable enzymatic assay for the determination of formic acid in urine, Clin. Chim. Acta *108* (1980), 355–360
33. Vigliani, E. C., Zurlo, N.: Erfahrungen der Clinica del Lavoro mit einigen maximalen Arbeitsplatzkonzentrationen (MAK) von Industriegiften, Arch. Gewerbepathol. Gewerbehyg. *13* (1955), 528–534
34. Wigaeus, E., Hom, S., Astrand, I.: Exposure to acetone, Scand. J. Work Environ. Health *8* (1981), 84–94
35. Thiess, D.: Zur Biotransformation Aceton (Propan-2-on)/Isopropanol (Propan-2-ol) in der Leber. Z. Gesamte Hyg. *31* (1985), 530–531
36. Deutsche Forschungsgemeinschaft: Analytische Methoden zur Prüfung gesundheitsschädlicher Arbeitsstoffe. Band 2: Analysen in biologischem Material, D. Henschler (Ed.), VCH-Verlagsgesellschaft, Weinheim
37. Kumagai and Matsunaga: Physiologically-based pharmacokinetic model for acetone, Occup. Environ. Med. *52* (1995), 344
38. Mizunuma, K., Yasugi, T., Kawai, T., Horiguchi, S., Ikeda, M.: Exposure-excretion relationship of styrene and acetone in factory workers: A comparison of a lipophilic solvent and a hydrophilic solvent. Arch. Environ. Contam. Toxicol. *25* (1993), 129–133

39. Satho, T., Omae, K., Takebayashi, T., Nakashima, H., Higashi, T. Sakurai, H.: Acetone excretion into urine of workers exposed to acetone in acetate fiber plants, Int. Arch. Occup. Environ. Health *67* (1995), 131–134
40. Seeber, A., Kiesswetter, E., Vangala, R. R., Blaszekewicz, M., Golka, K.: Combined exposure to organic solvents: an experimental approach using acetone and ethyl acetate. Appl. Psychol. Int. Rev. *41* (1992), 281–292
41. BEI: Notice of intent to establish – Acetone, Appl. Occup. Environ. Hyg. *8 (5)* (1993), 505–509
42. Wang, G., Maranelli, G., Perbellini, L., Raineri, E., Brugnone, F.: Blood acetone concentration in "normal people" and in exposed workers 16 h after the end of the workshift, Int. Arch. Occup. Environ. Health *65* (1994), 285–289
43. Greim, H., Lehnert, G. (Eds.): Biologische Arbeitsstoff-Toleranzwerte (BAT-Werte) und Expositionsäquivalente für krebserzeugende Arbeitsstoffe (EKA), 6th issue, VCH-Verlagsgesellschaft, Weinheim (1993)
44. Henschler, D., Lehnert, G. (Eds.): 2-Propanol, in: Biologische Arbeitsstoff-Toleranzwerte (BAT-Werte) und Expositionsäquivalente für krebserzeugende Arbeitsstoffe (EKA), 5th issue, VCH-Verlagsgesellschaft, Weinheim (1990)

Authors: K. H. Schaller, G. Triebig
Approved by the Working Group: 18th April 1995

Alkali chromates (Cr(VI))

EKA for exposure to soluble alkali chromates (Cr(VI)) apart from exposure to welding fumes

The correlation between external and internal exposure yields the following data:

Air ($mg\ CrO_3/m^3$)	Erythrocytes* (µg Cr/l whole blood)	Urine** (µg Cr/l)
0.03	9	12
0.05	17	20
0.08	25	30
0.10	35	40

* Sampling: with long-term exposure: after several shifts

** Sampling: end of exposure or end of shift

EKA for exposure to alkali chromates (Cr(VI)) exclusively through exposure to welding fumes

The correlation between external and internal exposure yields the following data:

Air ($mg\ CrO_3/m^3$)	Urine* (µg Cr/l)
0.03	12
0.05	20
0.08	30
0.10	40

* Sampling: end of exposure or end of shift

Date of evaluation 1988

Formula M_2CrO_4, $M_2Cr_2O_7$

M = alkali metal

Molecular weight

CrO_4^{2-} 116.0

$Cr_2O_7^{2-}$ 216.0

Essential BAT Value Documentations. DFG, Deutsche Forschungsgemeinschaft

ISBN 3-527-31477-6

MAK
for chromium (VI) compounds in the form of dusts/aerosols (except those which are insoluble in water, e.g. lead chromate, barium chromate) (but zinc chromate Category III A1)
[last established: 1987]

Carcinogenic substance: Category III A2 of the MAK and BAT Values List

The documentation refers both to soluble alkali chromates and chromates as found in welding fumes. In the general part of this documentation (sections 1–5) both aspects are dealt with together; the evaluation of the threshold values in biological material for the two areas is treated separately.

1 Metabolism and Kinetics

Toxic effects of chromium compounds are attributed mainly to the hexavalent form of the metal, which almost always occurs in the chemical form of the chromate anion. Industrially important among the soluble chromates are mono or dichromates ($Cr_2O_4^{2-}$; CrO_7^{2-}) which are interconvertible via a pH-dependent equilibrium (15). With physiological pH values as they occur in the blood or in tissues this equilibrium shifts entirely to the side of the monochromates (56). There are several recent reviews of the absorption, distribution, retention and excretion of chromates (19, 22, 23, 31, 35). At the moment there are still great uncertainties about the states of chromium and its compounds in welding fumes. The presently available data for the kinetics and the metabolism of the chromates can be summarised as follows:

1.1 Absorption

An absorption of the chromates can take place in humans both via the gastrointestinal tract (2–6% of the dose) (12, 32) and the skin ($1-10\ mg/cm^2 \cdot h$) (3). Both routes of absorption, however, play a lesser role in the industrial field than does the intake of chromates via the respiratory passages.

Chromates can be absorbed by humans relatively quickly via the lungs, as shown in occupational-medical examinations, which correlate the Cr(VI) content of the air in the breathing zone with the chromium excretion in the urine after the end of exposure (47, 50). Important parameters which determine the uptake from the lung into the organism are the size and the solubility of the inhaled particles (7, 24, 38). Animal-experimental investigations on rabbits after the instillation of sodium chromate in comparison to chromium (III) chloride show that initially after absorption the applied chromate continues to occur in the hexavalent form in the plasma (55). This is the prerequisite for the transport into the erythrocytes. Variable amounts of the chromate which penetrates into the organism can apparently be reduced to Cr(III) in the plasma (see section 4.2).

1.2 Distribution

Chromates which penetrate into the blood circulation do not remain in the plasma. According to animal experimentation approximately 70–80% of the hexavalent chromium initially present in the plasma can be incorporated into the erythrocytes (55). With employees exposed to chromates individually differing amounts were found (see section 4.2). The very fast active transport process is probably based on a special anion transport system in the erythrocyte membrane (42) which exchanges bicarbonate for chloride ions at the necessary speed for blood buffering (18). A few other anions such as sulphate, phosphate (10, 43) as well as chromate (59) can also pass the cell membrane via this transport system. As could be shown above all in animal experiments, a further part of the chromium (VI) present in the plasma is transferred into the cells of the liver and kidneys. The kidneys store chromium under these conditions to a particularly great extent (2, 6, 53, 55). Investigations into the mechanism of the chromium movement in the kidneys revealed glomerular filtration which is followed by an almost complete tubular reabsorption (8, 33). Small amounts of chromium could be detected in animal experiments after inhalational chromate exposure also in the spleen and the bone marrow (2, 6, 53, 55). The blood-brain barrier can, according to all the available results, not be crossed by chromate ions (55).

1.3 Metabolism and Retention

A rapid reduction of chromium (VI) to chromium (III) takes place intracellularly after the passage of chromate through the cell membrane. In the erythrocytes this is mediated by both haemoglobin and glutathione (GSH). Outside the erythrocytes (above all in liver and kidneys) GSH, due to its high concentration, is probably mainly responsible for the reduction as GSH can easily reduce chromium (VI) to chromium (III) in vitro (56). The chromium (III) formed is then bound, due to its chemical characteristics (41), in complexes with proteins and other cell components. In this form the chromium cannot leave the cell again but can probably only be released with the cell death during physiological cell recycling (57).

1.4 Excretion

Pulmonally absorbed chromates are almost exclusively eliminated via the kidneys. The kinetics of renal chromium excretion is determined mainly by the mechanism of the intracellular storage described above, particularly in the erythrocytes. With humans a two-phase course of renal chromium excretion is observed in which a relatively rapid initial elimination phase is followed by a much slower one (the biological half-life lies in the region of several weeks) (54). After chromium (VI) exposure, thus, first of all, only part of the incorporated chromium is eliminated quickly from the organism, while another part persists for a longer time. This slow elimination phase is probably determined above all by the life span and the cell recycling of the erythrocytes (60).

The excretion via the faeces plays only a minor role after pulmonary absorption. It is difficult to quantify this amount. In how far an excretion of chromium via the bile in the gastro-intestinal tract and a possible enterohepatic circulation plays a role has not yet been clarified in humans. In rats low-molecular-weight compounds containing chromium which were probably GSH chromium adducts (58) could be traced in the bile after the application of alkali chromates (30, 37).

A transplacental transfer of chromates has been proven in animal experiments (54); little is known as to whether this also applies for humans. Indications of placental passage of chromium compounds during pregnancy were provided by investigations which showed that foetal and neonatal human tissue can contain much more chromium than the corresponding tissue of adult human beings (44).

2 Critical Toxicity

Under the conditions of acute intoxication caused by high concentrations of alkali chromates, kidney damage, according to some authors also liver damage, was observed in animal experiments (23, 48). In addition, the formation of methaemoglobin occurred; damage to the bone marrow was also reported in animal experiments (21).

For the evaluation of chromate concentrations such as usually occur at workplaces the possible carcinogenic effect of chromium (VI) compounds is decisive. Here it is noticeable that the carcinogenicity of different chromates is dependent upon their solubility. In particular, according to animal experiments, chromates of medium solubility (e.g. zinc chromate, calcium chromate) show an especially high carcinogenic effect after inhalation (35, 36). Target organs after inhalational exposure are the bronchi and lungs. The carcinogenic effect is weaker with chromates with a very low solubility (e.g. lead chromate) or very high solubility (e.g. alkali chromates). Mutagenic effects of chromate ions are found in vitro in systems with intact cells (for details see MAK documentation).

The difference in the strength of carcinogenicity has led to a different grouping of individual chromium (VI) compounds in section III of the MAK and BAT Values List. At the moment (MAK and BAT Values List 1993) zinc chromate is listed in section A1; chromium (VI) compounds in the form of dusts/aerosols (except those that are practically insoluble in water, e.g. lead chromate, barium chromate) are grouped under section A2. The suspicion of a carcinogenic potential (section B) is given for lead chromate.

As chromium (VI) compounds apparently only differ in degree but not in principle in their carcinogenic effect it seems at present not justified to take individual substances out of a general evaluation of the chromium (VI) compounds.

Therefore, for chromates no figure for a BAT value can be given but merely correlations between exposure and concentrations in biological media (see section 6.3).

3 Exposure and Effects

According to the above explanations the chromium (VI) concentration in the air at the workplace is to be regarded as the external exposure. The internal exposure exists in the biologically relevant concentration in the target tissue, e. g. in the respiratory tract, where carcinogenic effects manifest themselves.

Exposure parameters in the wider sense are all the chromium concentrations in different biological media, such as blood, plasma and urine. Exposure parameters in the narrower sense are chromium concentrations in body compartments which are directly and exclusively accessible to the chromium (VI) compounds, e. g. cell components of the blood. That part of chromium (VI) taken up which is transferred into the blood cells (depending on the individual reduction capacity of the plasma) is bound there irreversibly (28).

Such irreversible chromium adducts in the erythrocytes or leucocytes can be understood as parameters of internal chromium (VI) effects. By monitoring the DNA strand-break frequency in the leucocytes of persons exposed to chromium (VI) a further (be it very unspecific) response parameter of internal chromium (VI) exposure is available (51, 52, 63). This can be applied mainly in the evaluation of acute chromium (VI) intoxications.

4 Selection of the Indicators

The chromium burden and effects which occur after contact with chromium (VI) can be assessed in principle via the chromium concentrations in the urine, whole blood and plasma, as well as in the blood cells.

4.1 Chromium in Urine

Most investigations available to date have involved stainless-steel welders. This will be dealt with in more detail in this documentation (see section 6.4). Mainly linear correlations between the exposure to welding fumes containing soluble chromium (VI) compounds and the urinary chromium excretion were found (4, 17, 49, 62).

For persons exposed to alkali chromates, preventive measures based only on measurement of the urinary chromium excretion could not completely prevent the reddening of the nasal mucous membranes by the chromate. With the introduction of the chromium determination in erythrocytes improved surveillance has become possible for this group of persons.

4.2 Chromium in Erythrocytes

Data from the investigation of chromium concentrations in the blood and their correlation with external chromium (VI) exposure has been gained in occupational medical practice from time to time since about 1960. The cell penetration capability of chromium (VI) compounds (16) can be used in this context for the differentiation and evaluation of internal chromium exposures (28).

It was found that with exposures to Cr(VI) up to the level of the TRK value valid at present (0.1 mg CrO_3/m^3 air) the physiological reduction capacity of the plasma (20) prevents a considerable accumulation of chromium in the erythrocytes in approx. 70% of those exposed to chromium (VI). The other persons exposed to chromium (VI) accumulate a significant erythrocyte burden under the same workplace conditions. Such formally weak chromium (VI) reducers are thus recognisable via the chromium content in the erythrocytes. Compared to that of the rest of the population, their urinary chromium excretion is generally reduced.

Additional chromium determination in whole blood or plasma does not furnish any further diagnostic information. The chromium concentrations in the serum of healthy unexposed persons amount to 0.16 µg Cr/l (mean value) with a range of 0.04 – 0.35 µg Cr/l (52).

4.3 Chromium in Leucocytes

Part of the internal chromium (VI) exposure after the uptake of chromium (VI) can be bound in the leucocytes by the nucleic acids they contain (9, 11, 45, 51). A genotoxic effect of this chromium burden on the leucocytes can be determined by monitoring the frequency of DNA strand-breaks (45, 46).

5 Methodology

5.1 Chromium in Urine

The DFG Commission for the Investigation of Health Hazards of Chemical Compounds in the Work Area have developed a reliable method for the determination of the chromium concentration in urine and published it in their loose-leaf collection "Analysen in biologischem Material" and in the English edition "Analyses of Hazardous Substances in Biological Materials" (14).

5.2 Chromium in Erythrocytes

For the determination of chromium in erythrocytes a method has been described which, after the isolation and washing of the erythrocytes, employs electrothermal atomic absorption spectrometry with direct determination of the chromium in the graphite furnace (25, 28). The chromium concentrations determined in the erythrocytes are expressed in terms of the initial volume of blood under consideration of the packed cell volume of the whole blood (PCV_{Blood}) and that of the washed erythrocytes ($PCV_{Suspension}$) (see formulas under 5.4).

5.3 Chromium in Leucocytes

The determination of chromium in leucocytes can take place by the method of determination described for erythrocytes. Leucocytes isolated from the blood by a density-gradient centrifugation are washed and concentrated like erythrocytes (46).

The monitoring of the frequency of DNA strand breaks in the leucocytes can take place with the methodology of alkaline DNA elution (5, 46).

5.4 Calculation of the Chromium Concentration in Erythrocytes and Leucocytes

Bearing in mind possible losses during sample preparation due to the individual packed cell volumes (PCV_{Blood}, $PCV_{Suspension}$) the chromium concentration in erythrocytes c_{Ery} $\left(\frac{\mu g\ chromium}{l\ blood}\right)$ or in leucocytes c_{Leuco} $\left(\frac{\mu g\ chromium}{l\ blood}\right)$ can be calculated as follows:

$$c_{Ery/Leuco}\left(\frac{\mu g\ chromium}{l\ blood}\right) = \frac{PVC_{Blood}}{PCV_{Suspension}} \cdot c_{Suspension}\left(\frac{\mu g\ chromium}{l\ suspension}\right)$$

$c_{Ery/Leuco}$ = chromium concentration in the erythrocytes or leucocytes per blood volume

$c_{Suspension}$ = measured chromium concentration of the erythrocyte or leucocyte suspension

PCV_{Blood} = packed cell volume of the whole blood

$PCV_{Suspension}$ = packed cell volume of the erythrocyte or leucocyte suspension

The chromium determination in biological material must be carried out in accordance with the TRGS 410 (Technical Guideline for Dangerous Chemicals) under the conditions of the statistical quality control according to the regulations of the Bundesärztekammer.

6 Evaluation of the Biological Exposure Equivalents for Carcinogenic Substances (EKA)

The actual chromium concentrations in the target tissue after inhalation of chromium (VI) cannot be directly determined. But the concentrations can be deduced from the chromium concentrations in biological material because of the pharmacokinetic situation (see section 1).

6.1 Chromium in Urine

Statistical analyses of the correlation data gained in numerous investigations on welders exposed to chromium (VI) show that an exposure to welding fumes of about 8 hours with (on average) approx. 100 μg CrO_3/m^3 leads to an average urine level of about 30–55 μg Cr/l (see section 6.4). Interindividual variations in the chromium excretion rates were attributed first of all to a differing basic chromium burden on the organism (47). A further important cause of interindividual correlation differences are the individual differences in the ability to reduce chromium (VI) (28).

6.2 Chromium in Erythrocytes

After contact with chromium (VI) within the range of the TRK value valid at present (0.1 mg CrO_3/m^3) significantly increased chromium levels in the erythrocytes are to be observed in some employees (see section 4.2) (27, 28). The amounts of chromium also detectable in the leucocytes under these circumstances neither lead to obvious cytotoxic effects (29), nor to a statistically significantly increased frequency of DNA strand-breaks (5, 11, 45).

6.3 Exposure to Soluble Alkali Chromates: Correlation between External Exposure and Biological Parameters

The above discussion indicates that the erythrocytic chromium levels after Cr(VI) exposure are increased particularly in persons with a low spontaneous reduction ability of the plasma (weak reducers) and the urinary excretion levels (measured after the shift) of those with a good reduction capacity (strong reducers) are increased. This relationship was investigated in employees who were exposed to soluble alkali chromates, on average to an air concentration of 40 μg CrO_3/m^3 (24 "weak reducers"; 52 "strong reducers"). In practice biological monitoring must be geared to these circumstances (26). According to the data available so far, the following relationship, expressed in table form, between the external exposure and the two biological parameters under discussion is apparent:

Chromium concentration in air (mg CrO_3/m^3)	Maximum chromium level in the erythrocytes** (μg Cr/l*)	Maximum excretion in urine at end of shift*** (μg Cr/g creatinine)
0.03	9	12
0.05	17	20
0.08	25	30
0.10	35	40

* The chromium content in erythrocytes is given by μg Cr per l initial blood volume. The content is determined from the measured concentration in the erythrocyte suspension, the packed cell volume of the whole blood (PCV_{Blood}) and the packed cell volume of the suspension ($PCV_{Suspension}$).

** with "weak" reducers

*** with "strong" reducers

6.4 Exposure to Welding Fumes: Correlation between External Chromium/Chromate Exposure and Biological Parameters in Welders

The relationship between the chromate concentration in the air of welding workplaces and the chromium excretion in urine is amply documented in the literature. Table 1 shows that with manual metal arc welders chromium concentrations in the urine between 29 and 55 μg/l correspond to a chromium/chromate exposure of 100 μg chromium trioxide per m^3 ambient air. If onc expresses the chromium excretion in terms of the creatinine content in the urine one obtains values between 18 and 38 μg chromium per g creatinine. (For the conversion between the dimensions μg/l and μg/g creatinine a creatinine content in the urine of 1.5 g/l was taken as a basis).

With the evaluation of a relationship between the external and internal chromium exposure of manual metal arc welders it must furthermore be taken into account that only part of the chromium present in the ambient air occurs in the form of hexavalent chromium. For the calculation of a relationship between the external chromium concentration and the chromium excretion in the urine it was assumed that 50% of the chromium in the ambient air was chromate. On the other hand the molecular weight of the chromium trioxide is almost twice as high as the atomic weight of the chromium. It can therefore be assumed for the sake of simplicity in the interpretation of the ambient air concentrations given in table 1 that with manual metal arc welders a chromium concentration of 100 μg total chromium per m^3 ambient air corresponds to a numerically similar value for the chromium trioxide concentration.

The assumption that 50% of the chromium is present as chromate is, however, uncertain. Often in the literature a much higher level is stated. On the other hand significantly less chromate was found by Zober et al. (61, 63) in the welding fumes of stainless-steel welders (MMA). A review of the chromate level in the welding fumes of various welding processes has been published (39).

Differentiation according to welding methods has been carried out in table 2. With the welding methods metal inert gas welding (MIG), metal active gas welding (MAG) and tungsten inert gas welding (TIG) the level of the hexavalent chromium in the total chromium concentration in the ambient air is much lower than with manual metal arc welding. Emmerling et al. (13) state that the chromium share in the ambient air with MAG and TIG welding is 5.4 and 22.1% respectively. If one considers these relatively low chromium levels in the ambient air compared to those for the manual metal arc welders arithmetically, then the chromium excretions of the MAG and TIG welders fit the framework provided by the manual metal arc welders. It is particularly remarkable that the chromium excretion in the urine is almost exclusively determined by the external exposure to hexavalent chromium compounds. Exposures to other valencies of this metal are of hardly any importance in the chromium amounts excreted in the urine. This means that predominantly the share of the metal taken in in the chromate form is reflected in the chromium excretion in the urine. Metallic chromium or chromium (III) compounds accordingly do not seem to be absorbed quickly enough to be noticeable after the end of a workshift in a significant increase in the chromium excreted in the urine. On the other hand equally high chromate exposures, regardless of how they arose, seem to be reflected in the same chromium ex-

Tab. 1: Investigations of the chromium/chromate concentration in the ambient air at the workplace and the chromium concentration in the urine of welders; Welding process: manual metal arc welding (MMA) of high-alloyed chromium/nickel-steels. Values in ( ) converted according to a creatinine content in the urine of 1.5 g/l.

Total chromium concen-tration Air	Chromate concen-tration Air	Chromium concentration Urine		Chromium concentration in urine for exposure to 100 µg CrO_3/m^3		Correlation between external and internal exposure	Type of welding	Number of persons ex-amined	References
(µg Cr/m^3)	(µg CrO_3/m^3)	(µg Cr/l)	(µg Cr/g creat.)	(µg Cr/l)	(µg Cr/g creat.)				
89.4	96.6	28.0	–	29	19		MMA	26	13
100		–	23.9	(37.3)	24.9	+	MMA	19	54
100		40	–	55	(36.3)	+		5	17
	100	–	38	48	38	+		5	49
103		37.3	–	32	(21)		MMA	53	47
	100	–	30.8	(46.2)	30.8	+	MMA	5	40
	100	–	33	(44.7)	29.8	+	MMA	36	34
	100	17.5	–		18		MMA	20	62

Tab. 2: Investigations of the chromium/chromate concentration in the ambient air at the workplace and the chromium concentration in the urine of welders who use differing welding processes; MIG = metal inert gas welding, MAG = metal active gas welding, TIG = tungsten inert gas welding.

Total chromium concentration Air	Chromate concentration Air	Chromium concentration Urine		Chromium concentration in urine for exposure to 100 µg CrO_3/m^3		Correlation between external and internal exposure	Type of welding	Number of persons examined	References
(µg Cr/m^3)	(µg CrO_3/m^3)	(µg Cr/l)	(µg Cr/g creat.)	(µg Cr/l)	(µg Cr/g creat.)				
62	23	–	12.1	29.6	26.4	+	MIG	12	34
179	15	14.8	–	Basic excretion + 20		+	MAG	33	13
37.8	14.4	8.7		Basic excretion + 8			TIG	24	13

Tab. 3: Correlations between the chromate concentration in the workplace air (µg CrO_3/m^3) and in urine (µg/l) in welders, as well as the calculated urine value for an exposure to 100 µg CrO_3/m^3.

Regression equation Cr_{Urine} = a $Chromate_{Air}$ + b Cr_{Urine} (µg/l); $Chromium_{Air}$ (µg CrO_3/m^3)	Correlation coefficient r	Chromium concentration in urine for exposure to 100 µg CrO_3/m^3 (µg Cr/l)	Welding type	Number of persons examined	Comments	References
Cr_{Urine} = 0.20 $Chromate_{Air}$ + 12.57	0.573	34	MMA, MAG, TIG	68		13
Cr_{Urine} = 0.19 $Chromate_{Air}$ + 12.28	0.672	31	MMA-Rutile welding	17		13
Cr_{Urine} = 0.034 $Chromate_{Air}$ + 15.34	0.580	18	MMA, MAG, TIG	20	42 pairs of values; Sampling: end of shift	62
Cr_{Urine} = 0.139 $Chromate_{Air}$ + 11.91	0.677	26		20	32 pairs of values; Sampling: next morning	62
Cr_{Urine} = 0.1 $Chromate_{Air}$ + 25.8	0.91	36 µg Cr/g creat.; 18 µg Cr/g creat. for ambient air concentrations in µg Cr/m^3	MMA	5	Air concentration: there is an uncertainty whether the Cr(VI) values were given as µg CrO_3/m^3 or as µg Cr/m_3	40

cretion level in the urine. Mutti et al. (34) found highly significant relationships between the chromate concentration in the ambient air and the chromium excretion in the urine which have proved independent of whether the chromate was present in the form of potassium dichromate or chromic anhydride or occurred as a component of welding fumes.

These observations suggest that the chromium concentration in the urine is a suitable parameter for the chromate exposure at the workplace. It is probably of less importance how high the concentration of chromium of other valancies in the ambient air is.

The studies listed in table 1 show the relationships between the chromium/chromate exposure in the ambient air and the chromium concentration in the urine. This relationship between the external and internal exposure is based on measurements of the contaminants through personal air sampling and the chromium concentrations in urine samples which were taken at the end of the shift. On the basis of this data a generally valid relationship between the external chromate exposure and the chromium concentration in the urine can be evaluated which corresponds more or less with the data (section 6.3) found for the level of the urinary excretion of chromium after alkali chromate exposure.

The data in table 1 can be supplemented by the correlations given in the literature (Tab. 3). The data from Emmerling et al. (13) allow differentiation according to the welding method used. From the studies listed in table 3, with an ambient air value of 100 µg CrO_3/m^3 a urinary excretion of chromium of about 30–40 µg/l would be derived.

There is little data in the literature on the chromium content of erythrocytes after exposure to welding fumes. Emmerling et al. (13) have given a relationship between the chromate content of the ambient air and the chromium content of erythrocytes. With the examination of 80 stainless-steel welders they ascertained a highly significant relationship between the two parameters. These values have been supported at least in their magnitude by the results by Angerer et al. (1). According to this study there is a statistically highly significant relationship between the chromium concentration of the urine and that of the erythrocytes. From these provisional data an erythrocyte burden in the region of 4–5 µg Cr/l and a renal excretion of approx. 30 µg Cr/l can be derived for an ambient air concentration of 100 µg CrO_3/m^3.

With both investigations the accumulation of chromium in the erythrocytes after exposure to welding fumes is much lower than with a comparable alkali chromate exposure. This may be the result of the form of the particles in which the chromium occurs in the welding fumes. On the other hand the proportion of chromium (VI) may vary. As these questions still remain unanswered it does not yet seem possible to determine threshold values for the chromium content in the erythrocytes for the exposure to welding fumes.

6.5 Evaluation of the Biological Exposure Equivalents

After rounding the data given in section 6.3 the following Biological Exposure Equivalents result.

a) Exposure to soluble alkali chromates (Cr(VI)) and/or to welding fumes

Chromium concentration in the air ($mg\ CrO_3/m^3$)	Threshold value excretion in urine at the end of the shift (μg Cr/l)
0.03	12
0.05	20
0.08	30
0.10	40

b) Exposure to soluble alkali chromates (Cr(VI))

Chromium concentration in the air ($mg\ CrO_3/m^3$)	Threshold value chromium level in the erythrocytes (μg Cr/l whole blood)*
0.03	9
0.05	17
0.08	25
0.10	35

* For calculation see section 5.4 and 6.3

7 Interpretation of the Data

For chromates, at the time of compilation of this documentation (1987/88), a TRK value of 0.1 mg CrO_3 in total dust was valid; for "manual metal arc welding with covered electrodes" a TRK value of 0.2 mg CrO_3 was given. The latter value is of a size for which there is no sufficient recent literature on the excretion of chromium in urine which would allow the continuation of the correlation table in section 6.5 under a).

It should be taken into account that in contrast to monitoring by measuring the air concentration, effective biological monitoring of those exposed to the chromate is much simpler as the total body burden is indicated by biological monitoring while air measurements only allow an incomplete statement.

With the biological monitoring of persons occupationally exposed to soluble alkali chromates, the determination of chromium exposure levels in the urine and in the erythrocytes are not to be judged as equally valuable preventive measures. The high cellular chromium burden of those individuals who are only able to reduce chromates weakly can only be diagnosed in the erythrocytes. For routine examinations of those exposed to chromium (VI) the checking of the chromium concentrations in erythrocytes should therefore be given priority if possible, particularly as with this method not only the effects of current chromium exposure but also those of up to

3 weeks previously can be reproduced (28). Chromium-urine examinations are more appropriate with persons exposed to soluble alkali chromates for checking after occasional or only slight exposure to chromium (VI) (see section 6.4).

The investigation of chromium in erythrocytes is not bound to any particular sampling time (28). In contrast to this, results of chromium determination in the urine only then allow a reliable evaluation if these samples are taken at the end of exposure periods (28).

8 References

1. Angerer, J., Amin, W., Heinrich-Ramm, R., Szadkowski, D., Lehnert, G.: Int. Arch. Occup. Environ. Health *59* (1987), 503–512
2. Baetjer, A. M., Damron, C., Budacz, V.: The distribution and retention of chromium in men and animals. AMA Arch. Ind. Health *20* (1959), 136–150
3. Baranowska-Dutkiewicz, B.: Absorption of hexavalent chromium by skin in man. Arch. Toxicol. *47* (1981), 47–50
4. Berode, M., Guillemine, M.: Evaluation d'une exposition professionelle au chrome par le dosage du chrome urinaire. Med. Soc. Prev. *22* (1977), 201–202
5. Bianchi, V., Celotti, L., Lanfranchi, G., Majone, F., Marin, G., Montaldi, A., Sponza, G., Tamino, G., Venier, P., Zantedeschi, A., Levis, A. G.: Genetic effects of chromium compounds. Mutat. Res. *117* (1983), 279–300
6. Bragt, P. C., van Dura, E. A.: Toxicokinetics of hexavalent chromium in the rat after intratracheal administration of chromates of different solubilities. Ann. Occup. Hyg. *27* (1983), 315–322
7. Campbell, K. I.: Inhalation toxicology. Clin. Toxicol. *9* (1976), 849–921
8. Collins, R. J., Fromm, P. O., Collins, W. D.: Chromium excretion in the dog. Am. J. Physiol. *201* (1961), 795
9. Cupo, D. Y., Wetterhahn, K. E.: Binding of chromium to chromatin and DNA from liver and kidney of rats treated with sodium dichromate and chromium (III) chloride in vivo. Cancer Res. *45* (1985), 1146–1151
10. Deuticke, B.: Über die Kinetik der Phosphat-Permeation in den Menschen-Erythrocyten bei Variation von extracellulärer Phosphat-Konzentration, Anionen-Milieu und Zell-Volumen. Pflügers Archiv *296* (1967), 21–38
11. Doerjer, G., Bedell, M. A., Oesch, F.: DNA adducts and their biological relevance. In: G. Obe (ed.) Mutations in man. Springer Verlag, Berlin 1984, pp. 20–34
12. Donaldson, R. M., Barreras, R. F.: Intestinal absorption of trace quantities of chromium. J. Lab. Clin. Med. *68* (1966), 484
13. Emmerling, G., Zschiesche, W., Schaller, K. H., Weltle, D., Valentin, H., Zober, A.: in: Verhandlungen der Deutschen Gesellschaft für Arbeitsmedizin. 27. Jahrestagung. Gentner, Stuttgart 1987, pp. 497–501
14. Fischer, M.: Chrom: Bestimmung im Harn. In: D. Henschler (ed.) Analytische Methoden zur Prüfung gesundheitsschädlicher Arbeitsstoffe. Bd. 2: Analysen in biologischem Material. 9. Lfg, VCH Verlagsgesellschaft, Weinheim 1988
15. Freier, R. K.: Gebiete des relativen Überwiegens von Ionen von sechswertigem Chrom bei 25 °C. In: Freier (ed.) Aqueous Solution. Vol. 2, de Gruyter Verlag, Berlin 1978, p. 622
16. Gray, S. J., Sterling, K.: The tagging of red cells and plasma proteins with radioactive chromium. J. Clin. Invest. *29* (1950), 1604–1613
17. Gylseth, B., Gundersen, N., Langard, S.: Evaluation of chromium exposure based on a simplified method for urinary chromuim determination. Scand. J. Work. Environ. Health *3* (1978), 28–31
18. Hladky, S. B., Rink, T. J.: ph equilibrium across the red cell membrane. In: Ellory/Lew (ed.) Membrane transport in red cells. Academic Press, London 1977, pp. 115–135
19. International Agency for Research on Cancer: IARC Monographs on the evaluation of the carcinogenic risk of chemicals to humans. Vol. 23: Some Metals and Metallic Compounds. Lyon 1980, pp. 205–325

20. Korallus, U., Harzdorf, C., Lewalter, J.: Experimental bases of ascorbic acid therapy of poisoning by hexavalent chromium compounds. Int. Arch. Occup. Environ. Health *53* (1984), 247 – 256
21. Langard, S.: Chromium. In: Waldron (ed.) Metals in the environment. Academic Press, London 1980, pp. 111 – 132
22. Langard, S.: Absorption, transport and excretion of chromium in man and animals. In: S. Langard, (ed.), Biological and environmental aspects of chromium. Elsevier, Amsterdam 1982, pp. 149 – 169
23. Langard, S., Hensten-Pettersen, A.: Chromium toxicology. In: Williams (ed.) Systemic aspects of biocompatibility. Vol. 1. CRC Press, Boca Raton FL 1981, pp. 143 – 161
24. Laskin, S., Sellakumar, A.: Models in chemical respiratory carcinogenesis. In: Karbe/Park (eds.) Experimental lung cancer. Carcinogenesis and Bioassays, Springer, Berlin 1974, pp. 7 – 19
25. Lewalter, J., Domik, D., Weidemann, H.: Chrom in stabilisiertem Vollblut, Plasma und Erythrozyten. In: D. Henschler (ed.) Analytische Methoden zur Prüfung gesundheitsschädlicher Arbeitsstoffe. Bd. 2: Analysen in biologischem Material. 10. Lfg., VCH Verlagsgesellschaft, Weinheim 1993.
26. Lewalter, J., Korallus, U., Toxicol. Lett. *33* (1986), 153
27. Lewalter, J., Korallus, U.: Correlation of hexavalent chromium stress and strain in isolated erythrocytes and leukocytes (in preparation)
28. Lewalter, J., Korallus, U., Harzdorf, C., Weidemann, H.: Chromium bound detection in isolated erythrocytes: a new principle of biological monitoring of exposure to hexavalent chromium. Int. Arch. Occup. Environ. Health *55* (1985), 305 – 318
29. Littorin, M., Hoegstedt, B., Stroembaeck, B., Karlsson, A., Welinder, H., Mitelman, F., Skerfving, S.: No cytogenetic effects in lymphocytes of stainless steel welders. Scand. J. Work Environ. Health *9* (1983), 259 – 264
30. Manzo, L., di Nucci, A., Edel, J., Gregotti, C., Sabbioni, E.: Biliary and gastrointestinal excretion of chromium after administration of Cr-III and Cr-VI in rats. Res. Commun. Chem. Pathol. Pharmacol. *42* (1983), 113 – 125
31. Mertz, W.: Chromium occurrence and function in biological systems. Physiol. Rev. *49* (1969), 163 – 239
32. Mertz, W., Roginski, E. E., Reba, R. C.: Biological activity and fate of trace quantities of intravenous chromium (III) in the rat. Am. J. Physiol. *209* (1965), 489 – 494
33. Mutti, A., Cavatorta, A., Borghi, L., Canali, M., Giaroli, C., Franchini, I.: Distribution and urinary excretion of chromium. Studies on rats after administration of single and repeated doses of potassium dichromate. Med. Lav. *3* (1979), 171 – 179
34. Mutti, A., Pedroni, C., Arfini, G., Franchini, I., Minoia, C., Micoli, G., Baldi, C., Int. J. Environ. Anal. Chem. *17* (1984), 35 – 41
35. National Institute for Occupational Safety and Health: Criteria for a Recommended Standard for Occupational Exposure to Chromium VI. U.S. Dept. of Health, Education and Welfare, Public Health Service (1975)
36. Nettesheim, P., Hanna, M. G., Doherty, D. G., Newell, R. F., Hellmann, A.: Effect of calcium chromate dust, influenza virus, and 100 R whole-body X radiation on lung tumor incidence in mice. J. Nat. Cancer Inst. *47* (1971), 1129 – 1144
37. Norseth, T., Alexander, J., Aaseth, J., Langard, S.: Biliary excretion of chromium in the rat: A role of glutthione. Acta Pharmacol. Toxicol. *51* (1982), 450 – 455
38. Pavia, D., Bateman, J. R. M., Sheahan, N. F., Agnew, J. E., Newman, S. P., Clarke, S. W.: Techniques for measuring lung mucociliary clearance. Eur. J. Respir. Dis. *110* (1980), 157 – 177
39. Pfeiffer, W.: Nickel- und Chromatexposition an Schweißarbeitsplätzen. Empfehlung für die meßtechnische Überwachung. In: Berufsgenossenschaftliches Institut für Arbeitssicherheit., 7. Lfg. (ed.) BIA-Handbuch, E. Schmidt, Berlin 1987
40. Rahkonen, E., Junttila, M. L., Kalliomäki, P. L., Olkinonora, M., Koponen, M., Kalliomäki, K.: Int. Arch. Occup. Environ. Health *52* (1983), 243 – 255
41. Rollinson, C. L.: Problems of chromium reactions. In: Andrews/Kniseley/Wagner (eds.), Radioactive pharmaceuticals. U.S. Atomic Energy Commission, Oak Ridge, Tenn., Conf-651111, Springfield, Ill.: U.S. Dept. of Commerce, AEC Symposium Series 6 (1966)
42. Rothstein, A., Cabantchik, Z. I., Kraut, P.: Mechanism of anion transport in red blood cells: role of membrane proteins. Fed. Proc. *35* (1976), 3 – 10
43. Schnell, K. F., Gerhardt, S., Schöppe-Fredenburg, A.: Kinetic characteristics of the sulfate self-exchange in human red blood cells and red blood cell ghosts. J. Membrane Biol. *30* (1977), 319 – 150

44. Schroeder, H. A., Balassa, J. J., Tipton, I. H.: Abnormal trace metals in man – chromium. J. chron. Dis. *15* (1962), 941–964
45. Sina, J. F., Bean, C. L., Dysart, G. R., Taylor, V. I., Bradley, M. O.: Evaluation of the alkaline elution; rat hepatocyte assay as a predictor of carcinogenic/mutagenic potential. Mutat. Res. *129* (1983), 357–391
46. Skare, J. A., Schrotel, K. R.: Alkaline elution of rat testicular DNA: Detection of DNA strand breaks after in vivo treatment with chemical mutagens. Mutat. Res. *130* (1984), 283–294
47. Sjoergren, B., Hedstroem, L., Ulfvaeson, U.: Urine chromium as an estimator of air exposure to stainless steel welding fumes. Int. Arch. Occup. Health *51* (1983), 347–354
48. Tandon, S. K.: Organ toxicity of chromium in animals. In: Langard (ed.), Biological and environmental aspects of chromium. Elsevier Biomedical Press, Amsterdam 1982, pp. 209–220
49. Tola, S., Kilpio, J., Virtamo, M., Haapa, K.: Urinary chromium as an indicator of the exposure of welders to chromium. Scand. J. Work Environ. Health *3* (1972), 192–202
50. Tossavainen, A., Nurminen, M., Mutanen, P., Tola, S.: Application of mathematical modelling for assessing the biological half-times of chromium and nickel in field studies. Br. J. Ind. Med. *37* (1980), 285–291
51. Tsapakos, M. J., Wetterhahn, K. E.: The interaction of chromium with nucleic acids. Chem.-Biol. Interactions *46* (1982), 265–277
52. Versieck, J., Hoste, J., Barbier, F.: Determination of chromium and cobalt in human serum by neutron activation analysis. Clin. Chem. *24* (1978), 303–308
53. Weber, H.: Long-term study of the distribution of soluble chromate-VI in the rat after a single intratracheal administration. J. Toxicol. Environ. Health *11* (1983), 749–764
54. Welinder, H., Littorin, M., Gullberg, B., Skerfving, S.: Elimination of chromium in urine after stainless steel welding. Scand. J. Work Environ. Health *9* (1983), 397–403
55. Wiegand, H. J., Ottenwaelder, H., Bolt, H. M.: Disposition of intratracheally administered chromium (III) and chromium (VI) in rabbits. Toxicol. Lett. *22* (1984), 273–276
56. Wiegand, H. J., Ottenwaelder, H., Bolt, H. M.: Toxicology *33* (1984), 341
57. Wiegand, H. J., Ottenwaelder, H., Bolt, H. M.: Arbmed. Sozmed. Prävmed. *20* (1985), 109
58. Wiegand, H. J., Ottenwaelder, H., Bolt, H. M.: Arch. Toxicol *57* (1985), 31
59. Wiegand, H. J., Ottenwaelder, H., Bolt, H. M.: Arch. Toxicol. Suppl. *8* (1985), 319
60. Wiegand, H. J., Seelemann, I., Ottenwälder, H., Bolt, H. M. in: Verhandlungen der Deutschen Gesellschaft für Arbeitsmedizin. 27. Jahrestagung. Gentner, Stuttgart 1987, pp. 503–506
61. Zober, A., Schaller, K. H., Weltle, D.: Staub Reinh. Luft *44* (1984), 465
62. Zober, A., Schaller, K. H., Weltle, D.: DVS-Berichte. Bd. 95. Düsseldorf: Deutscher Verlag für Schweißtechnik, 1985
63. Zober, A., Weltle, D., Schaller, K. H., Valentin, H.: Schweißen und Schneiden, Nr. 10 (1984), 1–4

Authors: H. M. Bolt, J. Lewalter
Approved by the Working Group: 15th March 1988

Aniline

BAT

free aniline	1 mg/l urine
aniline released from aniline-haemoglobin conjugate	100 µg/l blood

Date of evaluation	1985
Addendum	1993
Synonyms	aminobenzene phenylamine
Formula	C_6H_7N

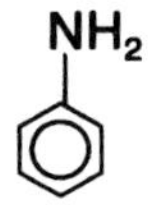

Molecular weight	93.13
Melting point	−6.3 °C
Boiling point	184.13 °C
Vapour pressure at 20 °C	64 Pa (0.48 torr)
MAK	2 ml/m^3 (ppm) 8 mg/m^3

1 Metabolism and Kinetics

Toxic effects of aniline are observed after inhalation and after oral or cutaneous exposure (6). It is quickly absorbed and its metabolites are excreted within 24 to 48 hours, predominantly via the kidneys. An accumulation of metabolites bound to haemoglobin is observed and, as a consequence of erythrocyte degradation, in the spleen (18, 22). Recent investigations on various species of animal have shown that the main route of metabolism takes place via acetylation to acetanilide and further to *N*-acetyl-

Essential BAT Value Documentations. DFG, Deutsche Forschungsgemeinschaft

ISBN 3-527-31477-6

p-aminophenol (13, 27). In addition O-conjugates of *o*-aminophenol and *p*-aminophenol are found in the urine (14). Phenylhydroxylamine and nitrosobenzene are only excreted in small amounts. The main metabolic pathways of aniline are shown in figure 1. Furthermore, additional metabolic pathways of aromatic amines have been discussed recently, e. g. co-oxidation by prostaglandin synthetase (21) and conjugation reactions of hydroxamic acids (12). The relationship of *o*-hydroxylation to *p*-hydroxylation depends to a great extent upon the kind of animal and in humans, moreover, is subject to great individual variation (24). *m*-Aminophenol is only formed in small amounts. With increasing exposure to aniline the formation of aminophenol increases significantly (25).

In addition to acetylation N-oxidation takes place to a small extent. This leads to the formation of methaemoglobin mainly because phenylhydroxylamine is formed from aniline in the liver and then oxidised in the erythrocytes to nitrosobenzene (7). In the presence of oxygen in coupled oxidation reactions the bivalent iron in the haemoglobin is simultaneously oxidised to the trivalent form.

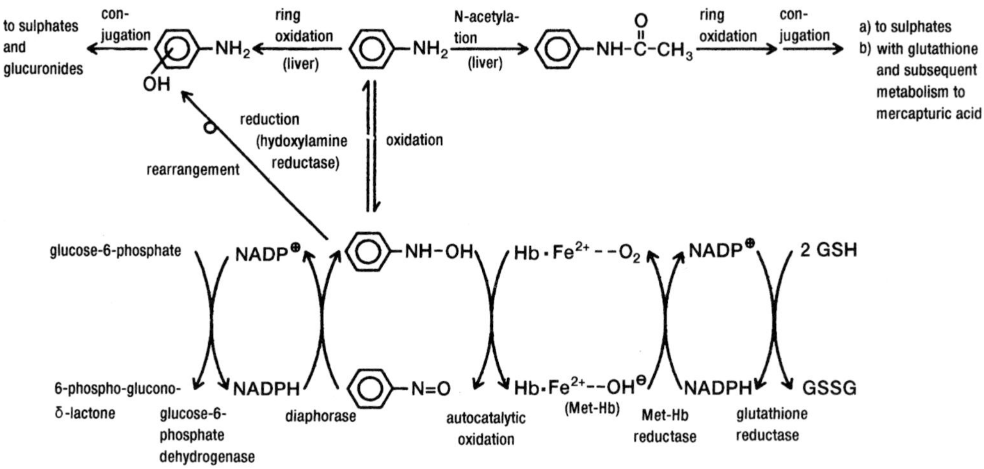

Fig. 1: Metabolism of aniline (4, 5, 7, 8)

This cycle can repeat itself several times as nitrosobenzene can be reduced to phenylhydroxylamine again by NADPH-dependent diphorases. The transformation of phenylhydroxylamine to *o*-aminophenol and *p*-aminophenol and the conjugation of the intermediates involved are considered to be detoxifying mechanisms (10). The intermediate, nitrosobenzene, can also bind covalently to SH-groups of haemoglobin and glutathione (1, 23, 28, 31) forming a sulphinic acid amide. These reactions are shown in figure 2.

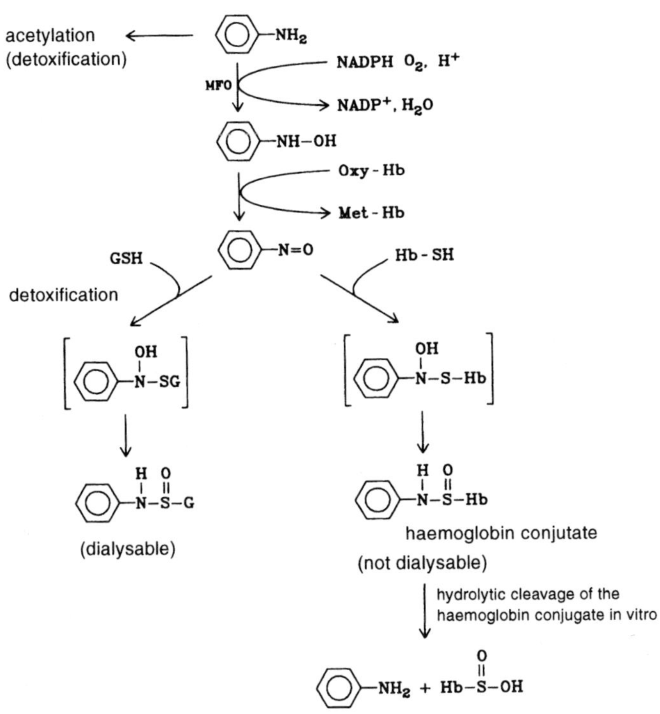

Fig. 2: Formation of aniline conjugates with glutathione and haemoglobin (according to (28)); MFO = mixed function oxygenases

2 Critical Toxicity

High concentrations of aniline in the workplace air quickly lead, i. e. within 10–30 minutes, first to central nervous effects, then via dizziness and clouding of consciousness to unconsciousness. The formation of methaemoglobin is recognisable by the blue colouring of the lips, nose, ears and nail bed. These acute toxic effects can be prevented by observance of the MAK value.

Sub-acute aniline exposures are also supposed to have effects on liver metabolism (25). The type and extent are, however, not described in any more detail. With large-scale destruction of the erythrocytes kidney damage can occur. In isolated cases changes in the white blood count and damage to the bone marrow have been described (29).

Chronic aniline exposures can lead after only slight formation of methaemoglobin and correspondingly only slight cyanosis to the formation of Heinz (inclusion) bodies and anaemia. With slow progression often only subjective complaints occur until finally occasionally hypochromic anaemia and isolated inclusion bodies can be found, usually with only slightly increased methaemoglobin levels. Manifest clinical symptoms do not occur until the methaemoglobin level is more than 10 %. Known effects in humans are described in detail in the MAK documentation for aniline (3).

2.1 Methaemoglobin Formation

For details of the pathophysiology of methaemoglobinaemia reference can be made to the current MAK documentation for aniline (3). Notes and information on the practical use of methaemoglobin determination in biological monitoring can be found in a publication by the Working Group on the problem of establishing BAT values for aromatic amines (6).

2.2 Other Effects of Aniline

In addition to the formation of methaemoglobin, exposure to aniline also causes other effects. The formation of Heinz bodies has been observed, inclusion bodies resulting from denaturation of haemoglobin. Chronic uptake of aniline can cause haemolysis and lead to anaemia. In addition to these effects on erythrocytes, neurotoxic effects can be expected.

2.3 Possible Carcinogenic Effects

For a discussion of potential carcinogenic effects of aniline and aromatic amines reference can be made to a review compiled by the Commission (6). On the basis of experiments in which aniline was fed to rats in very high doses for a prolonged period this substance is suspected of having carcinogenic potential. Therefore it is listed in category III B of the List of MAK and BAT Values (19a). The ability of aniline metabolites to react with macromolecules is of relevance in this context.

3 Exposure and Effect

In the sense of the exposure-effect concept the aniline concentration in the workplace air is defined as the external aniline exposure. Its permissible level is set by the MAK value. The internal exposure is the actual amount of aniline absorbed. It governs the extent to which phenylhydroxylamine and nitrosobenzene are formed metabolically. The effects include the pathophysiological changes in erythrocytes caused by these metabolites. These correlate even after acute intoxication only to a certain extent with the excretion of particular metabolites in the urine. The effects caused by aniline are conventionally evaluated via the changes in the blood methaemoglobin level. This question has been discussed by the Working Group elsewhere (6).

More recently the effects of aniline have been evaluated by measuring the levels of stable protein conjugates. The aniline-haemoglobin conjugate in a blood sample is cleaved hydrolytically and the released aniline determined quantitatively. Bound aniline can be detected even days after exposure. This is possible even in cases in which free aniline and its metabolites have already been completely eliminated. Unlike the determination of methaemoglobin, the results gained by this method are much less dependent on the time of sampling.

4 Selection of the Indicators

There is an extensive publication on this subject (18). Information on exposure and effect relationships on the basis of extensive monitoring of occupationally exposed persons can be found there. Internal exposure can be determined routinely by the measurement of the concentrations of aniline, acetanilide or aminophenols in whole blood or urine. The analysis of aniline should be preferred. The effect can be determined via the level of methaemoglobin or aniline-haemoglobin conjugate.

The importance of the methaemoglobin determination is the possibility it provides of being able to evaluate the extent of acute intoxication quickly. A considerable disadvantage for the setting of a BAT value is the dependency of the findings on the sampling time. The evaluation of the aniline-haemoglobin conjugate is therefore more suitable, in particular for intermittent or chronic exposure.

5 Methodology

Methods to determine the aniline concentration in the blood and urine as well as the analysis of aniline-haemoglobin conjugates have been published in the loose-leaf collection "Analysen in biologischem Material" (Analyses of Hazardous Substances in Biological Materials) (17). This also applies to the determination of methaemoglobin and *p*-aminophenol (2).

6 Evaluation of the BAT Value

Threshold limit values are not established for acute intoxications, which are rare today, but for chronic exposure at the workplace. There are only few investigations on the excretion of aminophenols (9, 26). A tolerance value of 5 mg *p*-aminophenol per l urine was published by Linch (19). Lauwerys (15), on the other hand, recommended permitting internal exposures up to levels causing excretion of 10 mg *p*-aminophenol per l urine. He based his conclusions on investigations in which manifest damage after exposure to aniline was only observed after excretion at *p*-aminophenol concentrations of more than 50 mg/l (20).

In recent reviews (16, 17, 30) the tolerance levels are based almost exclusively on methaemoglobin determinations, seldom on the specific detection of aniline or aminophenol in the body fluids. Generally a methaemoglobin level of 5 % is regarded as tolerable (6).

In accordance with recent results the determination of aniline-haemoglobin conjugates for the monitoring of occupationally exposed persons has gained in importance. In investigations of 1000 employees exposed regularly to aniline and more than 50 employees with acute aniline intoxication it was found that at methaemoglobin levels of less than 5 % also less than 100 µg aniline was released from the haemoglobin conjugate per l whole blood (18). For aniline a BAT value of

100 µg aniline released from the aniline-haemoglobin conjugate/l whole blood

has therefore been set.

When this effect value is observed, damage caused by restriction of the oxygen transport capacity of the erythrocytes can be avoided. In the investigations mentioned above (18) aniline excretion in the urine was also measured. In all cases in which the methaemoglobin level was over 5 % and the aniline level in the haemoglobin conjugate was over 100 µg/l whole blood, aniline excretion was greater than 1 mg/g creatinine. The concentrations of free aniline in the blood were then over 1 mg/l blood. A urine concentration of

1 mg free aniline/l urine

is therefore set as a BAT value for aniline.

7 Interpretation of the Data

After contact with aniline at the level of the MAK value a satisfactory correlation between aniline values in the urine and the aniline-haemoglobin conjugate is only found after three consecutive working days (18). The aniline-haemoglobin conjugate can thus be measured after at least 3 previous working days at any time within a shift period. Also for the determination of free aniline, sampling should take place after at least 3 previous working days.

Simultaneous determination of the blood and urine parameters defined above has been shown to be necessary only at the first examination or immediately after accidents. Routinely the monitoring of persons exposed occupationally to aniline can be limited to the urine investigation. Sampling should be carried out under contamination-free conditions, as far as possible after washing and in private clothes in an occupational medical department.

The aniline concentration in the urine should in the case of high-temperature workplaces be expressed in terms of the creatinine level. For information on the principle of creatinine relativisation reference is made to the special foreword in the loose-leaf collection.

For the intervals between follow-up examinations the "berufsgenossenschaftlicher Grundsatz" G33 (guidelines issued by the Employers' Liability Insurance Association) for occupational-medical health surveillance (11) should be referred to.

8 References

1. Albrecht, W., Neumann, H.-G.: Biomonitoring of aniline and nitrobenzene. Hemoglobin bindings in rats and analysis of adducts. Arch. Toxicol. *57* (1985), 1–5
2. Lewalter, J., Biedermann, P.: Aromatic amines. In: Angerer, J., Schaller, K. H. (eds.): Analyses of Hazardous Substances in Biological Materials, Vol. 4. VCH Verlagsgesellschaft, Weinheim 1994, pp. 67–105
3. Henschler, D. (ed.): Anilin. Gesundheitsschädliche Arbeitsstoffe. Toxikologisch-arbeitsmedizinische Begründung von MAK-Werten, 18th issue. VCH Verlagsgesellschaft, Weinheim 1982
4. Atlas, S. A., Nebert, D. W.: Pharmacogenetics and human disease. In: Parke, D. V., Smith, R. L.: Drug Metabolism from Microbe to Man, Taylor and Francis, London 1976, pp. 393–430
5. Beckett, A. H., Belanger, P. M.: Metabolic N-oxidation of secondary and primary aromatic amines as a route to ring hydroxylation to various N-oxygenated products, and to dealkylation of secondary amines. Biochem. Pharmacol. *25* (1976), 211–214
6. Bolt, H. M., Neumann, H. G., Lewalter, J.: Arbeitsmed. Sozialmed. Präventivmed. *20* (1985), 197–201
7. Cartwright, G. E.: Methemoglobinemia and sulfhemoglobinemia. In: Thorn, G. W. et al. (eds.): Harrison's Principles of Internal Medicine, 8th ed. McGraw-Hill, New York 1977, pp. 1710–1713
8. Damani, L. A.: Oxidation at nitrogen centers. In: Jakoby, W. B., Bend, J. B., Caldwell, J. (eds.): Metabolic Basis of Detoxication. Academic Press, New York 1982, pp. 127–149
9. Dutkiewicz, T., Piotrowski, J.: Experimental investigations on the quantitative estimation of aniline absorption in man. Pure Appl. Chem. *3* (1961), 319–323
10. Evans, E. E, Dinman, A. L., Leech, A. M. A.: Arch. Ind. Health *18* (1958), 422; cited in: Fassett, D. W., Irish, D. D. (eds.): Patty's Industrial Hygiene and Toxicology, 2nd rev. ed. Vol. 2, Toxicology. Wiley & Sons, New York 1958, p. 2110
11. Grundsatz G 33: Aromatische Nitro- und Aminoverbindungen. Berufsgenossenschaftlicher Grundsatz für arbeitsmedizinische Vorsorgeuntersuchungen. Hauptverband der gewerblichen Berufsgenossenschaften e.V. (ed.), 2nd ed. Stuttgart 1981
12. Hanna, P. E., Banks, R. B. in: Anders, M. W. (ed.): Bioactivation of Foreign Compounds. Academic Press, New York 1985, pp. 375–402
13. Irons, R. D., Gross, E. A., White, E. L.: Aniline: evidence for an enterogastric cycle in the rat. Fd. Cosmet. Toxicol. *18* (1980), 393
14. Kao, J., Faulkner, J., Bridges, J. W.: Metabolism of aniline in rats, pigs and sheep. Drug Metab. Disp. *6* (1978), 549
15. Lauwerys, R. R.: Biological criteria for selected industrial toxic chemicals, a review. Scand. J. Work Environ. Health *1* (1975), 139–172
16. Lauwerys, R. R.: Occupational toxicology. In: Doull, J., Klaasen, C. D., Amdur, M. O. (eds.): Toxicology: The Basic Science of Poisons. Macmillan, New York 1980, pp. 699–709
17. Lauwerys, R. R.: Industrial chemical exposure, guidelines for biological monitoring. Biochemical Publication, Davis, California 1983, pp. 97–100
18. Lewalter, J., Korallus, U.: Hemoglobin conjugation and acetylation of aromatic amines – new knowledges for biological monitoring. Int. Arch. Occup. Environ Health. *56* (1985), 179–196
19. Linch, A. L.: Biological monitoring for industrial exposure to cyanogenic aromatic nitro and amino compounds. Am. Ind. Hyg. Assoc. J. *35* (1974), 426–432

19a. Deutsche Forschungsgemeinschaft (DFG): Maximale Arbeitsplatzkonzentrationen und Biologische Arbeitsstofftoleranzwerte 1985. Mitteilung XXI der Senatskommission zur Prüfung gesundheitsschädlicher Arbeitsstoffe. VCH Verlagsgesellschaft, Weinheim 1985

20. Michaux, P., Boiteau, H. L., Tolot, F.: Valeur et limite du depistage clinique et biologique en pathologie professionelle. Arch. mal. prof. med. tra. secur. soc. *32* (1971), 1
21. Nelson, S. D. in: Anders, M. W. (ed.): Bioactivation of foreign compounds. Academic Press, New York 1985, pp. 349–374
22. Neumann, H. G.: Analysis of hemoglobin as a dose monitor for alkylating and arylating agents. Arch. Toxicol. *56* (1984), 1–6
23. Neumann, H. G.: Dosimetry and doseresponse relationships. International seminar on methods of monitoring human exposure to carcinogenic and mutagenic agents. Finland 1983

24. Parke, D. V., Williams, R. T.: Species differences in the *o*- and *p*-hydroxylation of aniline. Biochem. J. *63* (1956), 12
25. Piotrowski, J.: Exposure tests for organic compounds. Industrial Toxicology. US Government Printing Office, Washington D. C. 1977, pp. 70–75
26. Piotrowski, J.: Quantitative estimation of aniline absorption through the skin in man. J. Hyg. Epid. Microbiol. Immunol. *1* (1957), 1–23
27. Smith, J. N., Williams, R. T.: The fate of aniline in the rabbit. Biochem. J. *44* (1959), 242–250
28. Tannenbaum, S. R., Skipper, P. L., Green, L. C., Turesky, R. J., Kadlubar, F. F.: Monitoring exposure to 4-aminobiphenyl via blood protein adducts. International seminar on methods of human exposure to carcinogenic and mutagenic agents. Finland 1983
29. Valentin, H., Lehnert, G., Petry, H., Weber, G., Wittgem, H., Woitowitz, H. J.: Arbeitsmedizin. Band 2: Berufskrankheiten. Thieme Verlag, Stuttgart 1979
30. Valentin, H., Schaller, K. H., Triebig, G. in: Arbeitsmedizin aktuell, Labordiagnostik, Praktische Hinweise für die Durchführung arbeitsmedizinisch-toxikologischer Untersuchungen. G. Fischer Verlag, Stuttgart 1983, pp. 55–70
31. Wieland, E., Neumann, H. G.: Methemoglobin formation and binding to blood constituents as indicators for the formation, availability and reactivity of activated metabolite derived from trans-4-aminostilbene and related aromatic amines. Arch. Toxicol. *40* (1978), 17–35

Author: J. Lewalter
Approved by the Working Group: 10th May 1985

9 Addendum

Evaluation of the aniline concentration in erythrocytes and in the haemoglobin or globin adduct

Metabolism and Kinetics

Aromatic amines can be oxidised during liver metabolism to hydroxylamine compounds and stabilised by conjugation. The glucuronidated aromatic amines are generally eluted via urine. Only small amounts of the conjugates probably penetrate cell membranes such as those of the erythrocytes, and are cleaved there by β-glucuronidase back to the hydroxylamine (1, 2). Some of the phenylhydroxylamine released from various precursors is reduced by hydroxylamine reductase to aniline which can leave the erythrocytes again by diffusion. Some of the hydroxylamine can reach the haem in Hb and be oxidised there to the nitroso compound forming Met-Hb. Only this reactive nitroso intermediate can react with the SH-groups of glutathione (GSH) and globin to yield sulfinamides.

In the blood there is approx. 160 g Hb/l, i. e. approx. 24 mmol SH-groups and approx. 350 mg GSH/l, which corresponds to 1.2 mmol SH-groups. First of all the SH-groups of globin react and then approx. in the ratio of 20 to 1 also those of glutathione (3).

In practice there are two typical forms of exposure:

1. Acute, mainly high aniline exposure
2. Chronic or intermittent (usually low-level) aniline exposure

The two forms of exposure differ in the elimination speed of the products. According to the experience of the Commission (3) transitions are observed between the following extreme types of elimination:

1. Free aromatic amines and aromatic amines released from instable adducts (glutathione conjugates) are excreted with biological half-lives <5 hours.
2. Hb-conjugates are stable and are eliminated during the life cycle of the erythrocytes of approx. three months.

Casuistic Evaluation of the Dominant Processes in Erythrocytes

The consequences of chronic low-level aniline exposures have been observed to date particularly in smokers and those of higher level exposures to aniline particularly after accidental intoxication. In smokers predominantly the accumulated Hb-conjugates of amino aromatics and practically no GSH-conjugates or free aniline are found in the erythrocytes. On the other hand aniline intoxication can lead to erythrocyte concentrations which are degraded in several phases.

After aniline intoxication leading to Met-Hb values of around 40 %, up to 80 % of the aniline in the erythrocytes is eliminated from the erythrocytes in the first 24 hours. A further 10 to 20 % follows in the next 24 hours. Only the last 10 to 20 % of the original erythrocyte aniline can be determined in the erythrocytes in the form of Hb adducts, and that even after a further 10 days (3).

Conclusions and Recommendations

The present BAT value for aniline of 100 µg aniline/l blood released from Hb is based on an evaluation of Hb-adduct formation in several hundred cases of aniline intoxication with Met-Hb values around 5 %. This procedure has proved itself in practice and is recommended for correct occupational-medical surveillance.

Furthermore, for differential diagnosis of unknown levels of aniline comparative evaluation of the total aniline in the erythrocytes and the Hb conjugate formation is recommended. It provides information not only as to the extent of the adduct formation but also as to its cause. Acute aniline intoxication can be recognised by the temporarily increased total aniline levels in the erythrocytes which usually consists of free aniline metabolites and GSH conjugates of nitrosobenzene in addition to considerably smaller amounts of Hb-adducts of aniline. Chronic aniline exposure with Met-Hb values below 5 % or aniline exposure without Met-Hb formation can be recognised above all by the cumulative Hb-adduct formation. In these cases the small amounts of the free aniline metabolites and the GSH-conjugates can no longer be determined with the presently available methods of analysis.

10 References (Addendum)

1. Turesky, R. J., Lang, N. P., Butler, M. A., Teitel, C. H., Kadlubar, F.: Metabolic activation of carcinogenic heterocyclic amines by human liver and colon. Carcinogenesis *12* (1991), 1839–1845
2. Goldstein, J. A., Faletto, M. B.: Advances in mechanisms of activation and deactivation of environmental chemicals. Environ. Health Perspect. *100* (1993), 169–176
3. Lewalter, J.: unpublished investigations (1984–1993)

Author: J. Lewalter
Approved by the Working Group: 27th May 1993

Arsenic and inorganic arsenic compounds

(with the exception of arsenic hydride and its salts)

BLW	50 µg arsenic and methylated metabolites/ l urine[1] Sampling time: end of exposure or end of shift after several previous shifts
Date of evaluation	2002

Substance	CAS No.	Formula	Molecular weight	Melting point (°C)
arsenic	7440-38-2	As	74.92	817
arsenic trioxide	1327-53-3	As_2O_3	197.82	193
arsenous acids	36465-76-6 13464-58-9	$HAsO_2$ and H_3AsO_3	125.94	not stated
and their salts, e.g.[2]				
sodium arsenite	7784-46-5	$Na AsO_2$	191.89	not stated
arsenic pentoxide	1303-28-2	As_2O_5	229.82	315
arsenic acid	7778-39-4	H_3AsO_4	141.94	35
and its salts, e.g.				
lead arsenate	7778-39-4	$Pb_3(AsO_4)_2$	899.43	382
calcium arsenate	7778-44-1	$Ca_3(AsO_4)_2$	398.07	1

MAK [last established: 1971, 2002]	Carcinogen category 1

(See also the documentation for carcinogenic substances for arsenic trioxide in Vol. 2)

Arsenic, arsenic trioxide and pentoxide, arsenous acids, arsenic acid and their salts (arsenites and arsenates) are carcinogenic substances (Carcinogen category 1) and do not, therefore, have MAK and BAT values (Greim 2002). The former TRK value (technical exposure limit) for arsenic and its inorganic compounds was 0.10 mg arsenic/m^3 (measured as the inhalable fraction of the aerosol; calculated as arsenic). This arsenic concentration in air correlated with an arsenic concentration in urine of 130 µg/l at the end of exposure or the end of the shift after several previous shifts (see the EKA documentation for arsenic trioxide in Volume 2 of this series; Greim and Lehnert 1995). The inorganic arsenic and methylated metabolites are analysed together.

---

1 volatile arsenic compounds determined by means of direct hydrogenation with hydride-AAS

2 with the exception of gallium arsenide

Essential BAT Value Documentations. DFG, Deutsche Forschungsgemeinschaft

ISBN 3-527-31477-6

In addition to their carcinogenic effects in man, arsenic and the above-named arsenic compounds have toxic effects on the skin, the nervous system and the vascular system. Even with internal exposure values to arsenic below those corresponding to external exposure to arsenic trioxide at the level of the TRK value (EKA_{TRK}), such toxic effects have been described, so that with exposure at the level of the EKA_{TRK} value protection against these effects is not guaranteed (Wichmann and Lehnert 1987).

1 Metabolism and Kinetics

1.1 Absorption and distribution

Man is exposed to different forms of organic and inorganic arsenic in foodstuffs, water and other matrices. Studies of the kinetics and metabolism of arsenic and its compounds are, therefore, complex. Inhalation exposure to inorganic arsenic occurs mainly at the workplace. In air, arsenic and its inorganic compounds are particle-bound and respiratory absorption therefore takes place in a two-phase process. After deposition of the particles in the respiratory tract and lungs, the arsenic is desorbed from the deposited particles. The extent to which the particles are deposited and the resulting exposure to arsenic therefore also depend on the size of the particles. Desorption of the arsenic compounds from the particles, however, depends on their solubility in water. For the reasons named, pulmonary retention cannot be estimated or quantified with sufficient certainty.

All water-soluble inorganic arsenic compounds are absorbed after ingestion to a considerable extent (up to 95 %) in the gastrointestinal tract (Marquardt 1997). The bioavailability depends, however, among other things also on the matrix of the foodstuff. Dermal absorption can be regarded as low compared to absorption after inhalation and gastrointestinal absorption (Wester *et al.* 1993).

Inhaled and ingested inorganic arsenic compounds first of all enter the blood. With a half-time of two hours, inorganic arsenic is rapidly eliminated from the blood. The arsenic compounds are distributed, as investigations with radioactively labelled arsenic compounds showed, in all the organs investigated. In addition to renal elimination, biliary excretion takes place. Experiments showed that elimination occurs in three phases in man. About 66 % of the administered doses is renally eliminated with a half-time of 2.1 days, around 30 % with a half-time of 9.4 days and the rest (4 %) with a half-time of 38.4 days (Marquardt 1997).

1.2 Metabolism

The metabolism of arsenic in man and in many species of animal takes place in two steps; first of all arsenic(V) is usually reduced to arsenic(III), which is then methylated to form monomethylated and dimethylated arsenic compounds. A detailed overview of the metabolism of arsenic compounds can be found in the IPCS programme (WHO 2001) and in the EKA documentation for arsenic trioxide in Volume 2 of this series (Greim and Lehnert 1995).

2 Critical Toxicity

A detailed description of the symptoms of acute and chronic intoxication with arsenic can be found in the current WHO monograph on arsenic and arsenic compounds (WHO 2001).

2.1 Acute toxicity

The symptoms of intoxication after short-term and long-term absorption of inorganic arsenic compounds are similar and depend on the dose and bioavailability of the substance. The trivalent arsenic compounds are three to four times more toxic than the corresponding pentavalent compounds. The oral LD_{50} values for inorganic arsenic compounds, depending on the arsenic species and the experimental animal, are in the range from 7 to 100 mg/kg body weight (Marquardt 1997).

The clinical symptoms after the ingestion of arsenic compounds occur within 30 to 60 minutes. Described are cardiovascular collapse, CNS depression and severe gastrointestinal symptoms. Death takes place within a few hours. With less dramatic cases of intoxication the main symptoms are gastrointestinal complaints including a metallic taste, a dry mouth, burning lips, dysphagia, vomiting attacks and occasional haematemesis.

2.2 Chronic toxicity

The carcinogenic effects of inorganic arsenic compounds have been demonstrated in epidemiological studies in man. In addition to tumours of the bronchi and the lungs, in particular the skin tumours (basaliomas situated on the trunk) are pathognomonic.

In addition to the carcinogenic effects, inorganic arsenic compounds cause damage in particular to the cardiovascular system and the nervous system. Long-term exposure to inorganic arsenic compounds is associated with cardiovascular diseases and cerebrovascular impairment. In particular the impairment of the peripheral vascular muscle-coat, even as far as gangrene of the affected extremities, has been consistently observed (WHO 2001). The neurotoxic effects can affect both the peripheral nervous system (Feldman *et al.* 1979, WHO 2001) and the central nervous system (WHO 2001).

Arsenic and its compounds are sensitizing to the skin only in exceptional cases and the described association between exposure to arsenic and diabetes mellitus needs further clarification (Rahman *et al.* 1995).

3 Exposure and Effects

Peripheral vascular diseases were described in persons who consumed spring water with a high arsenic concentration. Symptoms such as acrocyanosis and Raynaud's phenomenon were described after cumulative absorption of 8 g arsenic (Borgono *et al.* 1977). After cumulative absorption of 20 g arsenic, gangrene of the feet developed (Pershagen and Vahter 1979).

In occupationally exposed copper smelters, vasospastic changes in the arteries of the fingers were reported (Lagerkvist *et al.* 1986, 1988). The workers were mainly exposed to arsenic trioxide. The exposure was determined by analysing the inorganic arsenic and its metabolites in urine. The mean arsenic concentration in the urine of the exposed workers was 71 µg/l (range 10–340 µg/l), that of the asymptomatic controls 7 µg/l (range 5–20 µg/l). There were statistically significant differences between the exposed persons and the controls in the systolic blood pressure of the finger after cooling and the anamnesis of Raynaud's syndrome. It cannot be excluded, however, that in the past the exposure of the workers was much higher than at the time of the investigation. In the same group exposed to arsenic, the peripheral nervous system was investigated by means of electromyography and determination of the sensory nerve conduction velocity in the arms and legs. The exposed workers were found to have a slightly reduced nerve conduction velocity, which was interpreted as a subclinical sign of neuropathy (Blom *et al.* 1985). In another study, an increased incidence of clinically manifest and subclinical neuropathy in copper smelters was reported when the arsenic concentration in urine reached 250 µg/l (Feldman *et al.* 1979). One publication describes peripheral neuropathy in 51 persons with arsenic concentrations in urine above 100 µg/l (Heyman *et al.* 1956). Engel *et al.* (1994) give an overview of the vascular effects after long-term exposure to arsenic in their review based on 177 publications.

In studies of the nephrotoxic (Foà *et al.* 1987) and hepatotoxic effects (Kodama *et al.* 1976), statistically significant changes were found in exposed workers who excreted mean concentrations of arsenic in the urine of 102 µg/l and 82 µg/l, respectively.

To conclude, there are sufficient data from occupational-medical studies (see Table 1) which show adverse effects can occur at relatively low arsenic concentrations in urine, i.e. even below the former EKA_{TRK} of 130 µg/l.

Table 1. Relationship between adverse effects on health and the arsenic concentrations in occupationally exposed persons (modified from ACGIH (2001)

Observed effects	Arsenic in urine (µg/l) median (range)	Author
vasospastic tendency	71 (10–340)	Lagerkvist *et al.* 1986
peripheral neuropathy	71 (10–340)	Blom *et al.* 1985
peripheral neuropathy	< 250	Feldman *et al.* 1979
peripheral neuropathy	> 100	Heyman *et al.* 1956
impaired kidney function	103	Foà *et al.* 1987
increase in liver enzymes	82 ± 49 (SD)	Kodama *et al.* 1976

4 Selection of the Indicators

After exposure to inorganic arsenic there is a significant and specific increase in the arsenic species monomethylarsenic acid, dimethylarsinic acid and inorganic arsenic excreted in urine. The determination of these three arsenic species in urine is therefore the preferred method for the biological monitoring of workers exposed to inorganic arsenic. The determination of these arsenic species is not influenced by organic arsenic compounds, such as arsenobetaine and arsenocholine, taken up with food. Determination of the total amount of arsenic excreted in urine is not suitable for monitoring investigations because organic arsenic compounds of maritime origin are also determined (see the EKA documentation for arsenic trioxide in Volume 2 of this series; Greim and Lehnert 1995).

Inorganic arsenic and its metabolites are rapidly excreted after the beginning of exposure. The arsenic concentration in urine increases slowly and remains at a relatively constant level during the first three days of exposure. During the working day and from the end of work to the beginning of the next shift there are no notable changes in the concentration. The elimination kinetics show that during the working week there is significant accumulation of arsenic and its metabolites. Sampling should therefore take place at the end of the working week (see Section 1.1).

The determination of arsenic in blood and the arsenic concentrations in hair and finger nail samples have not acquired any importance in the biomonitoring of occupationally exposed persons (see the EKA documentation for arsenic trioxide in Volume 2 of this series; Greim and Lehnert 1995).

5 Methods

Inorganic and methylated organic arsenic compounds in urine are transformed for quantitative analysis into volatile hydrides and determined by atomic absorption spectroscopy. As a result of this method of direct hydrogenation of the urine sample only inorganic arsenic compounds and their metabolites monomethylarsenic acid and dimethylarsinic acid are transformed into volatile hydrides and quantified. A tested method can be found in "Analyses of Hazardous Substances in Biological Materials" (Angerer and Schaller 1991). If the urine sample is digested wet or dry the total arsenic content is determined. Therefore preparation of the urine samples should on no account be carried out. The following refers to the determination of inorganic arsenic and its methylated metabolites. In biological monitoring this arsenic fraction should be determined (Angerer and Schaller 1991).

6 Background Exposure

In persons not occupationally exposed, the diet is the main route of absorption for inorganic arsenic compounds. Food, with the exception of sea-food, contains less than 0.25 mg arsenic/kg; various kinds of fish between 1 and 10 mg/kg, and shell fish more than 100 mg/kg. In food of maritime origin the arsenic is in organic form, usually as arsenobetaine and arsenocholine. The daily uptake with food is estimated to be between 0.04 (without fish) and 0.19 mg arsenic (with fish). In comparison, in Germany, insignificant amounts of arsenic are taken up from the drinking water and air. With the hydride-AAS method suggested in Section 5 the aromatic arsenic compounds excreted unmetabolized in the urine are not determined. Under these analytical conditions the background exposure is below 25 µg/l urine. Recent investigations have shown, however, that also the level of excretion of the named arsenic fraction (inorganic arsenic, monomethylarsonic acid and dimethylarsinic acid) can be influenced by the consumption of large amounts of food of maritime origin. These foods can already contain the methylated substances, in particular dimethylarsinic acid (Apostoli *et al.* 1999). It is therefore recommended that in future only the inorganic arsenic fraction be determined. Separation of the arsenic species is, however, a time-consuming and complicated analytical procedure. Reference values for the various arsenic species in urine samples from the general population of northern Germany have been published (Heinrich-Ramm *et al.* 2001).

7 Evaluation of the BLW Value

The former TRK value for arsenic trioxide and pentoxide, arsenous acids, arsenic acid and their salts was 0.10 mg arsenic/m^3 air. In 1994 an EKA correlation was established for arsenic trioxide, in which an arsenic concentration in the air of 0.10 mg/m^3 corresponds to the excretion of 130 µg arsenic/l urine. The TRK value was not toxicologically grounded and observation of the value did not provide sufficient protection against the toxic effects named in Section 2.2.

For the prevention of (non-carcinogenic) toxic effects of arsenic, irrespective of the carcinogenic potency of arsenic, exposure should remain below 50 µg arsenic/l urine. Taking into account the literature cited, it is to be expected that arsenic-induced effects can develop at arsenic concentrations in urine in the range of 100 µg/l. Changes in the peripheral nerves of occupationally exposed persons were detected even at a mean arsenic concentration of 71 µg/l urine (Blom *et al.* 1985). The BLW value has therefore been set at

50 µg arsenic/l urine

This value is also compatible with the American BEI value (Biological Exposure Indices) (35 µg arsenic/l urine, sampling at the end of the working week), as this refers to the collective median and does not represent an individual ceiling value (ACGIH 2001).

8 Interpretation of Data

The toxicologically relevant arsenic concentration in urine is determined with the method described in "Analyses of Hazardous Substances in Biological Materials" (Angerer and Schaller 1991). The arsenic taken up with food of maritime origin is not determined. The use of the so-called hydride method is therefore imperative. The total amount of arsenic renally excreted must not be determined after preparation of the urine sample as the results can be greatly influenced by the food consumed. Fish and other sea-food can contain a high level of organic arsenic compounds. These compounds are rapidly absorbed by the gastrointestinal tract and can lead to the increased excretion of arsenic in urine. Arsenic concentrations in urine in the range of the BLW value can be reached and even exceeded (Mindt-Prüfert *et al.* 1999).

It should also be noted that also with the use of the hydride-AAS method, the excretion of inorganic arsenic and its methylated metabolites can be influenced by high fish consumption (Apostoli *et al.* 1999). Fish can also frequently contain methylated arsenic compounds (in particular dimethylarsinic acid). The total amount of arsenic in urine can, therefore, be increased.

If the BLW is exceeded, the individual should be specifically asked about his fish consumption over the last few days, and if necessary the arsenic concentration should be redetermined after a period without fish. After a single meal containing sea-food contaminated with organic arsenic compounds, the amount of arsenic excreted within 24 hours was 50 % to 70 % of the total amount of arsenic taken up (Marquardt 1997). Short-term control investigations can therefore be useful.

In some countries, such as Bangladesh, Argentina, Chile and India, considerable amounts of arsenic are taken up by the general population with the drinking water from contaminated wells. This causes amounts of arsenic to be excreted in urine which are above the BLW value (WHO 2001).

9 References

ACGIH (American Conference of Governmental Industrial Hygienists) (2001) Arsenic and soluble inorganic compounds: BEI® 7th edition, Documentation. Publication # 7DOC-665, ACGIH®, Cincinatti

Angerer J, Schaller KH (1991) Arsenic. in: Henschler D (Ed.) Analyses of hazardous substances in biological materials, Vol. 3, VCH, Weinheim

Apostoli P, Bartoli D, Alessio L, Buchet JP (1999) Biological monitoring of occupational exposure to inorganic arsenic. Occup Environ Med 56: 825–832

Blom S, Lagerkvist B, Linderholm H (1985) Arsenic exposure to smelter workers. Clinical and neurophysiological studies. Scand J Work Environ Health 11: 265–269

Borgono JM, Vincent P, Venturino H, Infante A (1977) Arsenic in the drinking water of the city of Antofagasta: epidemiological and clinical study before and after the installation of a treatment plant. Environ Health Perspect 19: 103–105

Engel RR, Hopenhayn-Rich C, Receveur O, Smith AH (1994) Vascular effects of chronic arsenic exposure: a review. Epidemiol Rev 16: 184–209

Feldman RG, Niles CA, Kelly-Hayes M, Sax DS, Dixon WJ, Thompson DJ, Landau E (1979) Peripheral neuropathy in arsenic smelter workers. Neurology 29: 939–944

Foà V, Colombi A, Maroni M, Barbieri F, Franchini I, Mutti A, De Rosa E, Bartolucci GB (1987) Study of kidney function of workers with chronic low level exposure to inorganic arsenic. in: Foà V, Emmett EA, Maroni M, Colombi A (Eds) Occupational and environmental chemical hazards, Cellular and biochemical indices for monitoring toxicity, Ellis Horwood Limited Publishers, Chichester, 362–367

Greim H (Ed.) (2002) Arsen und anorganische Arsenverbindungen (mit Ausnahme von Arsenwasserstoff). Gesundheitsschädliche Arbeitsstoffe, Toxikologisch-arbeitsmedizinische Begründungen von MAK-Werten, 35. Lieferung, Wiley-VCH, Weinheim

Greim H, Lehnert G (Eds) (1995) Arsenic trioxide. in: Biological exposure values for occupational toxicants and carcinogens – Critical data evaluation for BAT and EKA values, Vol. 2, VCH, Weinheim, pp. 123–136

Heinrich-Ramm R, Mindt-Prüfert S, Szadkowski D (2001) Arsenic species excretion in a group of persons in northern Germany – Contribution to the evaluation of reference values. Int J Hyg Environ Health 203: 475–477

Heyman A, Pfeiffer JB Jr., Willett RW, Taylor HM (1956) Peripheral neuropathy caused by arsenical intoxication. A study of 41 cases with observations on the effect of BAL (2,3, dimercapto-propanol). N Engl J Med 254: 401–409

Kodama Y, Ishinishi N, Kunitake E, Inamasu T, Nobutomo K (1976) Subclinical signs of the exposure to arsenic in a copper refinery. in: Nordberg GF (Ed.) Effects and dose-response relationships of toxic metals, Elsevier Scientific Publishing Company, Amsterdam, 464–470

Lagerkvist B, Linderholm H, Nordberg GF (1986) Vasospastic tendency and Raynaud's phenomenon in smelter workers exposed to arsenic. Environ Res 39: 465–474

Lagerkvist BE, Linderholm H, Nordberg GF (1988) Arsenic and Raynaud's phenomenon. Vasospastic tendency and excretion of arsenic in smelter workers before and after the summer vacation. Int Arch Occup Environ Health 60: 361–364

Marquardt H (Ed.) (1997) Lehrbuch der Toxikologie, Spektrum Akademischer Verlag, Heidelberg–Berlin, 510

Mindt-Prüfert S, Heinrich-Ramm R, Szadkowski D (1999) Zum alimentären Einfluß auf die Arsenausscheidung im Urin bei arbeitsmedizinischen Vorsorgeuntersuchungen. in: Rettenmeier AW, Feldhaus C (Ed.) Dokumentationsband über die 39. Jahrestagung der Deutschen Gesellschaft für Arbeitsmedizin und Umweltmedizin e.V., Druckerei Rindt, Fulda, 591–593

Pershagen G, Vahter M (1979) Arsenic: A toxicological and epidemiological appraisal. 071-SNV Rapporter från SNV, Statens naturvårdverk, Solna, Sweden

Rahman M, Wingren G, Axelson O (1995) Diabetes mellitus among Swedish art glass workers – an effect of arsenic exposure? Scand J Work Environ Health 22: 146–149

Wester RC, Maibach HI, Sedik L, Melendres J, Wade M (1993) *In vivo* and *in vitro* percutaneous absorption and skin decontamination of arsenic from water and soil. Fundam Appl Toxicol 20: 336–340

WHO (World Health Organization) (2001) Arsenic and arsenic compounds. Environmental Health Criteria 224, Geneva

Wichmann N, Lehnert G (1987) Arbeitsmedizinische Erfahrungen und TRK-Wert für Arsen. Arbeitsmed Sozialmed Präventivmed 22: 18–20

Author: H. Drexler

Approved by the Working Group: 10.02.2002

Arsenic trioxide

EKA	The correlation between external and internal exposure yields the following data:

Air Arsenic trioxide mg As/m³	Urine Arsenic µg As/l
0.01	50
0.05	90
0.10	130

Sampling: end of exposure or end of shift after several consecutive shifts

Date of evaluation	1993
Synonyms	–
Formula	As_2O_3
Molecular weight	197.84
Melting point amorphic or glassy form crystalline cubic form	 312.3 °C 274.0 °C
Solubility in water amorphic or glassy form crystalline cubic form	 37 g/l (20 °C) 18 g/l (20 °C)
MAK [last established: 1975]	Carcinogenic substance: Category III A1 of the MAK and BAT Values List
TRK [1993]	0.1 mg/m³ (calculated as arsenic in total dust) for arsenic trioxide and pentoxide, arsenous acids, arsenic acid and its salts (arsenites, arsenates)

In 1986 the working group "Setting of Threshold Limit Values in Biological Material" of the DFG Commission for the Investigation of Health Hazards of Chemical Compounds in the Work Area published a relationship between the arsenic concentration in the air and the level of arsenic excretion in biological material for exposure to

Essential BAT Value Documentations. DFG, Deutsche Forschungsgemeinschaft

ISBN 3-527-31477-6

arsenic trioxide at the workplace (Exposure Equivalents for Carcinogenic Working Materials, EKA). The volatile arsenic compounds in the urine sample which can be determined after direct hydrogenation were defined as the arsenic excretion in urine. These are inorganic arsenic and its products of metabolism monomethylarsonic acid and dimethylarsinic acid. The correlation determined between the external and internal exposure is based on the data from two field studies (31, 36).

The TRK value valid at the time of the evaluation was 0.2 mg/m^3. Not least thanks to a publication by the working group "Setting of Threshold Limit Values in Biological Material" the TRK value was reduced in 1988 to 0.1 mg/m^3 (39).

In the meantime the availability of new scientific data allows reassessment of the relationship between external and internal exposure to arsenic. Of particular relevance is a study on the external and internal exposure to arsenic trioxide by Offergelt et al. (30). Arsenic concentrations in the air are shown to correspond to lower renal excretion levels than described in the relationship between exposure equivalents. The reasons for this difference include the fact that the method of determination of arsenic in the air at the workplace used to ascertain the external exposure has been improved. A method published by the ISO allows the efficient determination of arsenic trioxide dusts and fumes in the air. This is achieved by the use of specifically prepared filters. It can be assumed that in most previous investigations the published arsenic concentrations in the air were too low with the consequence that the arsenic excretion levels given in the correlation tables should be assigned to higher air concentrations.

This new data from the literature and the improvements in the methods make a reevaluation of the EKA values for arsenic excretion in urine necessary.

1 Metabolism and Kinetics

Arsenic compounds can be taken up by man both via the lungs and also via the gastrointestinal tract. At the workplace inhalation is the dominant route of absorption. It should be borne in mind that in addition to inhalation, gastrointestinal absorption of arsenic from contaminated hands must also be assumed to take place (36).

The pulmonary deposition of inhaled arsenic compounds is above all determined by the size of the particles (32, 34). Non-inspirable particles are transferred with the mucous into the gastro-intestinal canal. From there, transfer of arsenic trioxide or the arsenic acid via the intestinal mucous membranes to the blood and lymph vessels is possible (34). The absorption in the lungs depends to a great extent upon the solubility of the arsenic compounds. Foa et al. (18) have suggested that pulmonary clearance is biphasic. 75 % is eliminated with a half-time of four days, 25 % with a half-time of ten days. Studies on persons who were investigated 2 to 19 years after the end of exposure provided indications of considerably longer retention times (8).

Gastrointestinal absorption is the most important route of absorption of arsenic from non-occupational exposure. Absorption takes place above all with food, in particular when sea-food is eaten, and with drinking water. The absorption of inorganic arsenic compounds from the gastrointestinal tract is determined mainly by the solubility of the compounds. The proportion of the dose absorbed in humans is more than 90 % if water-soluble compounds are ingested. In the case of arsenic trioxide which is only slightly soluble in water the gastro-intestinal absorption is slower and depends on the size of the particles and the pH of the hydrochloric acid in the stomach. Organic arsenic compounds from sea-food are almost completely absorbed after ingestion (18).

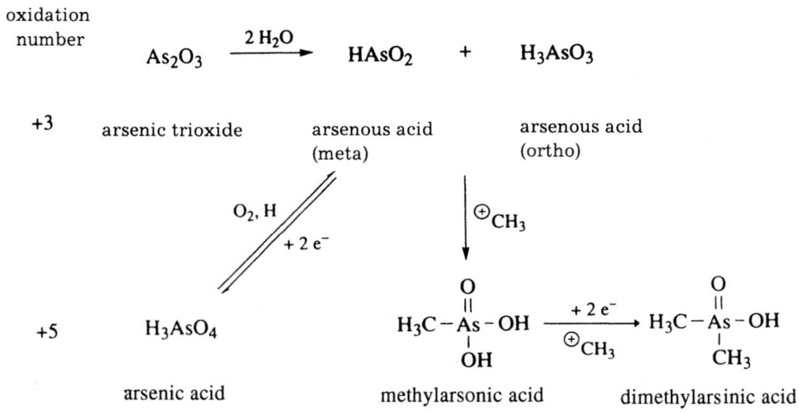

Fig. 1: Metabolism of arsenic trioxide in mammals and humans; metabolites in the urine: arsenic (III), arsenic (V), methylarsonic acid (MA) and dimethylarsinic acid (DMA)

The metabolism of arsenic in the human organism is shown in figure 1. Animal experimental and human investigations have shown that arsenic (III) is metabolised to arsenic (V), monomethylarsonic acid (MMA) and dimethylarsinic acid (DMA). The main metabolite is dimethylarsinic acid which accounts for 50–80 % of the urinary metabolites. It is in principle true that occupationally exposed persons show the same spectrum of metabolites as non-exposed persons. However, there are quantitative differences which depend on the level of exposure. After high exposures the metabolism to dimethylarsinic acid decreases which is probably to be interpreted as a saturation of the methylation process (5, 6, 15, 24). Methylation is the most important natural detoxification mechanism. Both monomethylarsonic acid and dimethylarsinic acid are less toxic than the inorganic acid.

Organoarsenic compounds such as occur in food are not biologically transformed and thus form no inorganic or methylated arsenic compounds in the human organism.

Buchet et al. (4) investigated the changes with time in the concentration of arsenic metabolites in the urine after ingestion (3 persons) of 6.67 µmol sodium arsenate (III). The total arsenic content was determined by dry ashing, the metabolites arsenous acids and arsenic acid as well as monomethylarsonic acid (MMA) and dimethylarsinic acid (DMA) according to a modified method from Braman et al. (7). After one day, 22 % of the dose had been excreted, 38 % in the form of inorganic arsenic, 23 % as MMA and 39 % as DMA. After four days, 50 % of the arsenic taken up had been excreted with the urine, whereby the proportion of inorganic arsenic was reduced to 11 % and that of dimethylarsinic acid had increased to 76 %. After 14 days the persons showed normal arsenic values.

Mappes (26) obtained the following results after ingestion of 13.40 µmol arsenic trioxide in an experiment on himself: 52 % of the arsenic taken up had been excreted in the urine after 24 hours. Pharmacokinetic investigations demonstrated that for arsenic trioxide there are two different compartments.

2 Critical Toxicity

Chronic arsenic intoxication is of importance from an occupational medical point of view. A detailed description of the symptoms can be found in the occupational-medical toxicological documentation of the MAK value (19) as well as in Landrigan (22), Arnold (3) and Vahter (35).

Due to its carcinogenic properties in humans, arsenic trioxide as well as arsenic pentoxide, arsenous acid, arsenic acid and its salts have been classed in category A1 of section III "Carcinogenic Substances" of the MAK and BAT Values List (13). A review of the human carcinogenicity can be found in the documentation of the IARC (21) and the WHO (38).

3 Exposure and Effects

The DFG Commission for the Investigation of Health Hazards of Chemical Compounds in the Work Area have given their detailed opinion on the question of the body burden and effect on persons occupationally exposed to arsenic trioxide both in the occupational-medical toxicological documentation of MAK Values and also in the publication by Wichmann and Lehnert (39). Due to the carcinogenic effects of inorganic arsenic in man the chronic effects of arsenic cannot be used to evaluate a threshold limit value.

Enterline found in an epidemiological study a significant linear relationship between the standardised mortality ratio (SMR) for lung cancer and the renal arsenic excretion (14). On the basis of the regression equation of SMR = 86.1 + 0.590 As in urine (µg/l) the SMR for an arsenic concentration in the urine of 100 µg/l is 145, for 500 µg/l the SMR is 380.

The US American BEI documentation (2) is based on the relationship between internal exposure, determined as arsenic excretion in the urine, and the corresponding effects on health. As relevant effects peripheral neuropathy, peripheral angiopathy and liver and kidney function disorders are listed.

4 Selection of the Indicators

After exposure to inorganic arsenic there is a significant and specific increase in the arsenic species monomethylarsonic acid, dimethylarsinic acid and inorganic arsenic excreted in the urine. The *determination* of these three arsenic species *in the urine* is therefore the preferred method for the biological monitoring of workers who are exposed to inorganic arsenic. The measurement of these species of arsenic is not influenced by organic arsenic compounds taken up with food.

Inorganic arsenic and its metabolites are rapidly excreted after the beginning of exposure. The urine concentration increases slowly and remains at a relatively constant level during the first days of exposure. During the working day and from the end of work to the beginning of the next shift there are no great changes in the concentration (30, 36). The elimination kinetics result in a significant accumulation of arsenic and its metabolites during the working week. Sampling should therefore take place at the end of the working week.

The determination of *arsenic in blood* is of no importance in the biological monitoring of occupationally exposed persons (22, 28). The reason for this is that the biological half-life in blood both for inorganic and organic arsenic is relatively short. This means that the blood concentration is only at an increased level for a short time after absorption. Furthermore, there are no routine methods available for the specific determination of inorganic arsenic and its metabolites in blood.

The arsenic concentrations in *hair and finger nail samples* are usually higher than in other compartments of the human organism. The reason for this is the high content of cystine whose thiol groups bind trivalent inorganic arsenic. The measurement of the arsenic content of hair and finger nail samples has not acquired any importance in occupational medical practice, the reasons being the non-standardised sampling, difficulties in analysis as well as a considerable danger of contamination. Moreover, there are no relevant studies for the evaluation of threshold limit values.

5 Methodology

Inorganic and organic arsenic compounds in urine are transformed for quantitative measurement into volatile hydrides and determined by atomic absorption spectroscopy (hydride method) (16, 17). Using the method of direct hydrogenation of a urine sample only inorganic arsenic compounds and their metabolites monomethylarsonic acid and dimethylarsinic acid are transformed into volatile hydrides and quantified. Organic arsenic compounds, which are taken up during consumption of sea-foods and excreted renally, are not determined (29, 37). A tested method can be found in the loose-leaf collection "Analysen im biologischen Material" (20) and in its English edition "Analyses of Hazardous Substances in Biological Materials" (1).

If the urine sample is digested wet or dry the total arsenic content is determined. Therefore wet or dry digestion should not be carried out.

The following explanations refer to the measurement of inorganic arsenic and its metabolites. In biological monitoring this "arsenic fraction" should be measured. Table 1 gives an overview of the published data for non-exposed persons. Only studies which distinguish between the various arsenic species were taken into account. Column Σ shows the "fraction" determined by the hydride AAS method.

Tab. 1: Arsenic values in the air and urine in non-exposed persons and percentage distribution of the various arsenic species

Air	Urine							Literature
	As (III)	As (V)	Methylarsonic acid (MA)	Dimethylarsinic acid (DMA)	Σ As (III), As (V), MA, DMA	Total As	spec. weight	
(µg As/m³)	(µg/l)	(µg/l)	(µg/l)	(µg/l)	(µg/l)	(µg/l)	urine	
	8.4 % 1.9	17.3 % 3.9	8.0 % 1.8	66.4 % 15.0	100 % 22.6	–	–	4[1)]
			3.6 ± 2.4	15.5 ± 6.8				4[2)]
	6 % 3.7 ± 1.4 6 %	5 % 3.0 ± 1.3 5 %	20 % 11.3 ± 5.3 19 %	68 % 39.2 ± 18.2 67 %	100 % 57.3 ± 21.3 98 %	58.4 100 %	1.024	48[3)]
3.6 ± 1.56[a)]	7 % 1.3 ± 1.58 6 %	7 % 1.3 ± 1.59 6 %	19 % 3.4 ± 1.63 16 %	66 % 11.5 ± 1.47 54 %	100 % 17.5[b)] 83 %	21.2 100 %	1.018	38[4)]
	11 % 1.6 ± 1.2 11 %		12 % 1.7 ± 1.2 11 %	77 % 11.2 ± 5.9 74 %	100 % 14.5 ± 7.5[a)] 96 %	15.1[b)] 100 %	–	6[5)]

[1)] n = 4.3 ♂ + 1 ♀, 34 ± 7.8 years
[2)] x ± s, n = no data
[3)] Ibd. p. 51, Tab. 2, x ± s, n = 20; total arsenic was calculated on the basis of a given correlation: $y_{\text{wet digestion}}$ (µg/l) = 0.915 · $x_{\text{separation method}}$ (µg/l) + 6
[4)] a) geom. mean ± s, 56 % <1.2 µg/m³ (detection limit), n = 41; urine values: geom. mean ± s, n = 41; b) calculated; total arsenic determined by wet digestion
[5)] Ibd. p. 22, Tab. 10, x ± s, n = 5; a) calculated b) dry ashing; geom. mean because an outlier is included (arithm. mean 18.7 ± 14.3)

As the measurement of arsenic in the air is also of great importance for the evaluation of a correlation between the external and internal exposure the method is briefly described here. The determination of arsenic in particle and vapour form should take place according to the sampling method AGSA-AA I No. 15-90 of the ISO. Cellulose acetate membrane filters impregnated with sodium carbonate and glycerine are used as sampling phases. The filters prepared in this way guarantee an extremely efficient separation of the arsenic compounds, independent of the state of aggregation (10, 30). For the quantitative determination of arsenic the filters are digested by wet oxidative digestion and the arsenic quantified using hydride AAS or GF-AAS. This method represents the present state of the art.

6 Background Exposures

Arsenic can be taken up by man in drinking water, food and from the air. Food is the main route of absorption. Food, with the exception of sea-food, contains less than 0.25 mg arsenic/kg; various kinds of fish between 1 and 10 mg/kg and shell fish more than 100 mg/kg. In food of maritime origin the arsenic is in organic form (arsenobetaines and arsenocholines). The daily uptake via food is estimated to be between 0.04 (without fish) and 0.19 mg arsenic (with fish). The daily arsenic uptake via the drinking water and the air is not significant.

With the hydride AAS method suggested in chapter 5 the aromatic arsenic compounds excreted unmetabolised in the urine are not determined. Under these conditions of measurement the "normal" arsenic excretion is below 25 µg/l (see also Tab. 1). Thus, it must be ensured that the above-mentioned method of analysis is used for the monitoring of persons occupationally exposed to arsenic. After the digestion of urine samples and the consumption of crustaceans arsenic can be measured in the urine in the mg range.

7 Evaluation of the Biological Exposure Equivalents for Carcinogenic Substances (EKA)

Various field studies on humans can be referred to for the evaluation of correlations between the external arsenic exposure and the renal excretion of arsenic. The correlation evaluated in 1986 is based mainly on two studies (31, 36).

The meaningfulness of the field study carried out by Pinto et al. (31) on 24 workers from a smelting works is limited by the fact that the total arsenic excretion in the urine was analysed without any further specification. It was checked anamnestically that no fish was eaten in the period of investigation. Nevertheless, it cannot be excluded that the results were influenced by the uptake of organoarsenic compounds. Furthermore, it must be assumed that the arsenic concentrations given for the air were too low as arsenic oxide vapours were probably not determined.

This assumption also applies to the study by Vahter et al. (36). According to investigations by Costello et al. (10) only approx. 42 % of the arsenic trioxide in the vapour phase is determined when untreated cellulose acetate filters are used. There was a highly significant correlation of r = 0.92 between the arsenic concentration in the air measured by personal air sampling and the renal excretion of organic arsenic and its metabolites (36). However, with four persons the urinary excretion values were much greater than were to be expected from the external exposure. The authors suspected that the persons had been exposed to arsenic taken up directly from contaminated hands, cigarettes or snuff. Therefore this study was not included in the present evaluation.

The study carried out by Landrigan et al. (23) was also not included in the evaluation. This working group investigated 48 lead battery workers who were exposed both to arsine and arsenic trioxide. According to the currently available data it seems that the relationship between the arsenic content of the air and the renal excretion of inorganic arsenic and its metabolites is influenced by the chemical form of the arsenic species at the workplace. It is known e.g. that lead arsenate, calcium arsenate, gallium arsenide and to a certain extent arsenic trisulphide are absorbed more slowly in the lungs than arsenic trioxide. Arsine, however, is absorbed considerably better than arsenic trioxide. Due to this mixed exposure and the fact that the total arsenic content of the urine was determined, this study can also not be used for the evaluation.

Roels at al. (33) investigated persons exposed to arsenic in a glass factory. As, on the one hand, only a small fraction of the dust was able to enter the alveoli and, on the other, the urinary excretion levels were relatively high, the authors assumed that oral uptake from contaminated hands had had a considerable influence on the results.

The studies described below were taken into account for the evaluation of the EKA value. The data presented there are used for the compilation of table 2.

Tab. 2: Calculated arsenic concentration in the urine (arsenic, inorganic and metabolites) at various arsenic concentrations in the air at the workplace

	Arsenic concentrations in the air (mg/m^3)			
Study	0.01	0.05	0.10	Reference
82 smelters As_2O_3 exposure	25 µg/l	76 µg/l	139 µg/l	Smith 1977
28 smelters As_2O_3 exposure	44 µg/l	101 µg/l	127 µg/l	Enterline 1987
11 smelters As_2O_3 exposure	68 µg/l	102 µg/l	146 µg/l	Yamauchi 1989
22 employees of sulphuric acid production Exposure to As_2O_3 dust and fumes	30 µg/g creatinine	54 µg/g creatinine	69 µg/g creatinine	Offergelt 1992

In a comprehensive study Smith et al. (34) investigated the excretion of inorganic arsenic and its metabolites in the urine of 82 smelters employed in a copper works. The external exposure was determined by personal air sampling, urine sampling took place in the morning on two consecutive days. There was a statistically significant correlation between the external exposure and the concentration of various arsenic species in the urine. A regression equation was only given for the relationship between the arsenic in the air and the dimethylarsinic acid excretion in urine. As dimethylarsinic acid represents approx. 65 % of the arsenic metabolites and the ratio of the arsenic species to one another was relatively constant and independent of the exposure concentration, for the fraction inorganic arsenic and its metabolites in the urine a concentration of about 70 µg/l can be estimated for external exposure to 50 µg/m³. In addition the authors quoted values for external and internal exposure for four exposure groups:

	Arsenic in air	Arsenic in urine
Controls	3.6 µg/m³	17.5 µg/m³
Group with low-level exposure	8.3 µg/m³	25.7 µg/m³
Group with medium-level exposure	46.1 µg/m³	49.6 µg/m³
Group with high-level exposure	52.7 µg/m³	96.6 µg/m³

The data yields the following relationship as a linear regression:

Arsenic in urine (µg/l) = 12.6 + 1.26 arsenic in air (µg/m³)

Within the framework of an epidemiological study of the frequency of lung cancer in the workers of a copper smelting works, a relationship between urine excretion and external exposure was established. The relationship was not linear: arsenic in urine [µg/l] = (arsenic in air [µg/m³]/0.0064)$^{0.515}$. The measurements were based on stationary air sampling (14).

Yamauchi et al. (40) published in 1989 a field study on 37 gallium arsenide workers and 11 smelters. The air concentrations measured by stationary air sampling were associated with urine values which resulted from two urine collections on 2 to 3 days. For gallium arsenide there were only small increases in the arsenic excretion. This can be attributed to the fact that gallium arsenide can only be absorbed by the human organism to a very small extent (35, 40). For the smelters who were exposed to arsenic trioxide an average urine excretion of inorganic arsenic and its metabolites of 239 µg/l was associated with an average air concentration of 0.336 mg/m³.

In a field study that was published in 1992 by Offergelt et al. (30) 18 workers of a company producing sulphuric acid were investigated. The arsenic concentration in the breathing zone was determined by the sampling and analysis method described above. The air measurements took place during five days, the urine samples were collected after the shift and before the next shift. In biological material the inorganic arsenic as well as the monomethylarsonic acid and the dimethylarsinic acid were measured selectively. For 82 pairs of values there was a significant correlation of r = 0.48. The regression equation was log arsenic in urine (µg/g creat.) = 1.130 + 0.353 log arsenic in

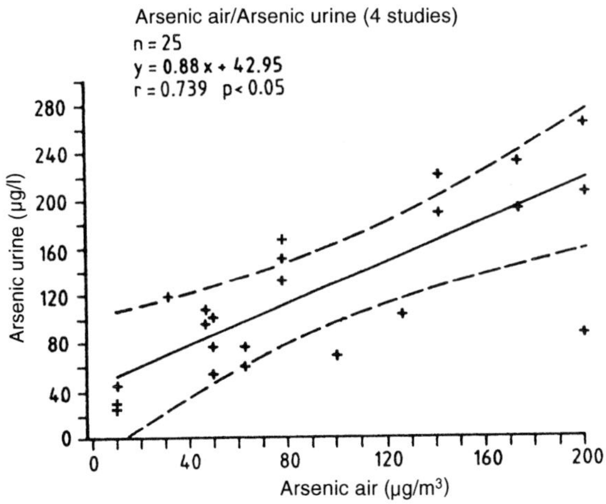

Fig. 2: Correlation diagram for the relationship between the arsenic concentration in the air and the renal arsenic excretion on the basis of the four studies used for the evaluation of the EKA values

air (µg/m^3). Table 3 shows the arsenic excretion (inorganic arsenic + metabolites) in the urine extrapolated for various arsenic concentrations in the air. The post shift values as well as the values before the next shift were taken into consideration.

The arsenic excretion levels in the urine listed in table 2 for defined arsenic concentrations in the air are calculated from linear and non-linear relationships between the data for the external and internal exposure. With the exception of the study by Enterline et al. (14), in which the arsenic fraction measured was not described, the urine excretion levels are based on the measurement of inorganic arsenic and its metabolites.

The correlates calculated show a high variance. This wide range can be explained, on the one hand, by the different methods of sampling and analysis of arsenic in the air. On the other hand the extrapolation from low external exposures to higher ones is critical with this database. As a rule the external exposures in the studies listed are below 0.05 mg/m^3. In the lower exposure range (0.01–0.05 mg/m^3) the calculated values correspond better than those in the upper range.

The lowest excretion values are to be found in the study by Offergelt et al. (30) in which great importance was laid on an exact and complete determination of the arsenic in the air. For a period of five days the external exposure was determined with a method of sampling and analysis recommended by the ISO, with personal air sampling during the whole of the shift. Of the persons investigated no-one wore personal breathing protection. An oral uptake of arsenic can be largely excluded. The arsenic levels in the urine measured at the end of the shift do not differ greatly from those in the urine samples which were collected before the next shift (see Tab. 3). The individual range of variation of the arsenic excretion is, however, considerable. It can be seen in table 3. The largest values measured in the lower range of exposure correspond in their order of magnitude with the extrapolated values from the other studies.

Tab. 3: Calculated renal arsenic excretion (inorganic arsenic and its metabolites MA + DMA) in the urine samples collected post-shift and before the next shift in relation to the arsenic concentration in the air at the workplace with exposure to As_2O_3 dusts and fumes (30)

Arsenic in air (mg/m^3)	Renal arsenic excretion (µg/g creatinine)	
	after the shift	before the next shift
0.0125	33 (26–42)	31 (24–40)
0.025	42 (36–50)	39 (33–47)
0.050	54 (47–62)	50 (43–58)
0.100	69 (56–84)	64 (52–79)
0.200	88 (65–117)	81 (60–111)
0.400	112 (75–166)	104 (68–158)

The results are given as geometric means with 95 % confidence intervals

The evaluation of the EKA values takes place on the basis of the four selected studies. The correlation analysis yields the relationship between air and urine values shown in figure 2. Only the data up to an external exposure to 0.20 mg/m^3 are included. The arsenic excretion in the urine (inorganic arsenic and metabolites) was determined by interpolation for external exposures of 0.01, 0.05 and 0.1 mg/m^3. The relationship between the arsenic concentration in the air at the workplace and the arsenic excretion in the urine is shown below:

Air Arsenic concentration	Urine Arsenic concentration
0.01 mg/m^3	51 µg/l
0.05 mg/m^3	87 µg/l
0.10 mg/m^3	131 µg/l

With regard to the criticism of the studies used, discussed in detail above, this correlation should be regarded as provisional.

Pretreatment of urine samples by wet or dry ashing techniques permits determination of the total arsenic content of the urine. In this way the arsenic taken up with food is included. In particular fish and other sea-foods contain high levels of organic arsenic compounds (9, 25, 27) which are quickly absorbed and excreted via the kidneys (11, 12). This can lead to a great increase in the total arsenic content of the urine (4, 17, 25, 37). For this reason pretreatment by wet or dry ashing should not be carried out.

The method of direct hydrogenation of the urine sample should be used. Even with this procedure it was observed that after ingestion of sea-food there is an increase in the level of arsenic compounds. The increase is small and can amount to 12 µg As/l urine (29, 37).

Occupational medical health examinations on persons exposed to inorganic arsenic must be carried out according to the berufsgenossenschaftlicher Grundsatz G 16 (guideline issued by the Employers' Liability Insurance Association).

9 References

1. Angerer, J., Schaller, K. H.: Analyses of Hazardous Substances in Biological Materials, Volume 3. Deutsche Forschungsgemeinschaft, VCH Verlagsgesellschaft, Weinheim 1991
2. American Conference of Governmental Industrial Hygienists (ACGIH): Threshold Limit Values for Chemical Substances and Physical Agents and Biological Exposure Indices. ACGIH, Cincinnati 1991–1992
3. Arnold, W.: Arsen, ein allgegenwärtiges Gift in der Umwelt des Menschen. Öff. Gesundh.-Wes. *49* (1987), 240–249
4. Buchet, J. P., Lauwerys, R., Roels, H.: Comparison of several methods for the determination of arsenic compounds in water and urine. Int. Arch. Occup. Environ. Health *46* (1980), 11–29
5. Buchet, J. P., Lauwerys, R., Roels, H.: Comparison of the urinary excretion of arsenic metabolites after a single oral dose of sodium arsenite, monomethylarsonate or dimethylarsinate in man. Int. Arch. Occup. Environ. Health *48* (1981), 71–79
6. Buchet, J. P., Lauwerys, R.: Study of inorganic arsenic methylation by rat liver in vitro: Relevance for the interpretation of observations in man. Arch. Toxicol. *57* (1985), 125 –129
7. Braman, R. S., Foreback, C. C.: Methylated forms of arsenic in the environment. Science *182* (1973), 1247–1249
8. Brune, D., Nordberg, G., Webster, P. O.: Distribution of 23 elements in the kidney, liver and lungs of workers from a smeltery and refinery in North Sweden exposed to a number of elements and of a control group. Sci. Tot. Environ. *16* (1980), 13–53
9. Chapmann, A. C.: On the presence of compounds of arsenic in marine crustaceans and shell fish. Analyst *51* (1926), 548–563
10. Costello, R. J., Eller, P. M., Hull, R. D.: Measurement of Multiple Inorganic Arsenic Species. Am. Ind. Hyg. Assoc. J. *44* (1983), 21–28
11. Coulson, E. J., Remington, R. E., Lynch, K. M.: Metabolism in the rat of the naturally occurring arsenic of shrimp as compared with arsenic trioxide. J. Nutrition *10* (1935), 255–270
12. Crecelius, E. A.: Changes in the chemical speciation of arsenic following ingestion by man. Environ. Health Perspect. *19* (1977), 147–150
13. Deutsche Forschungsgemeinschaft: List of MAK and BAT Values 1993, Maximum Concentrations and Biological Tolerance Values at the Workplace. VCH Verlagsgesellschaft, Weinheim 1993
14. Enterline, P. E., Henderson, V. L., Marsh, G. M.: Exposure to arsenic and respiratory cancer. A reanalysis. Am. J. Epid. *125* (1987), 929–938

15. Farmer, J. G., Johnson, L. R.: Assessment of occupational exposure to inorganic arsenic based on urinary concentrations and speciation of arsenic. Brit. J. Ind. Med. *47* (1990), 343–348
16. Fishbein, L.: Overview of analysis of carcinogenic and/or mutagenic metals in biological and environmental samples. I. Arsenic, beryllium, cadmium, chromium and selenium. Int. J. Environ. Anal. Chem. *17* (1984), 113–170
17. Fleischer, M., Schaller, K. H. in: Welz, B. (ed.): 4. Colloquium Atomspektrometrische Spurenanalytik. Überlingen 1987, pp. 577–585
18. Foa, V., Colombi, A., Maroni, M., Barbieri, F., Franchini, I, Mutti, A., De Rosa, E., Bartolucci, G. B.: Study of kidney function of workers with chronic low level exposure to inorganic arsenic. In: Foa, V., Emmett, E. A., Maroni, M., Calombi, A. (eds.): Occupational and environmental chemical hazards. Wiley & Sons, New York 1987, pp. 362–367
19. Henschler, D. (ed.): Gesundheitsschädliche Arbeitsstoffe. Toxikologisch-arbeitsmedizinische Begründung von MAK-Werten, 18th issue. VCH Verlagsgesellschaft, Weinheim 1992
20. Henschler, D. (ed.): Analytische Methoden zur Prüfung gesundheitsschädlicher Arbeitsstoffe. Band 2: Analysen in biologischem Material, 10th issue. VCH Verlagsgesellschaft, Weinheim 1991
21. International Agency for Research on Cancer (IARC): Some Metals and Metallic compounds. In: The evaluation of the carcinogenic risk of chemicals to humans. IARC Monograph No. 23. IARC, Lyon 1980, pp. 39–141
22. Landrigan, P. J.: Arsenic – State of the Art. Am. J. Ind. Med. *2* (1981), 5–14
23. Landrigan, P. J., Costello, R. J., Stringer, W. T.: Occupational exposure to arsine. An epidemiologic reappraisal of current standards. Scand. J. Work Environ. Health *8* (1982), 169–177
24. Lovell, M. A., Farmer, J. G.: Arsenic Speciation in Urine from Humans Intoxicated by Inorganic Arsenic Compounds. Human Toxicol. *4* (1985), 203–214
25. Lunde, G.: Occurrence and transformation of arsenic in the marine environment. Environ. Health Perspect. *19* (1977), 47–52
26. Mappes, R.: Versuche zur Ausscheidung von Arsen im Urin. Int. Arch. Occup. Environ. Health *40* (1977), 267–272
27. Munro, I. C.: Naturally occurring toxicants in foods and their significance. Clin. Toxicol. *9* (1976), 647–663
28. Nordberg, G. F., Pershagen, G., Lauwerys, R.: Inorganic arsenic. Toxicological and epidemiological aspects. Report to the Commission of European Communities. Department of Community Health and Environmental Medicine. Odense University, Odense 1979
29. Norin, H., Vahter, M.: A rapid method for the selective analysis of total urinary metabolites in inorganic arsenic trioxide exposure. Scan. J. Work Environ. Health *7* (1981), 38–44
30. Offergelt, J. A., Roels, H., Buchet, J. P., Boeckx, M., Lauwerys R.: Relation between airborne arsenic trioxide and urinary excretion of inorganic arsenic and its methylated metabolites. Brit. J. Ind. Med. *49* (1992), 387–393
31. Pinto, S. S., Varner, M. O., Nelson, K. W., Labbe, A. L., White, L. D.: Arsenic trioxide adsorption and excretion in industry. J. Occup. Med. *18* (1976), 677–660
32. Pinto, S. S., Enterline, P. E., Henderson, V., Varner, M. O.: Mortality experience in relation to a measured arsenic trioxide exposure. Environ. Health Perspect. *19* (1977), 127–130
33. Roels, H., Buchet, J. P., Truc, J., Croquet, F., Lauwerys, R.: The possible role of direct ingestion on the overall absorption of cadmium or arsenic in workers exposed to CdO or As_2O_3 dust. Am J. Ind. Med. *3* (1982), 53–65
34. Smith, T. J., Crecelius, E. A.: Airborne arsenic exposure and excretion of methylated arsenic compounds, Environ. Health. Perspec. *19* (1977), 89–93
35. Vahter, M.: Arsenic. In: Clarkson, T. W., Friberg, L., Nordberg, G. F., Sager, P. R. (eds.): Biological monitoring of toxic metals. Plenum Press, New York 1988, pp. 303–321
36. Vahter, M., Friberg, L., Rahnster, B., Nygren, A.: Airborne arsenic and urinary excretion of metabolites of inorganic arsenic among smelter workers. Int. Arch. Occup. Environ. Health *57* (1986), 79–91
37. Valkonene, S., Jarvisalo, J., Aitio, A.: Urinary arsenic in a Finnish population without occupational exposure to arsenic. In: Brätte/Schramel (eds): Trace Element-Analytical Chemistry in Medicine and Biology, Vol. 2, de Gruyter, Berlin 1983, pp. 611–621
38. World Health Organization (WHO): Environmental Health Criteria 18. Arsenic. IPCS International programme on chemical safety (1981)

39. Wichmann, N., Lehnert, G.: Arbeitsmedizinische Erfahrungen und TRK-Wert für Arsen, Arbeitsmed., Sozialmed., Präventivmed. *22* (1987), 18–20
40. Yamauchi, H., Takahashi, K., Mashiko, M., Yamamura, Y.: Biological monitoring of arsenic exposure of gallium arsenide- and inorganic arsenic-exposed workers by determination of inorganic arsenic and its metabolites in urine and hair. Am. Ind. Hyg. Assoc. J. *50* (1989), 606–612

Author: K. H. Schaller
Approved by the Working Group: 27th May 1993

Benzene

EKA The correlations between external and internal exposure yield the following data:

Air Benzene (ml/m³)	Air Benzene (mg/m³)	Whole blood Benzene (µg/l)	Urine *S*-Phenyl-mercapturic acid (mg/g creatinine)	Urine *trans,trans*-Muconic acid (mg/l)
0.3	1.0	0.9	0.010	—
0.6	2.0	2.4	0.025	1.6
0.9	3.0	4.4	0.040	—
1.0	3.3	5.0	0.045	2
2	6.5	14.0	0.090	3
4	13.0	38.0	0.180	5
6	19.5	—	0.270	7

Sampling time: end of exposure or end of shift

Date of evaluation 1993

CAS No. 71-43-2

Formula C_6H_6

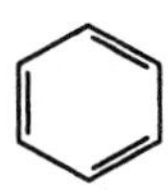

Molecular weight 78.11

Melting point 5.5 °C

Boiling point 80.15 °C

Vapour pressure at 20 °C 101 mbar

MAK [last established: 1971] Carcinogenic substance: Section III Category 1 of the List of MAK and BAT Values

Benzene is a key chemical which is used for a variety of syntheses. Global production is estimated at about 15 million tons per year (22). The most important compounds produced from benzene are: aniline dyes, alkyl benzenes (toluene, ethylbenzene, styrene),

Essential BAT Value Documentations. DFG, Deutsche Forschungsgemeinschaft

ISBN 3-527-31477-6

nitrobenzenes, halogenated benzenes (chlorobenzenes) and phenols. Benzene is used in the synthesis of insecticides, of components of washing powders, and of Nylon® and Perlon®. In addition, benzene is a component of petrol. According to the guidelines of the European Union, petrol may contain up to 5 % benzene. At present, an average concentration of 2.6 % (v/v) benzene is assumed for Europe. Contamination with up to 0.1 % benzene is permitted in solvents for paints and lacquers.

Due to its high vapour pressure benzene occurs at the workplace mainly as vapour. Additional exposure may occur via toluene which is contaminated with benzene. Such exposure is to be expected whenever technical grade aromatic solvents are used.

There are also considerable emissions of benzene in the general environment. Benzene emissions of 6000 tons per year caused by industry and commerce were estimated for the years 1988/89 for the Federal Republic of Germany. The benzene emissions caused by vehicles were estimated for the same period to be 41000 tons per year (23).

1 Metabolism and Kinetics

1.1 Absorption

Benzene is mainly taken up by inhalation. After reaching the blood-air equilibrium, approx. 50 % is retained (14). Equilibrium is attained after about 30 minutes. According to Angerer (3), the following relationship exists under steady-state conditions:

$$\log y = (0.71 \pm 0.77) \log x - (0.52 \pm 1.25)$$

where x designates the benzene concentration in blood (µg/l) and y the benzene concentration in ambient air (mg/m³).

In addition benzene absorption depends on the respiratory minute volume (11) and the amount of adipose tissue (19, 36), as benzene, a lipophilic substance, accumulates preferentially in the adipose and nerve tissue.

The dermal uptake of benzene is insignificant. After a single application of 50 µl ^{14}C-benzene to the forearm or the palm of the hand of rhesus monkeys less than 0.2 % is absorbed (26). Due to its importance as a carcinogenic substance, however, benzene is designated in the MAK documentation with an H for substances which can be absorbed in dangerous amounts through the skin. There are various data on gastro-intestinal uptake via drinking water and food. According to a report by the WHO (47), daily uptake of benzene with food amounts to 100–250 µg/day and in drinking water to 1–5 µg/day. As these data were estimated from calculations in the 70s they can no longer be accepted for the conditions prevailing in Germany today. According to Rosskamp and Seifert (32) the daily uptake of benzene with food and drinking water is in both cases less than 1 µg. Benzene uptake from the air (2–60 µg/day), indoors (150 µg/day), inside cars (25–400 µg/day), via tobacco smoke (400 µg/day) and passive smoking (7 µg/day) is of greater importance.

1.2 Elimination

After the end of exposure 16–50 % of the absorbed benzene is exhaled unchanged. The amount exhaled depends on the duration of exposure. The amount of benzene exhaled unchanged after 5 hours exposure only amounted to 16 % (46); after 2 hours exposure 30 % was found, however. These observations have also been confirmed by theoretical calculations using a 5-compartment model (15).

After the end of exposure the blood-benzene level decreases rapidly. At the end of a two-hour exposure period to 25 ml/m^3 benzene, a blood-benzene concentration of about 200 µg/l was measured, which 15 hours after the end of exposure had decreased to 10 µg/l (36). According to Angerer (3), the half-life of benzene in blood after the end of exposure is about 0.5 hours.

According to Low (24), elimination from various tissues is biphasic; at the beginning with a shorter half-life between 2.4 and 2.8 hours and then, in a slower phase dependent on the dose, with a half-life between 11 and 29 hours. At concentrations between 1 and 10 ml/m^3 there is a marked accumulation of the substance, however. In persons exposed long-term, elimination can therefore last for up to 150 hours (9).

In addition to being exhaled unchanged, benzene is metabolised in the liver. The main product of metabolism is phenol, which is eliminated renally in the form of its glucuronide or sulphate at a level of up to 45 % of the total amount of benzene absorbed (3). The biological half-life amounts to about 5 hours (38). By far the greatest amount is eliminated within 24 hours. Only after benzene exposures above 10 ml/m^3 does phenol accumulate in the course of the working week. This is no longer of importance today, however, as concentrations in this order of magnitude no longer occur.

In the course of benzene metabolism further metabolites are formed, which in humans, however, only make up about 1–3 % of the total amount of benzene taken up. Among these are diphenols, quinones, *trans-trans*-muconic acid and *S*-phenylmercapturic acid (19). In addition, adducts with guanine (21, 43), of DNA and with the cysteine of albumin (8) have been detected.

1.3 Metabolism and Biochemical Indicators

In a first stage, benzene is mainly oxidised in the liver to benzene epoxide, which can then react further in many ways. Transformation to the main metabolite, phenol, and to diphenols, which are mostly eliminated in the form of conjugates, mainly takes place spontaneously. Coupling to glutathione leads to the formation of *S*-phenylmercapturic acids, which are eliminated with the urine (34). Transformation via epoxide hydrolase yields a dihydrodiole, which can be further degraded to catechol, *o*-quinone, 1,2,4-trihydroxybenzene and *trans,trans*-muconic acid (20). Mercapturic acids can also occur (25). Furthermore, ring-expansion to benzene oxide (oxepin) is under discussion (16). In addition to indirect hydroxylation via the epoxide, direct hydroxylation of benzene seems to take place, possibly via free radicals. Detection of biphenyls seems to indicate this (40).

The reactions named above represent first and foremost a detoxification, but produce intermediates which are toxic or lead to metabolites via further metabolic stages which are responsible for the toxicity and carcinogenicity of benzene; in particular, *p*-benzoquinone and *trans-trans*-muconic aldehyde (18). A coupling product of guanine and benzoquinone was identified by Snyder (43) as an adduct with DNA. It was shown experimentally that benzene also reacts with haemoglobin to form adducts. This could not, however, be confirmed in humans. *S*-Phenylcysteine in albumin was identified as a coupling product (8).

There are only animal experimental results available on the influence of foreign substances on benzene metabolism. It is worth mentioning that benzene can induce its own metabolism (17, 41). Mixed exposure with the benzene homologue, toluene, inhibits benzene metabolism, but only at exposure levels above the MAK value. Ethanol influences metabolism in two ways: first of all inhibition takes place. After 16–18 hours, however, when the alcohol has been more or less degraded, the metabolism-increasing effect of CYP2E1 induction becomes effective (37). In addition, the metabolic phase is dependent on the uptake of carbohydrates. It increases linearly with decreasing carbohydrate uptake. According to Nakajima *et al.* (30) changes in diet or alcohol consumption lead to an acceleration in bioactivation, not, however, in detoxification. There is an increase in covalent binding to macromolecules. The benzene-induced haematotoxicity is amplified by ethanol.

2 Critical Toxicity

Due to the clastogenic and carcinogenic effect of benzene in humans and animals, data on critical toxicity cannot be given. An attempt has been made, however, at least to estimate roughly the carcinogenic risk for exposures in the range of the technical exposure limit (TRK). On the basis of animal experiments an attempt was made using pharmacokinetic calculations to extrapolate to the cancer risk in humans. According to these calculations the additional leukaemia risk after exposure to 1 and 10 ml/m^3 benzene during the whole work period is between 5 and 15, and between 44 and 152 cases, respectively, per 1000 exposed persons. The tumours taken as biological end points for the risk extrapolation were selected arbitrarily and are possibly not suitable for estimating the risk of leukaemia. The calculated risk data are therefore inexact. A detailed representation of this problem can be found in the occupational-medical–toxicological documentation for benzene in the 1992 supplement to the List of MAK and BAT Values. Swaen (44) tried to deduce the leukaemia risk from epidemiological data. According to him, at an exposure level of 10 ml/m^3 benzene and a working period of 30 years, the risk amounts to 5 cases per 1000 exposed persons.

3 Exposure and Effects

Internal exposure:
The benzene concentration which, under the given conditions of exposure, builds up in the organism. The parameter of internal exposure is the benzene concentration in blood.

Effect:
1. *S*-Phenylmercapturic acid as a product of degradation of glutathione metabolism which under given conditions of exposure is formed in the organism and is excreted in the urine.
2. *trans,trans*-Muconic acid as a final metabolite of oxidative metabolism which is also excreted renally.

3.1 Relationship Between External and Internal Exposure

The relationship between benzene exposure and the parameter benzene in blood is based on the results of a study by Angerer (3) with employees of an insecticide-producing company. The relationship between the benzene uptake and the excretion of *S*-phenylmercapturic acid in urine was deduced from two series of investigations on refinery workers and female workers in the shoe industry (28, 39). The EKA values for *trans,trans*-muconic acid were calculated from the study of Ducos *et al.* (13).

4 Selection of the Indicators

In addition to the determination of benzene in blood, all metabolites formed are suitable parameters for monitoring exposure to benzene. Determination of benzene in blood has the advantage of being highly specific (6). Analytical determination which is based on a head-space technique is comparatively simple and interference-free if contamination can be avoided during sampling and sample preparation. Due to the short biological half-life of benzene in blood, sampling should take place immediately after exposure.

The phenol excretion in urine, however, is not specific for exposure to benzene as it can be influenced by exogenous factors, e.g. components of food or medicines which contain phenyl groups. In an investigation, Angerer (3) was able to show that in 30 % of the persons in a collective exposed to an average concentration of 10 ml/m^3 benzene, the phenol concentration was below 35 mg/l, which corresponded to the maximum value of a non-exposed collective. This parameter is only suitable for benzene monitoring on a collective basis and in a concentration range greatly above the current TRK value and is therefore no longer used.

S-Phenylmercapturic acid, which is formed in amounts of about 0.1 % during the metabolism of benzene, represents a parameter suitable for indicating benzene exposure specifically and sensitively. Due to the small amount excreted, however, analysis is a complicated matter, so that this parameter cannot be determined in all occupational-medical laboratories (28).

Recently, excretion of *trans,trans*-muconic acid in urine has been discussed as a specific indicator metabolite for benzene (13). According to the most recent investigations by Angerer (6), this metabolite reacts very sensitively to benzene exposure even below 1 ppm.

In addition, oxidative products of benzene degradation can be considered for biological monitoring, such as catechol, hydroquinone, quinone and adducts with guanine or the cysteine of albumin. There is, however, little experience with regard to the validity of these parameters.

4.1 Benzene in Blood

Unlike the determination of phenolic benzene metabolites in urine, measurement of benzene in blood indicates the internal exposure not only of groups, but also of individuals. According to Docter and Zielhuis (11) and Täuber (45), it should be taken into account that during heavy physical work more benzene is taken up by the organism than during rest or light work. Under steady state conditions the equilibrium between benzene in the ambient air and benzene in the blood is reached after approx. 0.5 hours. After the end of exposure the concentration of benzene in blood decreases exponentially; the half-life is stated as being 0.5 hours. The time of blood sampling is therefore of great importance when monitoring benzene exposure by determination of the benzene concentration in blood. As the cited relationships between the benzene concentration in ambient air and the benzene concentration in blood are only valid under steady state conditions, blood sampling should take place immediately after the end of exposure. The requirements demanded of the sampling technique (3, 12) and storage should be taken into account.

4.2 *S*-Phenylmercapturic Acid in Urine

The *S*-phenylmercapturic acid concentration in urine increases continuously with exposure to benzene during the working day and reaches its maximum about 2 hours after the end of exposure. Afterwards it decreases again and at the beginning of the next shift it is within the normal range. It is a metabolite which indicates benzene exposure specifically and sensitively in the individual, even if benzene exposure is below 1 ml/m^3 (28). In practice it has been shown that there is a good correlation between benzene exposure and the *S*-phenylmercapturic acid excretion in urine at the end of the shift (39).

4.3 *trans,trans*-Muconic Acid in Urine

trans,trans-Muconic acid is a product of benzene metabolism. About 2 % of the benzene taken up is excreted with the urine as *trans,trans*-muconic acid. During occupational exposure to benzene the level of *trans,trans*-muconic acid in urine increases towards the end of the shift (31). The concentration of *trans,trans*-muconic acid in urine is a sensitive parameter for low level exposure to benzene (12, 13, 33, 39).

5 Methodology

5.1 Benzene in Blood

Various gas chromatographic methods are described for the determination of benzene in blood (1, 3). According to Snyder *et al.* (42), blood samples of 0.2–0.5 g are necessary. Up to 0.5 µg benzene/g blood can be detected. The analysis procedures described by Sato *et al.* (35) require 0.02–1 ml blood and have a detection limit of 0.02 µg benzene/ml blood.

According to Angerer (3), for the determination of the blood-benzene concentration 2 ml venous blood are taken and injected into a head-space vial sealed with a rubber stopper which contains about 50 mg ammonium oxalate as an anti-coagulant. After 30 minutes incubation at 60 °C, the benzene concentration is quantified by head-space gas chromatography.

The coefficient of variation (standard deviation as a percentage of the average value) for in-series precision is stated as being 2.6 % for this method. The detection limit is below 0.002 µg benzene/ml blood. This procedure has been validated by the working group "Analysen in biologischem Material" (Analyses of Hazardous Substances in Biological Materials) of the DFG Commission for the Investigation of Health Hazards of Chemical Compounds in the Work Area. It is possible to increase the sensitivity of the method by a factor of 10 by enrichment procedures, so that now benzene concentrations in the environmental range are accessible to determination (4, 5). Determination of benzene in blood is highly specific for detection of previous exposure to benzene, provided that contamination during sampling and preparation is avoided.

5.2 *S*-Phenylmercapturic Acid in Urine

Determination of *S*-phenylmercapturic acid in urine is carried out using gas chromatography/mass spectrometry. *S*-Fluoro-phenylmercapturic acid is added to 5 ml urine as an internal standard. The urine is extracted twice with 5 ml ethyl acetate. After evaporation of the extract, methylation is carried out with diazomethane. The *S*-phenylmercapturic acid is separated using gas chromatography and detected using mass spectrometry for the masses 194,042 and 212,032. The detection limit is 1 µg/l, in-series precision 8 % and day-to-day precision 10.5 % (28).

After acidification of the urine sample to a pH < 2 it can be transported at ambient air temperatures up to 25 °C and can be kept for at least three months at −18 °C.

5.3 *trans-trans*-Muconic Acid in Urine

The high-pressure liquid chromatographic procedure of Ducos (12) has proven internationally suitable for the determination of *trans,trans*-muconic acid in urine. A UV detector is used. During this procedure *trans,trans*-muconic acid is separated from the urine using an anion exchanger and at the same time enriched.

This procedure described by Ducos (12) has been optimised and tested with regard to its analytical reliability by the working group "Analyses of Hazardous Substances in Biological Materials" of the DFG Commission for the Investigation of Health Hazards of Chemical Compounds in the Work Area.

6 Background Exposures

According to Eikmann (14), environmentally-related exposure to benzene via air, water, food and passive smoking can be estimated at approx. 0.2 mg/day. The benzene level of tobacco smoke fluctuates between 20 and 90 µg per cigarette. If one assumes an average tobacco consumption of 20 cigarettes per day, the theoretical uptake amounts to 0.4 to 1.8 mg benzene per day. The benzene concentration inside cars is considerable. The benzene uptake is estimated at approx. 200 µg per day. This is reflected in the values of the blood-benzene concentration of the normal population. Brugnone *et al.* (10) found in employees from rural areas benzene levels of 200 ng/l (variation: 7–1003 ng/l) and in employees from urban areas values of 296 ng/l (variation: 7–2241 ng/l). The values for smokers and non-smokers were 381 ng/l (variation: 7–2241 ng/l) and 205 ng/l (variation: 7–924 ng/l). Angerer *et al.* (5) found for German non-smokers without occupational exposure a mean benzene level of 176 ± 62 ng/l, for smokers 211 ± 0.5 ng/l; immediately after smoking the concentration was 365 ± 178 ng/l.

In an investigation of 10 male and 10 female non-smokers and 20 male and 20 female smokers, phenylmercapturic acid concentrations of 0.2 µg/g creatinine (non-smokers) and 5 µg/g creatinine (smokers) were determined (29). The differences between smokers and non-smokers are considerably greater than those mentioned above. According to more recent investigations by van Sittert *et al.* 1993 (39), excretion of *S*-phenylmercapturic acid in smokers or non-smokers as a rule is below the analytical detection limit of 1–5 µg/g creatinine.

trans,trans-Muconic acid is also excreted in urine by persons not exposed to benzene occupationally. The reasons for this must include the environmental exposure to benzene in industrialised countries. In addition, other substances, such as sorbic acid, which is taken up with food, are being discussed as possible sources for the excretion of *trans,trans*-muconic acid. The *trans,trans*-muconic acid concentrations occurring in the urine of the normal population are quoted at values between not detectable and 3 mg/l. The *trans,trans*-muconic acid concentrations in the urine of the normal population are given with mean values between 0.13 and 1.11 mg/l (6, 7, 12, 13, 27, 33). From this data an upper norm limit (95th percentile) of 1 mg/l urine can be deduced for the *trans,trans*-muconic acid concentrations.

7 Evaluation of EKA Values

7.1 Benzene in Blood

From the published air/blood quotients of 1:8 to 1:10 a median value of approx. 280 µg benzene/l blood would be calculated to correspond to the air value of 10 ml/m^3. The empirically determined values from Angerer (3) and Angerer and Lehnert (2) correspond with these calculated values, however, only with regard to their order of magnitude. As median values they are subject to a degree of uncertainty and require the support of further investigations.

The following EKA values for benzene in blood have been evaluated:

Benzene in air ml/m^3	Benzene in whole blood µg/l
0.3	0.9
0.6	2.4
0.9	4.4
1.0	5.0
2	14.0
4	38.0
6	–

7.2 *S*-Phenylmercapturic Acid in Urine

Two studies were used for the evaluation. The collective investigated by Müller *et al.* (28) consisted of 20 women who worked for 8 hours a day in a shoe factory. Four were smokers and 16 non-smokers. They were exposed mainly to ethyl acetate and toluene which was contaminated with benzene.

The benzene concentrations at the workplace were determined simultaneously with active and passive personal dosimeters. The hazardous substances were quantified by gas chromatography/mass spectrometry. Values between 0.8 and 16.1 mg/m^3 (0.25 and 5 ppm) were measured for the exposure to benzene.

From the beginning of the shift to the next morning, urine from the women was sampled in portions and after derivatisation was evaluated using gas chromatography/mass spectrometry (28).

Correlations between benzene uptake and excretion of phenylmercapturic acid can be deduced from the values measured, expressed as µg/l, µg/g creatinine and the total amount.

Expressed as µg/l
PMA [µg/l] = 35.9 × benzene [ppm] – 1.4 r = 0.93

expressed as µg/g creatinine
PMA [µg/g creatinine] = 29.9 × benzene [ppm] + 5.4 r = 0.89

and expressed as the total amount
PMA [µg total] = 11.6 × benzene [ppm] + 1.1 r = 0.86

The EKA values can be calculated from these equations (Table 1).

Table 1: Phenylmercapturic acid excretion (*S*-PMA) after benzene exposure (37)

Benzene (ppm)	*S*-PMA (µg/l)	*S*-PMA (µg/g creatinine)	*S*-PMA (µg/24h)
1	40	35	12
2	80	70	24
3	120	100	36
4	160	130	48
5	200	160	60

A publication of van Sittert *et al.* (39) reports 12 studies carried out with employees from 10 factories who were exposed to benzene during the production and maintenance of machines in chemical plants and refineries. 31 male test persons were chosen for the evaluation of a relationship between the benzene level in the air and the excretion of *S*-phenylmercapturic acid in urine.

The benzene concentration at the workplace was determined with active personal dosimeters. The hazardous substances were determined gas chromatographically with a flame ionisation detector.

At the end of the shift urine was sampled from the male test persons and quantitative determination of *S*-phenylmercapturic acid took place using gas chromatography/mass spectrometry.

The following correlation between the benzene concentration in the air (up to 2 ppm) and the excretion of phenylmercapturic acid in urine was deduced from the values measured:

Benzene [mg/m^3] = 0.068 × PMA [µg/g creatinine] + 0.14 r = 0.963

The EKA values from this investigation can be seen in Table 2.

Table 2: Relationship between the benzene air exposure and *S*-PMA excretion (39)

Benzene air concentration (mg/m^3 eight hours TWA)	*S*-PMA urine concentration (µg/g creatinine) mean (95% CI)
1.0	12 (10–14)
2.3	27 (24–30)
3.0	42 (38–46)
3.25 (1 ppm)	46 (41–50)
4.0	56 (52–62)

For the evaluation of EKA values the relationship found in men by van Sittert *et al.* (39) can be taken as a basis and extrapolated for values above 2 ppm:

Benzene in air (ppm)	Phenylmercapturic acid in urine (mg/g creatinine)
0.3	0.010
0.6	0.025
0.9	0.040
1	0.045
2	0.090
4	0.180
6	0.270

7.3 *trans,trans*-Muconic Acid

Ducos *et al.* (13) investigated the excretion of *trans,trans*-muconic acid in workers exposed to benzene (n = 23) in 3 factories several times. These persons were exposed to benzene concentrations between 0.1 and 75 ppm. The air was sampled using personal air sampling. In these investigations in total 105 pairs of values were obtained (benzene/air–*trans,trans*-muconic acid/urine). There was a highly significant correlation ($p < 0.001$) between the benzene concentration in the air and the *trans,trans*-muconic acid excretion in urine. According to this, an increase in the benzene concentration in air by 1 ppm corresponds to an increase in the *trans,trans*-muconic acid concentration in urine of 1 mg/l. When evaluating EKA values it must be taken into account that excretion of *trans,trans*-muconic acid in non-occupationally exposed persons can be as much as 1 mg/l urine.

The following EKA values have been calculated on the basis of the relationship between the benzene concentration in ambient air and the excretion of *trans, trans*-muconic acid in urine:

Benzene in air ml/m^3	*trans,trans*-Muconic acid in urine mg/l
0.3	–
0.6	1.6
0.9	–
1.0	2
2	3
4	5
6	7

8 Interpretation of the Data

The determination of benzene in whole blood allows conclusions to be drawn about the internal exposure to benzene in individual workers. When interpreting the data, the amount of heavy physical work must be taken into consideration. The time of sampling also plays a decisive role. Blood should be sampled immediately after the end of exposure.

For the determination of *S*-phenylmercapturic acid it is sufficient to acidify urine sampled at the end of the shift with hydrochloric acid to a pH value < 2. It can be transported at ambient air temperatures up to 25 °C and kept at –18 °C for several months. Analysis can, however, only take place in laboratories equipped with a mass spectrometer.

Environmental influences affect the excretion of *S*-phenylmercapturic acid only to a limited extent. Smoking can represent exposure to 0.1 ml/m^3 benzene.

In the general population the amount of *trans,trans*-muconic acid excreted varies. The values are usually below 1 mg/l. Sorbic acid, which is added to various foods as a preservative, is suspected of being transformed into muconic acid.

As a result of this "normal excretion", *trans,trans*-muconic acid is diagnostically only a sufficiently reliable indicator of individual exposure for benzene concentrations of more than 1 ppm. In investigations with collectives, however, excretion of muconic acid also indicates very sensitively benzene concentrations below 1 ppm.

This means that with benzene air concentrations above 1 ppm, all 3 parameters are suitable for evaluation of individual exposure to benzene, whereas below 1 ppm only determination of benzene in blood and *S*-phenylmercapturic acid in urine allow reliable conclusions to be drawn.

9 References

1. Angerer, J.: Quantitative Bestimmung von Lösungsmitteln im Blut mit Hilfe der gaschromatographischen Dampfraumanalyse, Arbeitsmed. Sozialmed. Präventivmed. *11*, 116–118 (1976)
2. Angerer, J., Lehnert, G.: Biologische Grenzwerte für kanzerogene Arbeitsstoffe – Beispiel Benzol, in: Verhandlungen der Deutschen Gesellschaft für Arbeitsmedizin e.V., 22. Jahrestagung, Ed.: Stalder, Gentner Verlag, Stuttgart 427–431 (1983)
3. Angerer, J.: Prävention beruflich bedingter Gesundheitsschäden durch Benzol, Toluol, Xylole und Ethylbenzol, Schriftenreihe "Arbeitsmedizin, Sozialmedizin, Präventivmedizin", Gentner Verlag, Stuttgart (1983)
4. Angerer, J., Hörsch, B.: Determination of aromatic hydrocarbons and their metabolites in human blood and urine, J. Chromatogr. *580*, 229–255 (1992)
5. Angerer, J., Scherer, G., Schaller, K.H., Müller, J.: The determination of benzene in human blood as an indicator of environmental exposure to volatile aromatic compounds. Fresenius J. Anal. Chem. *339*, 740 (1991)
6. Angerer, J., Rauscher, D., Schaller, K.H., Letzel, S., Popp, W., Müller, G., Rüdiger, H.: Die t,t-Muconsäure als Untersuchungsparameter beruflich bzw. ökologisch bedingter Benzolexpositionen, in: Verhandlungen der Deutschen Gesellschaft für Arbeitsmedizin und Umweltmedizin e.V. 33. Jahrestagung, G. Triebig (Ed.) Gentner Verlag, Stuttgart, 191–195 (1993)
7. Bechtold, W.E., Lucier, G., Birnbaum, L.S., Yin, S.N., Li, G.L., Henderson, R.F.: Muconic acid determinations in urine as a biological exposure index for workers occupationally exposed to benzene, Am. Ind. Hyg. Assoc. J. *11*, 473–478 (1991)
8. Bechtold, W.E., Willis, J.K., Sun, J.D., Griffith, W.C., Reddy, T.V.: Biological Markers of Exposure to Benzene – S-Phenylcysteine in Albumin, Carcinogenesis *13*, 1217–1220 (1992)
9. Bittersohl, G.: Der gegenwärtige Stand der Kenntnisse über die Benzenwirkung – Metabolismus, Z. gesamte Hyg. *36*, 135–136 (1990)
10. Brugnone, F., Perbellini, L., Maranelli, G., Romeo, L., Guglielmi, G., Lombardini, F.: Reference values for blood benzene in the occupationally unexposed general population, Int. Arch. Occup. Environ. Health *64*, 179–184 (1992)
11. Docter, H.J., Zielhuis, R.L.: Phenol excretion as a measure of benzene exposure, Ann. Occup. Hyg. *10*, 317–326 (1967)
12. Ducos, P., Gaudin, R., Robert, A., Francin, J.M., Maire, C.: Improvement in HPLC analysis of trans,trans-muconic acid, a promising substitute for phenol in the assessment of benzene exposure, Int. Arch. Occup. Environ. Health *62*, 529–534 (1990)
13. Ducos, P., Gaudin, R., Bel, J., Maire, C., Francin, J. M., Robert, A., Wild, P.: t,t,-Muconic acid, a reliable biological indicator for the detection of individual benzene exposure down to the ppm level, Int. Arch. Occup. Environ. Health *64*, 309–313 (1992)
14. Eikmann, T., Kramer, M., Goebel, H.: Die Belastung der Bevölkerung durch Schadstoffe im Kraftfahrzeug-Innenraum – Beispiel Benzol, Zbl. Hyg. *193*, 41–52 (1992)
15. Fiserova-Bergerova, V., Vlach, J., Cassady, J.C.: Predictable "individual differences" in uptake and excretion of gases and soluble vapours simulation study, Brit. J. Ind. Med. *37*, 210–214 (1980)
16. Goldstein, B.D.: Introduction: Occam's razor is dull, Environ. Health Persp. *82*, 3–6 (1989)
17. Gollmer, L., Graf, H., Ullrich, V.: Characterisation of the benzene monooxygenase system in rabbit bone marrow, Biochem. Pharmacol. *33*, 3597–3602 (1984)
18. Huff, J.E., Hasemann, J.K., DeMarini, D.M., Eustis, S., Maronpot, R.R., Peters, A.C., Persing, R.L., Chrisp, C.E., Jacobs, A.C.,: Multiple-site carcinogenicity of benzene in Fisher 344 rats and B6C3F$_1$ mice, Environ. Health Persp. *82* (1989)
19. Hunter, C.G., Blair, D.: Benzene: Pharmacokinetic studies in men, Ann. Occup. Hyg. *15*, 193–199 (1972)
20. Inoue, O., Seiji, K., Nakatsuka, H., Watanabe, T., Yin, S.-N., Li, G.-L., Cai, S.-X., Jin, C., Ikeda, M.: Excretion of 1,2,4- benzenetriol in the urine of workers exposed to benzene, Brit. J. Ind. Med. *46*, 559–556 (1989)

21. Jowa, L., Witz, G., Snyder, R., Winkle, S., Kalf, G. F.: Synthesis and characterisation of deoxyguanosine benzoquinone adducts, J. Appl. Toxicol. *10*, 47–54 (1990)
22. Koch, R.(.H.).: Umweltchemikalien, physikalisch-chemische Daten, Toxizitäten, Grenz- und Richtwerte, Umweltverhalten, VCH- Verlagsgesellschaft, Weinheim (1989)
23. LAI – Länderausschuss für Immissionsschutz, Arbeitsgruppe "Krebsrisiko durch Luftverunreinigungen", Beurteilungsmasstäbe zur Begrenzung des Krebsrisikos durch Luftverunreinigungen. Abschlussbericht, LAI-Schriftenreihe, Erich Schmidt Verlag, Berlin (1991)
24. Low, L.K., Reddy, G.R., Blackburn, G.R., Mackerer,C.R.: Benzene mechanistic research project. Final report, Mobil Environmental and Health Sciences Laboratory, P.O. box 1209, Princeton NJ 08534–1029, USA, September, 1 (1991)
25. Lunte, S.M.L., Lunte C. E.: Electroanalytical approaches to understand benzene metabolism, J. Pharmaceutical Biomed. Analysis *8*, 131–136 (1990)
26. Maibach, H.I., Anjo, D.M.: Percutaneous penetration of benzene and benzene contained in solvents used in the rubber industry, Arch. Environm. Health *36*, 256–260 (1981)
27. Melikian, A.A., Prahalad, A.K., Hoffmann, D.: Urinary trans,trans-muconic acid as an indicator of exposure to benzene in cigarette smokers, cancer epidemiology, biomarkers & prevention *2*, 47–51 (1993)
28. Müller, G., Fahnert; R., Müller, Ch., Popp, W., Schmieding, W., Norpoth, K.: Biological Monitoring bei Benzolexpositionen bis zur Höhe des geltenden TRK- Wertes, in: Verhandlungen der Deutschen Gesellschaft für Arbeitsmedizin und Umweltmedizin e.V. 31. Jahrestagung, G. Schäcke, K. Ruppe, Ch. Vogel- Sührig (Eds.), Gentner Verlag, Stuttgart, 571–574 (1991)
29. Müller, G., Dibowski, A., Norpoth, K.: Die S-Phenylmerkaptursäure-Ausscheidung im Harn bei Rauchern und Nichtrauchern, in: Verhandlungen der Deutschen Gesellschaft für Arbeitsmedizin und Umweltmedizin e.V. 33. Jahrestagung, G. Triebig (Ed.), Gentner Verlag, Stuttgart, 467–471 (1993)
30. Nakajima, T., Okuyama, S., Yonekura, I., Sato, A.: Effects of ethanol and phenobarbital administration on the metabolism and toxicity of benzene, Chem. Biol. Interact. *55*, 23–38 (1985)
31. Popp, W., Müller, G., Angerer, J., Norpoth, K.: Benzol-Belastung und biologisches Monitoring bei Kfz-Mechanikern, in: Verhandlungen der Deutschen Gesellschaft für Arbeitsmedizin und Umweltmedizin e.V. 33. Jahrestagung, G. Triebig (Ed.) Gentner Verlag, Stuttgart (1993)
32. Rosskamp, E., Seifert, B.: Ausgewählte cancerogene Umweltschadstoffe. Gegenüberstellung der dem Menschen über verschiedene Belastungspfade zugeführte Mengen, Institut für Wasser-, Boden-, Lufthygiene des BGA, Berlin (1991)
33. Ruppert, T., Scherer, G., Rauscher, D., Angerer, J., Adlkofer, F.: Determination of urinary t,t-muconic acid by gaschromatography-mass spectrometry, J. Chromatogr. B. *66*, 71–76 (1995)
34. Sabourin, P.J., Bechtold, W.E., Griffith, W.C., Birnbaum, L.S., Lucier, G., Henderson, R.F.: Effect of exposure concentration, exposure rate and route of administration on metabolism of benzene by F344 rats and B6C3F_1 mice, Toxicol. Appl. Pharmacol. *99*, 421–444 (1989)
35. Sato, A., Nakajima, T., Fujiwara, Y.: Determination of benzene and toluene in blood by means of a syringe-equilibration method using a small amount of blood, Brit. J. Ind. Med., *32*, 210–214 (1975)
36. Sato, A., Nakajima, T., Fujiwara, Y., Muruyama, N.: Kinetic studies on sex difference in susceptibility to chronic benzene intoxication – with special reference to body fat content, Brit. J. Ind. Med. *32*, 321–328 (1975)
37. Sato, A., Nakajima, T., Koyama, Y.: Dose related effects of a single dose of ethanol on the metabolism in rat liver of some aromatic and chlorinated hydrocarbons, Toxicol. Appl. Pharmacol. *60*, 8–15 (1981)
38. Sherwood, R.J., Carter, F.W.G.: The measurement of occupational exposure to benzene vapour, Ann. Occup. Hyg. *13*, 125–146 (1970)
39. Sittert, N.J. van., Boogaard, P.J., Beulink, G.D.J.: Application of the urinary S-phenylmercapturic acid test as a biomarker for low levels of exposure to benzene in industry, Br. J. Ind. Med. *50*, 460–469 (1993)

40. Snyder, C.A.: Benzene, Ethels Browning's Toxicity and Metabolism of Industrial Solvents, 2nd edition. Vol. 1: Hydrocarbons, R. Snyder (Ed.), Elsevier Science Publishers B.V., 3–37 (1987).
41. Snyder, R., Uzuko, F., Gonasum, L., Bromfield, E., Wells, A.: The metabolism of benzene in vitro, Toxicol. Appl. Pharmacol. *11*, 346–360 (1967)
42. Snyder, R., Laskin, S., Goldstein, B.: An extractive method for determination of benzene in blood by gas chromatography, Am. Ind. Hyg. Assoc. J. *36*, 833–836 (1975)
43. Snyder, R., Jowa, L., Witz, G., Kalf, G., Rushmore, T.: Formation of reactive metabolites from benzene, Arch. Toxicol. *60*, 61 (1987)
44. Swaen, G., Meijers, J.: Risk assessment of leukaemia and occupational exposure to benzene, Brit. J. Ind. Med. *46*, 826–830 (1989)
45. Täuber, U.: Wirkung von Benzol auf Mensch und Tier. Deutsche Gesellschaft für Mineralölwissenschaft und Kohlechemie e.V., Forschungsbericht, 174–76 (1980)
46. Teisinger, J., Bergerova-Fiserova, V., Kurdna, J.: The metabolism of benzene in men, Pracovni Lakarstvi *4*, 175 (1952)
47. WHO (World Health Organization): Air quality guidelines for Europe. WHO Regional Publications, European Series No. 23 (1987)

Author: G. Müller, J. Angerer
Approved by the Working Group: 18.04.95

2-Butanone

BAT	5 mg 2-butanone/l urine Sampling time: end of exposure
Date of evaluation	1988
Synonyms	Methyl ethyl ketone MEK Ethyl methyl ketone
Formula	CH_3–CO–C_2H_5
Molecular weight	72.11
Melting point	–85.9 °C
Boiling point	79.6 °C
Vapour pressure at 20 °C	105 hPa
MAK	200 ml/m^3 (ppm) 590 mg/m^3

1 Metabolism and Kinetics

At the workplace 2-butanone (methyl ethyl ketone, MEK) is taken up predominantly via inhalation. The ketone is also able to enter the body in quite considerable amounts via the intact skin.

The metabolism of 2-butanone in the human body is only known in part (Fig. 1). Approx. 25 % of the ketone taken up by the body is eliminated unchanged via exhalation (1). The rest of the ketone is metabolised. Some is oxidised to 3-hydroxy-2-butanone which could be identified in the urine of exposed workers. Part of the 2-butanone absorbed is excreted unchanged in the urine. Together with the 3-hydroxy-2-butanone the amount of 2-butanone excreted in the urine accounts for only approx. 0.1 % of the dose taken in (2). In experimental animals, apart from the 3-hydroxy-2-butanone, 2,3-butanediol and 2-butanol were identified as products of 2-butanone metabolism (3).

It can be assumed that these metabolites are also formed in the human organism and then excreted in the urine. The hydroxy compounds are most probably partially bound to sulphates or glucuronic acid. The relation between the amounts of the various metabolites is at present unknown (Fig. 1).

Essential BAT Value Documentations. DFG, Deutsche Forschungsgemeinschaft

ISBN 3-527-31477-6

2-Butanone, as a fairly readily water-soluble solvent, is only eliminated to a relatively small extent, as already described, via exhalation. During the examination of persons occupationally exposed to 2-butanone it was found that the concentration of the toxic substance in the alveolar air (c_a) was approx. a quarter of the ambient air concentration (c_i) ($c_a/c_i = 0.27$) (4).

2-Butanone accumulates in blood at higher concentrations than in the ambient air. Persons occupationally exposed to 2-butanone show concentrations of the toxic substance in the blood during exposure which according to Perbellini et al. (2) are approx. 35 times higher than those in the ambient air (c_b/c_i).

According to this study the 2-butanone concentration in urine is lower. The ratio of the 2-butanone concentration in urine to that of ambient air (c_u/c_i) was determined as 1/4.8.

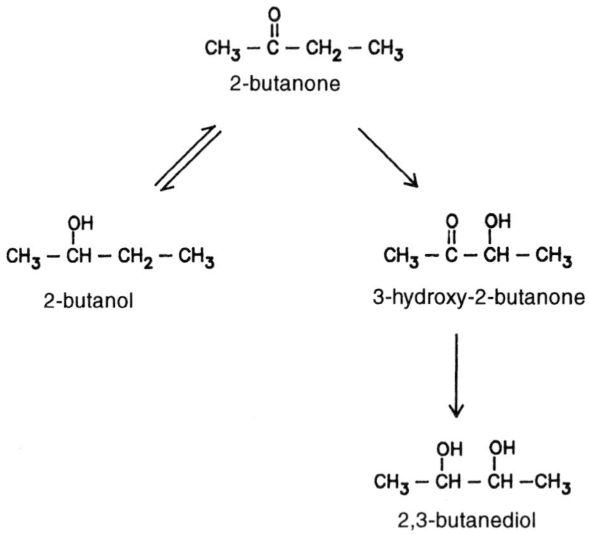

Fig.1: Metabolism of 2-butanone (3).

A close relationship has been found under workplace conditions between the 2-butanone concentration in ambient air on the one hand and the solvent concentration in alveolar air and in urine on the other (2). These authors did not reveal a correlation between the concentration of the toxic substance in blood and that in urine.

According to a mathematical model the 2-butanone concentration in the blood increases during the whole exposure period and after eight hours reaches approx. 16 % of the saturation value. After the end of exposure the 2-butanone is eliminated from the blood with a half-life of 270 min. 16 hours after the end of exposure the blood level has decreased to an insignificantly small value so that one can simply assume that after occupational exposure there is no accumulation of 2-butanone in the body.

The excretion of 2-butanone in urine follows the ketone level in the blood. Four hours after the start of exposure the butanone concentration in urine reaches values which even after continuing exposure increase only insignificantly.

An equilibrium between the ambient air concentration and the blood concentration of 2-butanone is reached much more slowly with 2-butanone than with less hydrophilic solvents such as e.g. aromatic hydrocarbons and to an even greater extent aliphatic hydrocarbons. This is probably mainly due to the fact that 2-butanone distributes itself relatively equally over the various compartments of the body. This can be seen from the distribution coefficients tissue/air which are very similar for the various tissues (2).

2 Critical Toxicity (see also MAK documentation)

Although 2-butanone is one of the most frequently used solvents only little is known about the systemic effects of this ketone on man. This is due not least to the fact that the irritating effects of the toxic substance on the eyes and mucous membranes prevent the uptake of higher doses at the workplace.

The odour threshold of 2-butanone is about 25 ppm (5). Concentrations in the ambient air of as little as 100 ppm can lead to slight irritation of the eyes. 2-Butanone concentrations above the currently valid MAK value of 200 ppm cause marked irritation of the eyes as well as mucous membranes, nose and throat (6).

With ambient air concentrations of more than 300 ppm the central depressive effects of 2-butanone come to the fore. Furthermore, with such concentrations headache (7) and "stomach ache" (8) were reported.

Whether 2-butanone also has neurotoxic properties cannot be clarified definitively at present. It can be regarded as certain that 2-butanone potentiates the neurotoxic effects of *n*-hexane and its metabolites 2-hexanol, 2-hexanone and 2,5-hexanedione. Spencer et al. (9) report about 79 cases of sensomotor polyneuritis in a factory where a mixture of 90 % 2-butanone and 10 % 2-hexanone (methyl-*n*-butyl ketone) was used as a solvent. In another case there was also an increase in the occurrence of sensomotor polyneuritis with the use of a 2-butanone/2-hexanone mixture (10). Here it should be particularly noted that the 2-butanone concentration in the ambient air was very low with values between 6 and 36 ppm. If 2-hexanone is present alone in the ambient air then about ten times higher concentrations are required to produce comparable effects.

The intensifying of the specific neurotoxic (peripheral) effect of *n*-hexane through 2-butanone has been studied in animal experiments. Two Japanese groups (11, 12) found greater changes in the neurophysiological parameters after simultaneous application of hexane and 2-butanone than were observed after exposure to pure hexane. This combination effect is apparently not due to metabolic interference, as Iwata et al. (13, 14) discovered no increase but rather a decrease in the 2,5-hexanedione excretion in the urine after simultaneous exposure to 2-butanone and *n*-hexane. 2,5-Hexanedione is regarded as the ultimate neurotoxic metabolite of *n*-hexane.

After simultaneous exposure to 2-butanone and toluene no additive effects on the CNS were discovered in an experimental study on volunteers. The 2-butanone concentration was 200 ppm, the toluene concentration 100 ppm (15).

3 Selection of the Indicators

At present especially the following parameters may be considered for the biological monitoring of persons exposed to 2-butanone:

- 2-butanone concentration in urine
- 2-butanone concentration in blood
- 2-butanone concentration in the alveolar air
- 3-hydroxy-2-butanone excretion in urine.

2-Butanone is sufficiently hydrophilic to enter the kidneys and be excreted in the urine. As has been shown in various studies, there is, therefore, also a close relationship between the 2-butanone concentration in the air at the workplace and the 2-butanone excretion in urine (see section 1). This proportionality makes the 2-butanone concentration in urine fundamentally a suitable parameter for the estimation of internal exposure. A further argument in favour of this parameter is that the irritant effects on the mucous membrane and also the central nervous effects of 2-butanone, i.e. the main toxic principle, are produced by the unchanged molecule of the toxic substance.

Practical and also analytical and methodological reasons speak in favour of the 2-butanone concentration in the urine as a parameter for the estimation of internal exposure. The determination of 2-butanone in urine is analytically and diagnostically specific which has led to there being sufficient data for the 2-butanone concentration in urine for the evaluation of a BAT value. A further advantage of this parameter is that the concentration of the toxic substance in urine reflects, as it were, the integral of the dose during the whole duration of exposure. As a disadvantage of this parameter the varying dilution of the urine samples and its influence on the 2-butanone concentration must be accepted.

Diagnostically even more sensitive and, unlike urine, the 2-butanone concentration in blood is not dependent upon the activity of the kidneys. As can be indirectly inferred from the results of Perbellini et al. (2) at steady state the 2-butanone concentration in the blood is approx. 7 times as high as that in urine. During investigation by members of the Commission of various collectives exposed to 2-butanone different results were found for the distribution of the ketone between blood and urine (Fig. 2). According to this investigation the relationship between the 2-butanone concentration in blood (c_b) and in urine (c_u) proved to be dependent upon the collective. The ratio c_b/c_u was between 0.5 and 2.5. A seven-fold higher concentration in the blood level than in the urine was not found even in a single case. From these results it can be concluded that the absorption and excretion kinetics of 2-butanone differ greatly in blood and urine. This means that the relationship of the ketone concentration in blood to that in urine depends markedly on the profile of the changes in the concentration of the 2-butanone in the air with time and on the time of taking the sample of biological material. It may be assumed that the steady state concentration of ketone in the blood is at least 2.5 times greater than that in urine. This was the largest value found in this investigation. Although it would be desirable in principle to define a BAT value for the 2-butanone concentration in blood the database described is not sufficient.

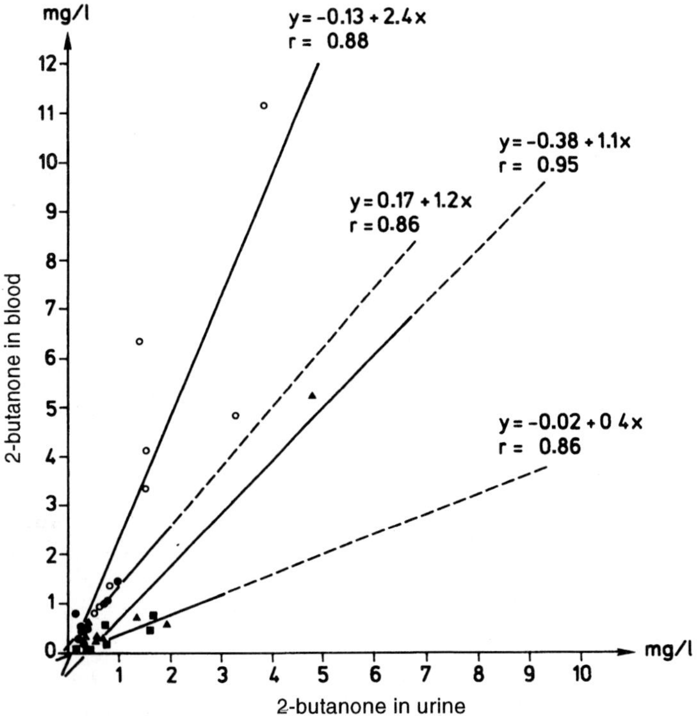

Fig. 2: Relationships between the concentrations of 2-butanone in the blood and urine under various conditions of exposure.

Fundamentally, the concentration of organic solvents in alveolar air represents a diagnostically specific and sensitive way of objectively determining internal exposure. The determination of this parameter is, however, accompanied by a series of problems. Among these are the difficulties and intrusiveness of taking samples of expired air. The transport and storage of alveolar air samples can also lead to errors in the measured values.

The disadvantage of 3-hydroxy-2-butanone in the urine as a parameter for the estimation of an internal 2-butanone exposure is that this metabolite is only formed in relatively small amounts from 2-butanone. The diagnostic sensitivity of this parameter is therefore not sufficient for health surveillance when monitoring persons with low level exposure. 3-Hydroxy-2-butanone is also said to be taken up with a normal diet. 3-Hydroxy-2-butanone excretion in urine therefore does not necessarily show an external occupational exposure to 2-butanone, which limits the diagnostic specificity of this parameter.

4 Methodology

The determination of 2-butanone in urine can be carried out simply and reliably by means of gas chromatographic head-space analysis (16). In particular the use of a fused silica capillary column with a chemically bound phase allows this head-space procedure to be used extremely selectively (17, 18).

The working group "Analytische Chemie" ("Analytical Chemistry") of the DFG Commission for the Investigation of Health Hazards of Chemical Compounds in the Work Area has developed a capillary gas chromatographic head-space procedure that allows the aliphatic ketones used as industrial solvents to be determined in biological matrices in a single analytical procedure.

5 Evaluation of the BAT Value

The evaluation of a BAT value for the 2-butanone excretion in urine is possible via the relationship between external exposure, internal exposure and effect. The present MAK value is 200 ppm (19). Central nervous effects occur first with still higher ambient air concentrations of 300 ppm or more. After exposure to concentrations below 200 ppm (corresponding to 590 mg/m^3) so far no detrimental effects of 2-butanone on the health of the employees have been observed.

With ambient air concentrations which meet the requirements of present-day occupational hygiene a significant correlation has been found between the external 2-butanone exposure and the excretion of 2-butanone in urine. On the basis of this relationship a BAT value can be established for this parameter. Table 1 contains the conversion factors known from the literature for external and internal 2-butanone exposure. With ambient air concentrations of 200 ppm 2-butanone concentrations in urine between 2.1 mg/l (2) and 5.3 mg/l (16) are to be expected. For the evaluation of a BAT value valid for the individual it must be noted that these values represent average values for collectives exposed to an ambient air concentration at the level of the threshold limit values. The results of members of the Commission on various collectives exposed to 2-butanone (Tab. 1) confirm the results of Perbellini et al. (2). For the 2-butanone concentration in the urine a BAT value of

5 mg 2-butanone per litre urine

has therefore been set.

A BAT value for the 2-butanone concentration of blood can at present not be established. The data available so far are not sufficient. The evaluation of such a value would seem, however, to be desirable.

Table 1: Relationship between the external exposure to 2-butanone and the excretion in urine

Collective and occupation	2-Butanone in air mg/m^3 $\bar{x} \pm s$ (range)	2-Butanone in urine µg/l $\bar{x} \pm s$ (range)	x2-butanone(a)-y2-butanone(u)	Authors
a) Published data				
27; shoe factory	101 ± 67 (8–272)	487 ± 277 (120–1120)	y = 3.2x + 196*	Perbellini et al. 1984 (2)
34; various industries	(up to 1000)		y = 3.2x + 320*	Ghittori et al. 1987 (20)
62; ♂ printing workers	(up to 300)		y = 26.3x + 53**	Miyasaka et al. 1982 (16)
b) Investigations by Commission members (in shortened form published by Angerer et al. (18))				
10; ♂ mechanics without respirators	12.4 ± 5 (5–21)	177 ± 64 (89–247)		
9; ♂ paint sprayers with respirators	161 ± 34 (16–210)	1249 ± 1451 (304–1936)		
8; ♂ paint sprayers with respirators	85 ± 136 (16–422)	805 ± 609 (146–1682)		
9; ♂ paint sprayers with respirators	84 ± 157 (22–472)	441 ± 299 (146–978)		

* x in µg/l; ** x in ppm

6 Interpretation of the Data

The urine samples for the determination of the 2-butanone concentration should be collected at the end of exposure. Immediately after urine collection, aliquots, as a rule 2 ml, should be pipetted into head-space vials (20 ml) which should then be sealed immediately with a gas-tight Teflon-coated rubber stopper. If this portioning into gas-tight head-space vials does not take place immediately and if the urine is left standing for longer periods after sampling at room temperature then, due to evaporation of 2-butanone, losses are to be expected. The samples can be transported and stored in these head-space vials. According to data available today, three-day storage at room temperature does not lead to errors. Storage of the urine samples for longer periods should take place in the deep-freezer at –18 °C.

The 2-butanone concentration in urine should be stated and evaluated as mass per volume, i.e. in mg/l. Relation to creatinine is not appropriate (16). Apparently 2-butanone excretion follows other mechanisms than those for creatinine. According to data from the same authors a relation of the mass of the excreted creatinine to the specific weight has not proved useful. According to the general procedure of the Commission (see Occupational-Medical Toxicological Documentation of BAT Values, special foreword: a) Creatinine as a Parameter in the Evaluation of the Concentration of Substances in Urine) the 2-butanone concentration should only be determined if the urine being analysed has a specific weight >1.010.

As already mentioned 2-butanone potentiates the neurotoxic effects of 2-hexanone and *n*-hexane. If *n*-hexane, 2-hexanol or 2-hexanone occur at the workplace together with 2-butanone then the BAT value established here for 2-butanone does not apply. If in such cases neither 2-butanone nor *n*-hexane (or 2-hexanol/2-hexanone) can be replaced at the workplace then, for practical reasons, according to the literature references quoted in the above documentation it can be assumed that below 1/10 of the BAT value mentioned here, even under conditions of mixed exposure, no peripheral neurotoxic effects are to be expected.

7 References

1. Tada, O., Nakaaki, K., Fukabori, S.: Rodo Kagaky *48* (1972), 305–310
2. Perbellini, L., Brugnone, F., Mozzo, P., Cocheo, V., Caretta, D.: Int. Arch. Occup. Environ. Health *54* (1984), 73–81
3. DiVicenzo, G. D., Kaplan, C. J., Dedinas, J.: Toxicol. Appl. Pharmacol. *36* (1976), 511–522
4. Brugnone, F., Perbellini, E., Gaffuri, E., Apostoli, P.: Int. Arch. Occup. Environ. Health *47* (1980), 245–261
5. Shell Chemical Corp.: Ind. Hyg. Bull. Toxicity Data Sheet, Methyl ethyl ketone, SC 57–109, 1959, quoted in: Clayton, G. D., Clayton, F. E. (eds.): Patty's Industrial Hygiene and Toxicology, 2nd. rev. Vol 2C, Toxicology. Wiley & Sons, New York 1962
6. Nelson, K., Ege jr., J. F., Ross, M., Woodman, L. E., Silverman, L.: J. Ind. Hyg. Toxicol. *25* (1943), 282
7. Elkins, H. B.: The Chemistry of Industrial Toxicology, 2nd ed. Wiley & Sons, New York 1962
8. Smith, A. R., Mayers, M. R.: Ind. Bull. N. Y. State Dept. Labor *23* (1944), 174; quoted in: Clayton, G. D., Clayton, F. E. (eds.): Patty's Industrial Hygiene and Toxicology, 2nd rev. ed. Vol. 2C. Toxicology. Wiley & Sons, New York 1962, p. 1733
9. Spencer, P. S., Schaumburg, H. H., Raleigh, R. L., Terhaar, C. H.: Arch. Neurol. (Chic.) *32* (1975), 219
10. Billmaier, D., Yee, H. T., Allen, N., Craft, B., Williams, N., Epstein, S., Fontaine, R.: J. Occup. Med. *16* (1974), 665
11. Misumi, J., Nagano, M.: Br. J. Ind. Med. *42* (1985), 155–161
12. Takeuchi, Y., Ono, Y., Hisagana, N., Iwata, M., Aoyama, M., Kitoh, J., Sugiura, Y.: Br. J. Ind. Med. *40* (1983), 199–203
13. Iwata, M., Takeuchi, Y., Hisagana, N., Ono, Y.: Int. Arch. Occup. Environ. Health *53* (1983), 1–8
14. Iwata, M., Takeuchi, Y., Hisagana, N., Ono, Y.: Int. Arch. Occup. Environ. Health *54* (1984), 273–281
15. Dick, R. B., Setzer, J. V., Wait, R., Hayden, M. B., Taylor, B. J., Tolos, B., Putz-Anderson, V.: Int. Arch. Occup. Environ. Health *54* (1984), 91–109
16. Miyasaka, M., Kumai, M., Koizumi, A., Watanabe, T., Kurasako, R., Sato, K., Ikeda, M.: Int. Arch. Occup. Environ. Health *50* (1982), 131–137
17. Kassebart, V., Angerer, J., Heinrich, R., Behling, K., Lehnert, G.: Kombinierte Lösungsmittelexposition bei Lackierarbeiten. In: Bolt, H. M., Piekarski, C., Rutenfranz, J. (eds.): Verhandlungen der Deutschen Gesellschaft für Arbeitsmedizin e. V., 25. Jahrestagung in Dortmund 1985. Gentner Verlag, Stuttgart 1985, pp. 449–453
18. Angerer, J., Kassebart, V., Wolf, D., Behling, K., Lehnert, G.: Kombinierte Lösungsmittelexpositionen bei Beizarbeiten. In: Bolt, H. M., Piekarski, C., Rutenfranz, J. (eds.): Verhandlungen der Deutschen Gesellschaft für Arbeitsmedizin e. V., 25. Jahrestagung in Dortmund 1985. Gentner Verlag, Stuttgart 1985, pp. 461–465
19. Deutsche Forschungsgemeinschaft: Maximale Arbeitsplatzkonzentrationen und Biologische Arbeitsstofftoleranzwerte. Mitteilung XXVI der Senatskommission zur Prüfung gesundheitsschädlicher Arbeitsstoffe. VCH Verlagsgesellschaft, Weinheim 1990
20. Ghittori, S., Imbriani, M., Pezzagno, G., Capodaglio, E.: Am. Ind. Hyg. Assoc. *48* (1987), 786–790

Author: J. Angerer
Approved by the Working Group: 15th March 1988

2-Butoxyethanol

BAT	100 mg butoxyacetic acid/l urine Sampling time: with long-term exposure after several consecutive shifts
Date of evaluation	1994
CAS No.	111-76-2
Synonyms	*n*-Butoxyethanol Butyl Cellosolve® *O*-Butyl ethylene glycol Butyl glycol Ethylene glycol n-butyl ether Ethylene glycol monobutyl ether Glycol butyl ether Monobutyl glycol ether 3-Oxa-1-heptanol
Formula	$C_6H_{14}O_2$ $CH_2{-}OH$ | $CH_2{-}O{-}CH_2{-}CH_2{-}CH_2{-}CH_3$
Molecular weight	118.17
Melting point	–70.4 °C
Boiling point	171.2 °C
Vapour pressure at 20 °C	about 1 mbar
MAK [last established: 1984]	20 ml/m^3 (ppm) 100 mg/m^3

1 Pharmacokinetics

1.1 Absorption

2-Butoxyethanol (BE) and 2-butoxyethyl acetate (BEAc) are absorbed at the workplace via the respiratory passages and the skin. Absorption through the skin occurs both on direct skin contact with the glycol ethers (1, 2, 3, 41) and directly from the gas phase.

Essential BAT Value Documentations. DFG, Deutsche Forschungsgemeinschaft

ISBN 3-527-31477-6

This is shown in a study by Johanson *et al.* (28). The importance of dermal absorption has been confirmed in *in vitro* experiments which investigated the permeation of various glycol ethers through human skin (5, 9).

As Johanson *et al.* (26) were able to show under experimental exposure conditions, 57 % of the inhaled amount of 2-butoxyethanol is absorbed. In the partition of 2-butoxyethanol between blood and air, at equilibrium the substance is found entirely in the blood. Johanson *et al.* (26) give a value of about 8000 for the distribution coefficient of 2-butoxyethanol between blood and air. This distribution equilibrium has the effect that under workplace conditions a steady state can virtually never be reached. This also leads to the situation that after exposure only a negligible amount of the absorbed glycol ether is eliminated via the respiratory passages.

Johanson *et al.* have carried out studies on the percutaneous absorption of 2-butoxyethanol. After dipping several fingers in pure 2-butoxyethanol the rate of absorption was found to be between 0.05 and 0.68 mg/cm^2 per hour. *In vitro*, absorption rates of between 0.17 mg/cm^2 per hour (5) and 0.20 mg/cm^2 per hour (9) were determined. These values correlate well with the data determined *in vivo*. 2-Butoxyethanol is therefore absorbed through the intact skin in smaller amounts than its lower homologues. For 2-methoxyethanol and 2-ethoxyethanol the rate of dermal absorption is given as 2.8 and 0.8 mg/cm^2 per hour, respectively.

There are no data available on percutaneous absorption of 2-butoxyethyl acetate. In analogy to ethoxyethanol, whose acetate is absorbed through the skin to a similar degree as the corresponding glycol ether, it can be assumed that this also applies for 2-butoxyethyl acetate.

More recent studies (28) show that 2-butoxyethanol is absorbed through the skin directly from the vapour phase. Percutaneous absorption can make up 75 % of the total uptake of the hazardous substance.

1.2 Elimination

In the study by Johanson *et al.* (28) the concentration of the substance in blood reached a plateau of 7.4 µmol/l after experimental exposure to 20 ppm for two hours. After exposure the substance is eliminated unchanged from the blood with a half-time of about 40 minutes. The amount of 2-butoxyethanol eliminated unchanged in urine was below 0.3 % of the absorbed dose. The half-time with which the unchanged glycol ether is eliminated with the urine was about 1.4 hours. If 2-butoxyethanol is absorbed percutaneously, it is eliminated, according to Johanson *et al.*, with a half-time of only 34 minutes (28).

Butoxyacetic acid is eliminated with urine with a half-time of 5.8 hours (23). This value correlates with the data from Knecht and Woitowitz, who determined a half-time for the excretion of butoxyacetic acid of 6 hours (31).

This means that the elimination of butoxyacetic acid as the ultimate toxic metabolite of 2-butoxyethanol takes place much more rapidly than that of ethoxyacetic acid and methoxyacetic acid, the metabolites of the homologous glycol ethers, ethoxyethanol and methoxyethanol. Half-times for the elimination of ethoxyacetic acid and methoxyacetic acid are given in the literature with values between 30 and 50 hours, and between 70 and 80 hours, respectively, so that under workplace conditions accumulation of the toxic metabolites can occur. Accumulation need not be feared during excretion of butoxyacetic acid.

In their experimental study on the effects on man of exposure to 2-butoxyethanol, Johanson *et al.* (29) were able to show that butoxyacetic acid is also detectable in blood. Between 2.9 and 7.9 mg butoxyacetic acid per litre blood was detected in the blood samples of exposed persons after exposure for two hours to a 2-butoxyethanol concentration in air of 20 ppm. This concentration is lower by at least one power of ten than that observed in urine after corresponding exposure. This metabolite is eliminated from the blood with a mean half-time of about four to five hours. This value therefore corresponds with the half-time for elimination of butoxyacetic acid in urine.

1.3 Metabolism

Most of the 2-butoxyethanol taken up by the human body is metabolised (see Figure 1). By the action of alcohol dehydrogenase (ADH), the primary alcohol group of the glycol ether is oxidised to a carboxyl group. Up to 55 % of the butoxyacetic acid formed is, according to Johanson (23), eliminated with the urine in free form. According to data from Rettenmeier *et al.* (36) between 16 % and 64 % of the butoxyacetic acid formed in the human body is excreted in the form of a glutamine conjugate as *N*-butoxyacetylglutamine. These results were recently confirmed in studies by Sakai *et al.* (37). During simultaneous uptake of ethanol and 2-butoxyethanol competitive antagonism occurs, which causes metabolism of 2-butoxyethanol to the toxic metabolite, butoxyacetic acid, to be inhibited.

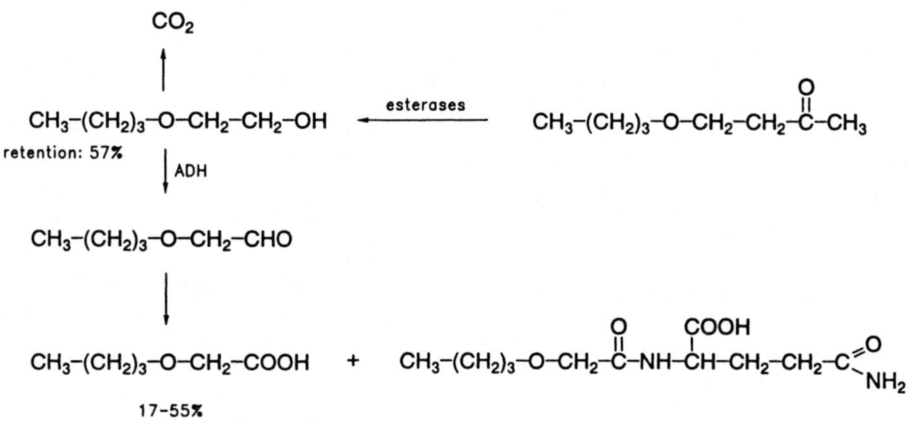

Fig. 1: Metabolism of 2-butoxyethanol and 2-butoxyethyl acetate

After absorption, 2-butoxyethyl acetate is rapidly and almost completely hydrolysed by the esterases in the mucous membranes of the nose, in blood, in the lungs, liver and kidneys (21, 42). The further metabolism of 2-butoxyethyl acetate is then identical to that of 2-butoxyethanol.

After acute intoxication, in addition to butoxyacetic acid, 2-butoxyethanol and oxalic acid were detected in urine in large amounts (35). Formation of oxalic acid was attributed to the increased hydrolysis of the ether bond, which occurs as a result of saturation of the oxidative route of degradation of 2-butoxyethanol.

Animal experiments have also shown metabolism of 2-butoxyethanol to be dose-dependent. In addition to butoxyacetic acid, ethylene glycol and both the glucuronide and sulphate of 2-butoxyethanol were found (13, 14, 17).

As demonstrated in animal experiments, part of the absorbed 2-butoxyethanol is oxidised to carbon dioxide and exhaled. After oral administration to rats of radioactively labelled 2-butoxyethanol in the drinking water, 50 % to 60 % of the radioactivity was recovered in the urine in the form of butoxyacetic acid, 8 % to 10 % was exhaled as CO_2 and 10 % of the dose was excreted in urine as ethylene glycol (33). The amount of the substance which is eliminated in the form of ethylene glycol and carbon dioxide decreases in the homologous series in the order methoxyethanol, ethoxyethanol and 2-butoxyethanol. The longer the chain length the larger the amount of alkoxyacetic acid eliminated in urine.

2 Critical Toxicity

The toxicological properties of 2-butoxyethanol and 2-butoxyethyl acetate are summarised in several monographs (7, 10, 22). In addition there are also a few recent studies available on the effects of 2-butoxyethanol and its metabolite, butoxyacetic acid. 2-Butoxyethanol mainly affects the haematopoietic system, followed by possible teratogenic and testicular effects. Effects on the central nervous system, the mucous membranes, and liver and kidneys have also been suggested.

After short-term exposure to concentrations between 100 and 200 ppm at the workplace or in experimental exposure systems, acute toxicity was observed on the mucous membranes of the eyes and nose and effects on the central nervous system. Long-term effects on the blood-forming system, on foetal tissue and on the germinative layer of the testes have only been described to date in animal experiments.

Animal experiments have shown for the glycol ethers derived from ethylene glycol that the toxic effects of the metabolites change systematically in the order 2-methoxyacetic acid, 2-ethoxyacetic acid and 2-butoxyacetic acid. Both the teratogenic and testicular effects decrease in this order. In animal experiments ten times higher doses of 2-butoxyethanol than of 2-methoxyethanol are necessary to achieve such effects. The differences in teratogenic and testicular effects between 2-butoxyethanol and the homologous 2-ethoxyethanol are smaller. While teratogenic effects are no longer observed with 2-butoxyethanol after exposure to 200 ppm, the corresponding threshold for 2-ethoxyethanol is 100 ppm. Toxic effects on the testes no longer occur with 2-butoxyethanol after doses of less than 500 mg/kg body weight, while the corresponding no observed effect level (NOEL) for 2-ethoxyethanol is considerably lower (< 100 mg/kg body weight).

With 2-butoxyethanol concentrations in air below 100 ppm, teratogenic effects were no longer observed. As embryotoxic effects only occur after maternally toxic effects have been observed, the Commission for the Investigation of Health Hazards of Chemical Compounds in the Work Area of the DFG has classified 2-butoxyethanol in group C with those substances for which there is no reason to fear a risk of damage to the developing embryo or foetus when MAK and BAT values are observed.

Unlike the teratogenic and testicular effects, the haematotoxic effects increase in the order 2-methoxyethanol to 2-butoxyethanol. In animal experiments a NOEL of 160 and 30 mg/kg body weight was found for 2-methoxyethanol and 2-butoxyethanol, respectively.

This means that under workplace conditions only haematotoxic effects are relevant. They are well documented in animal experiments (15, 16, 32). As shown in *in vivo* and *in vitro* studies (12, 15, 18), 2-butoxyacetic acid is the toxic agent.

The haemolytic effect of these glycol ether metabolites is considerably stronger than that of unchanged 2-butoxyethanol (5, 11). As shown in *in vitro* studies with erythrocytes, the rat seems to be the species most sensitive to the haemolytic effects of butoxyacetic acid. In order to produce haemolytic effects in human blood, butoxyacetic acid concentrations were necessary which were seven times the concentration necessary in rat blood (16).

Effects on the central nervous system and on the liver and kidneys were detected in animal experiments only after much higher doses than necessary to induce haemolytic effects (34).

After oral administration of up to 400 mg 2-butoxyethanol per kg body weight no immunosuppressive effects were observed in rats (40). These doses are higher by about a factor of 10 than those which induce haemolytic effects. Immunosuppressive effects need not be feared at concentrations found at the workplace.

This also applies for genotoxic effects. In an investigation with exposed persons, who absorbed among other things 2-butoxyethanol, no increase was observed in either the number of micronuclei or in the incidence of sister chromatid exchange (41).

3 Exposure and Effects

3.1 Relationship between External and Internal Exposure

There are numerous studies available in which external exposure to 2-butoxyethanol is compared with the resulting internal exposure. The concentration of 2-butoxyethanol and 2-butoxyethyl acetate in ambient air is used to deduce external exposure. The amount of free butoxyacetic acid excreted in urine is usually used as the parameter for internal exposure. In some cases the concentration of 2-butoxyethanol in blood or urine is also measured. The butoxyacetic acid concentration in blood was only evaluated in one study.

The studies available must be differentiated according to whether exposure was experimental or at the workplace (see Tables 1 and 2). The studies allow relationships between external and internal exposure to 2-butoxyethanol and 2-butoxyethyl acetate to be evaluated.

Only relatively low glycol ether concentrations were found at the various workplaces. The highest single value measured was 8 ppm (3), the highest mean value was 1.7 ppm (37). This means that even under very different workplace conditions the MAK value of 20 ppm is never reached. This is attributed to the low vapour pressure of glycol ether, which prevents larger amounts of the substance being released into the air at workplaces.

Exposure at the level of the MAK value was therefore only possible under experimental conditions (see Table 1). After mainly inhalation exposure to 20 ppm for two hours almost identical levels of butoxyacetic acid were measured in urine by Dornow *et al.* (8) and Johanson *et al.* (24) of on average 71 mg/g creatinine and 65 mg/l urine. If one assumes an exposure period of eight hours, then at the end of this period an average butoxyacetic acid concentration in urine of 285 mg/g creatinine or 260 mg/l would be expected.

If the level of butoxyacetic acid excreted after very low workplace exposure (see Table 2) is extrapolated to MAK value conditions, values are obtained which are also of this order of magnitude. This can be interpreted as an indication that for a wide concentration range there is a linear relationship between external and internal exposure.

These data are surprising in view of the fact that according to the literature considerable dermal absorption of the substance is to be expected. The considerable dermal absorption of 2-butoxyethanol from the gas phase observed by Johanson *et al.* (28) (about 75 %), obviously has the same effect at all workplaces and in all employees and also in experimentally exposed persons.

4 Selection of the Indicators

In the studies published to date (see Table 1) the following parameters are used to evaluate the internal exposure to 2-butoxyethanol and 2-butoxyethyl acetate and the effects.

- 2-butoxyethanol in blood,
- 2-butoxyacetic acid in blood,
- 2-butoxyacetic acid in urine (unbound),
- 2-butoxyacetic acid in urine (conjugated).

Tab. 1: Experimental exposure to 2-butoxyethanol (BE) and 2-butoxyethyl acetate (BEAc)

Collective	Substance (sampling)	Air BE or BEAc (ppm)	Urine BAA (mg/l) $\bar{x} \pm s$ (range)	BE	Blood BE (mg/l) $\bar{x} \pm s$ (range)	BAA	References
Inhalation 7 ♂ (2 hours, 50 weeks)	BE (exhaled air, blood, urine)	20	65 mg		0.80		Johanson *et al.* (24)
Inhalation 10 ♂ (2 hours) without EtOH	BE (with and without EtOH) Blood 4 hours after exposure Urine after exposure	20	71.3 ± 62 mg/g creat.	0.11 ± 0.07 mg/g creat.	0.320 ± 0.07 2.3 ± 0.54		Dornow *et al.* (8)
Dermal from air 4 ♂ (2× 2 hours at rest)	BE – only inhalation – only dermal	50			0.28 (0.21–0.32) 0.40 (0.33–0.47) 0.74 (0.21–1.16) 1.42 (1.18–1.53)		Johanson and Bowman (28)
Inhalation 5 ♂ (2 hours, 50 weeks)	BE (Blood 1.0 h 3.0 h 4.9 h 7.1 h after exposure)	20				2.88 (2.57–3.41) 5.83 (4.65–7.05 5.19 (2.44–7.46) 3.71 (1.90–6.39)	Johanson and Bowman (29)
Dermal 5 ♂ (12× 2 hours)	BE (urine 24 hours)		12.51 mg (1.1–41.3 mg)				Johanson *et al.* (25)

BE = 2-butoxyethanol, BEAc = 2-butoxyethyl acetate, BAA = butoxyacetic acid, EtOH = ethanol

Tab. 2: Ambient monitoring and biological monitoring of occupational exposure to 2-butoxyethanol and 2-butoxyethyl acetate. The data on excretion of butoxyacetic acid are for the non-conjugated form.

Collective (n)	Substance (sampling)	Air BE or BEAc (ppm)	Urine BAA (mg/l) $\bar{x} \pm s$ (range)	Blood BE (mg/l) $\bar{x} \pm s$ (range)	References
Printers (19 ♂)	MEAc, EEAc, BEAc (TWA, end of shift)	0.4 (< 0.1–1.5)	1.1 mg (0.5–3.8)		Johanson *et al.* (27)
Formulation of paints	EE, EEAc, BE (personal air monitoring, urine preshift and end of shift)				Angerer *et al.* (2)
Production (12 ♂)		1.1 (< 0.1–8.1)	10.5 (0.6–30.3)	121.3 (< 5.0–570.0)	
Storage (3 ♂)		< 0.1	4.5 (1.1–8.8)	49.4 (< 5.0–143.1)	
Laboratory (2 ♀)		< 0.1	4.2 (3.9–4.4)	< 0.5	
Formulation of paints (15 ♂, 4 ♀)	EE, EEAc, BE (Mon. urine beginning of shift, Tues. urine end of shift; personal air monitoring)				Söhnlein *et al.* (41)
	BE, Monday				
Production (12)		0.5 (< 0.1–1.4)	0.2 (< 0.02–1.3)		
Storage (2)		< 0.1 (0.05–0.12)	0.09		
Laboratory (4)		< 0.1 (< 0.02–0.12)	0.04		
Foreman (1)		< 0.1	< 0.02		
	BE, Tuesday				
Production (12)		0.6 (< 0.1–1.0)	16.4 (0.8–60.6)		
Storage (2)		< 0.1 (0.1–0.2)	0.9 (0.4–1.4)		
Laboratory (4)		< 0.1	1.6 (0.1–5.1)		
Foreman (1)		< 0.1	0.9		

Table 2: (continued)

Collective (n)	Substance (sampling)	Air BE or BEAc (ppm)	Urine BAA (mg/l) $\bar{x}$ ± s (range)	Blood BE (mg/l) $\bar{x}$ ± s (range)	References
			mg/g creatinine		Sakai *et al.* (37)
Control subjects (40)	BE, BEAc glycol ether		0.08 ± 0.14		
Solvent workers (70)	(urine end of shift)		(0.0–0.6)		
B (21)			0.67 ± 0.57 (0.0–2.0)		
C (19)			0.51 ± 0.32 (0.0–2.0)		
D (15)			0.12 ± 0.18 (0.0–1.5)		
E (6)			0.10 ±0.12 (0.0–0.8)		
F (9)		0.64 ± 0.14 (0.4–0.8)	3.92 ± 2.75 (1.3–9.9)		
Painters (6 ♂)	BE (urine Fri. end of shift, Mon. preshift)		194.28 (17.18–790.32)		Rettenmeier *et al.* (36)
Use of dispersion paints (5)	BE	0.84 ± 0.69	27.0 ± 15.4		Knecht *et al.* (31)
Ceramics industry (5 ♂)	BE	< 0.1	6.46 ± 5.52 (< 0.02–12.52)		Söhnlein *et al.* (41)
(19 ♂, ♀)		< 0.1	0.65 ± 0.87 (< 0.02–2.61)		

BE = 2-butoxyethanol
BEAc = 2-butoxyethyl acetate
BAA = butoxyacetic acid
MEAc = 2-methoxyethyl acetate
EE = 2-ethoxyethanol
EEAc = 2-ethoxyethyl acetate
TWA = time weighted average

Detection of the glycol ether in blood seems less suitable for biological monitoring. First of all, the unchanged substance is not responsible for the ultimate toxic effect and, secondly, the 2-butoxyethanol concentrations in blood under workplace conditions are only in the range of 1 µg/l (ppb). The analytical determinability and the diagnostic validity of this parameter both suffer as a result.

If the butoxyacetic acid concentration in blood is determined, not only is the ultimate toxic metabolite evaluated, but also the focus is on the actual target organ. However, there are also analytical reasons against using this parameter. The concentration of butoxyacetic acid in blood is about two powers of ten below that in urine (3). In addition, occupational-medical experience with this parameter is limited.

The concentration of butoxyacetic acid excreted in urine on the other hand has proved in numerous studies to be a reliable parameter for estimating internal exposure. The most important argument in favour of using this parameter for biological monitoring is that free 2-butoxyacetic acid is the ultimate toxic metabolite. Also the concentrations of butoxyacetic acid in urine occurring under workplace conditions are in the mg/l range and can therefore be reliably determined with the methods of instrumental analysis usual today.

Recent studies (36, 38) have shown that between 16 % and a maximum of 92 % of the total butoxyacetic acid excreted in urine occurs in the form of a conjugate, as *N*-butoxyacetylglutamine. The great fluctuations in the proportion of the substance excreted which appears as the conjugate mean that it makes sense to determine this conjugate in addition to free butoxyacetic acid.

These are the reasons for suggesting free butoxyacetic acid as a parameter for determining exposure to 2-butoxyethanol. In addition the database also recommends the choice of free butoxyacetic acid as a monitoring parameter. Only on the basis of relatively extensive occupational-medical experience in determining butoxyacetic acid excreted in urine can a BAT value be set at all.

Up until 1992 only the concentration of free butoxyacetic acid in urine was determined for monitoring persons exposed to 2-butoxyethanol and 2-butoxyethyl acetate.

It must be borne in mind that the amount excreted in the form of the glutamine conjugate seems to be quantitatively less important the higher the exposure level. This means that only with relatively low level external exposure to 2-butoxyethanol and 2-butoxyethyl acetate is the capacity of glutamine conjugation sufficient to detoxify the butoxyacetic acid. With increasing external 2-butoxyethanol concentrations which are of occupational-medical relevance, excretion of free butoxyacetic acid in urine becomes progressively more important.

Above all, however, it must be decided whether the concentration of free butoxyacetic acid in urine is of greater diagnostic importance than that of the total metabolites excreted. Free butoxyacetic acid, as the ultimate toxic agent, seems to be better suited for estimating the effects of exposure than its detoxification product, *N*-butoxyacetylglutamine.

Further investigations are necessary to clarify this question.

5 Methodology

In the literature a series of gas chromatographic methods are described for determining free butoxyacetic acid in urine (19, 20, 24, 27, 30, 39). These analytical procedures are unsatisfactory for various reasons. This applies in particular to shortcomings during sample preparation and during separation of butoxyacetic acid from the matrix. In some cases considerable loss of analytes occurs when using liquid/liquid extraction. Use of less suitable derivatisation aids, such as silylation, leads among other things to considerable interference.

The working group "Analytical Chemistry" has therefore selected (6), tested and published (4) a procedure in which butoxyacetic acid is separated from interfering urinary components and at the same time enriched using ion exchange and reversed-phase chromatography. After methylation of butoxyacetic acid, the derivative is separated by capillary gas chromatography and detected in a flame-ionisation detector. With this procedure it is possible to determine specifically, sensitively and exactly the butoxyacetic acid in urine in the whole exposure range relevant to occupational medicine. This procedure also has the advantage that it allows a series of further alkoxy carbonic acids in urine to be determined.

6 Evaluation of the BAT Value

According to the data published in the literature (see Tables 1 and 2) external exposure to 2-butoxyethanol and 2-butoxyethyl acetate at the level of the MAK value corresponds to a level of 2-butoxyacetic acid excreted in urine of 250 and 300 mg/l. Experimental and occupational exposure lead to comparable results (see Section 3).

It must be remembered that according to data from Johanson *et al.* (28), up to 75 % of the 2-butoxyethanol taken up is absorbed dermally directly from the gas phase. This also applies for exposure conditions on which the correlation between external and internal exposure is based (see Section 3). The risk evaluation on which the MAK value is based only considers, however, the dose taken up by inhalation. Therefore, in the above-mentioned evaluation for the excretion of butoxyacetic acid, the amount of the dose must be accounted for that is absorbed through the skin.

The effects resulting from external and internal exposure represent the most important parameters for the evaluation of a BAT value. The haemolytic effect on erythrocytes is the most important toxicological end point. In animal experiments (rat) a NOEL of 30 mg/kg body weight was found for butoxyacetic acid. An approximate calculation reveals that after purely inhalation exposure at the level of the MAK value, 14 mg 2-butoxyethanol per kg body weight is retained by an adult (70 kg body weight) (retention 57 %). This corresponds to about 19 mg butoxyacetic acid per kg body weight. This does not take into consideration simultaneous skin absorption. This means that under MAK value conditions, doses of the hazardous substance are to be expected at or above the level of the NOEL determined in animal experiments.

It seems that human erythrocytes are much more resistant than those of rats (5). On the other hand, these results were obtained in *in vitro* experiments and need to be confirmed *in vivo*. The fact that no haemolytic effects have been observed to date under workplace conditions is probably not least due to the fact that the 2-butoxyethanol concentrations occurring at the workplace are far below the MAK value.

Due to the experimentally determined haematotoxicity of butoxyacetic acid and the relationship deduced between external and internal exposure, and taking into account the high and variable skin absorption, a BAT value has been set of

100 mg butoxyacetic acid/l urine.

The sample should be taken at the end of several consecutive shifts. The creatinine level of the urine or its specific weight should also be determined.

7 References

1. Angerer, J., Begerow, J.: Untersuchungen zur äußeren und inneren Schadstoffbelastung bei berufsbedingter Glykolether-Exposition, Verh. D. Ges. Arb. Med., *29*. Jahrestagung, Gentner Verlag Stuttgart (1989), pp 339–344
2. Angerer, J., Lichterbeck, E., Begerow, J., Jekel, S., Lehnert, G.: Occupational chronic exposure to organic solvents XIII. Glycolether exposure during the production of varnishes, Int. Arch. Occup. Environ. Health *62* (1990), 123–126
3. Angerer, J., Rüdiger, H., Schaller, K.H., Söhnlein, B., Weltle, D., Lehnert, G.: Berufliche Glykoletherexposition – Untersuchungen zu genotoxischen Wirkungen und zur Evaluierung von BAT-Werten, Verh. D. Ges. Arb. Med., 31. Jahrestagung, Gentner Verlang Stuttgart (1991), pp 539–542
4. Angerer, J., Schaller, K.-H. (Eds.): Analyses of hazardous substances in biological materials, VHC Verlagsgesellschaft Weinheim (1994), Vol. 4
5. Bartnik, F.G., Reddy, A.K., Klecak, G., Zimmermann, V., Hostynek, J.J., Kunstler, K.: Percutaneous Absorption, Metabolism, and Hemolytic Activity of n-Butoxyethanol, Fundam. Appl. Toxicol. *8* (1987), 59–70
6. Begerow, J., Heinrich-Ramm, R., Angerer, J.: Determination of butoxyacetic acid in urine by capillary gas chromatography, Frensenius Z. Anal. Chem. *331* (1988), 818–820
7. Deutsche Forschungsgemeinschaft (D. Henschler, Ed.): Gesundheitsschädliche Arbeitsstoffe, toxikologisch-arbeitsmedizinische Begründung von MAK-Werten, VCH Verlag Chemie, Weinheim (1983 and 1984), 9th and 10th issue
8. Dornow, R., Knecht, U., Matulla, Ch., Woitowitz, H.-J.: Einfluß von Ethanol auf das Biomonitoring nach standardisierter Butyl-Glykol-Entwicklung, Verh. D. Ges. Arb. Med., 30. Jahrestagung, Gentner Verlag Stuttgart (1990), 273–277
9. Dugard, P.H., Walker, M., Mawdsley, S.J., Scott, R.C.: Absorption of some Glycol Ethers Through Human Skin in vitro, Environ. Health Perspect. *57* (1984), 193–197
10. ECETOC: Technical Report No. 17, The Toxicology of Glycol Ethers and its Relevance to Man: An Up-Dating of ECETOC Technical Report No. 4. (1985)
11. Foster, P.M.D., Lloyd, S.C., Blackburn, D.M.: Comparison of the in vivo and in vitro testicular effects produced by methoxy-, ethoxy- and n-butoxyacetic acid in the rat, Toxicology *43* (1987), 17–30
12. Ghanayem, B.J.,: Metabolic and Cellular Basis of 2-Butoxyethanol-induced Hemolytic Anemia in Rats and Assessment of Human Risk in vitro, Biochem. Pharmacol. *38/10* (1989), 1679–1684
13. Ghanayem, B.I., Blair, P.C., Thompson, M.B., Maronpot., R.R., Matthews, H.B.: Effect of Age on the Toxicity and Metabolism of Ethylene Glycol Monobutyl Ether (2-Butoxyethanol) in Rats, Toxicol. Appl. Pharamacol. *91* (1987), 222–234
14. Ghanayem, B.I., Burka, L.T., Sanders, J.M., Matthews, H.B.: Metabolism and Disposition of Ethylene Glycol Monobutyl Ether (2-Butoxyethanol) in Rats. Drug Metab. Dispis. *15/4* (1987), 478–484
15. Ghanayem, B.I., Burka, L.T., Matthews, H.B.: Metabolic basis of ethylene glycol monobutyl ether (2-butoxyethanol) toxicity: role of alcohol and aldehyde dehydrogenases. J. Pharmacol. Exp. Ther. *242* (1987), 222–231

16. Ghanayem, B.I., Burka, L.T., Matthews, H.B.: Structure-activity relationships for the in vitro hematotoxicity of n-alkoxyacetic acids, the toxic metabolites of glycol ethers, Chem. Biol. Interact. *70* (1989), 339–352
17. Ghanayem, B.I., Sanchez, I.M., Matthews, H.B.: Development of Tolerance to 2-Butoxyethanol Induced Hemolytic Anemia and Studies to Elucidate the Underlying Mechanisms, Toxicol. Appl. Pharamacol. (1992), 298–206
18. Ghanayem, B.I., Sullivan, C.A.: Assessment of the haemolytic activity of 2-butoxyethanol and its major metabolite, butoxyacetic acid, in various mammals including humans, Hum. Exp. Tocicol. *12/4* (1993), 305–311
19. Groseneken, D. van Vlem, E., Veulemans, H.: Gas chromatographic determination of methoxyacetic and ethoxyacetic acid in urine, Br. J. Ind. Med. *34* (1986), 62–65
20. Groseneken, D., van Vlem, H., Masschelein, R., van Vlem, E.: An improved method for the determination in urine of alkoxyacetic acids, Int. Arch. Occup. Environ. Health *61* (1989), 249–254
21. Guest, D., Hamilton, M. L., Deisinger, P.J., Di Vincenzo, G.: Pulmonary and Percutaneous Absorption of 2-Propoxyethyl Acetate and 2-Ethoxyethyl Acetate in Beagle Dogs, Environ. Health Perspect. *57* (1984), 177–183
22. Illing, H.P.A., Tinkler, J.J.B.: Glycol Ethers, Health and Safety Executive, Toxicity review *10* (1985)
23. Johanson, G.: Physiologically Based Pharmacokinetic Modelling of Inhaled 2-Butoxyethanol in Man, Toxicol. Lett. *34* (1986), 23–31
24. Johanson, G., Kronborg, H., Näslund, P.H., Byfält Nordqvist, M.: Toxicokinetics of inhaled 2-butoxyethanol (ethylene glycol monobutyl ether) in man, Scand. J. Work Environ. Health *12* (1986), 594–602
25. Johanson, G., Boman, A., Dynésius, B.: Percutaneous absorption of 2-butoxyethanol in man, Scand. J. Work Environ. Health *14* (1988), 101–109
26. Johanson, G., Dynésius, B.: Liquid/air partition coefficients of six commonly used glycol ethers, Br. J. Ind. Med. *45* (1988), 561–564
27. Johanson, G., Michel, I., Norbäck, D., Nise, G., Tillberg, A.: Biological Monitoring of Exposure to Ethylene Glycol Ethers, Arch. Toxicol., Suppl. *13* (1989), 108–111
28. Johanson, G., Boman, A.: Percutaneous absorption of 2-butoxyethanol vapour in human subjects, Br. J. Ind. Med. *48* (1991), 788–792
29. Johanson, G., Johanson, S.: Gas chromatographic determination of butoxyacetic acid in human blood after exposure to 2-butoxyethanol, Arch. Toxicol. *65* (1991), 433–435
30. Jönsson, A.K., Steen, G.: n-Butoxyacetic acid, a urinary metabolite from inhaled n-butoxyethanol (butylcellosolve), Acta Pharmacol. Toxicol. *42* (1978), 354–356
31. Knecht, U., Woitowitz, H.-J.: Glykol-Emissionen bei der handwerklichen Verarbeitung von Farben und Lacken, Verh. D. Ges. Arb. Med., 30. Jahrestagung, Gentner Verlag Stuttgart (1990), pp 317–320
32. Krasavage, W.J.: Subchronic Oral Toxicity of Ethylene Glycol Monobutyl Ether in Male Rats, Fundam. Appl. Toxicol. *6* (1986), 349–355
33. Medinsky, M.A., Singh, G., Bechtold, W.E., Bond, J.A., Sabourin, P.J., Birnbaum, L.S., Henderson, R.F.: Disposition of three Glycol Ethers Administered in Drinking Water to Male F344/N Rats, Toxicol. Appl. Pharmacol. *102* (1990), 443–445
34. National Institute for Occupational Safety and Health, (1990) Criteria for a recommended standard. Occupational exposure to ethylene glycol monobutyl ether and ethylene glycol monobutyl ether acetate, U.S. Department of Health and Human Services. Public Health Service. Center for Disease Control, Washington, D.C.
35. Rambourg-Schepens, M.O., Buffet, M., Bertault, R., Jaussaud, M., Journe, B., Fay, R., Lamiable, D.: Severe Ethylene Glycol Butyl Ether Poisoning. Kinetics and Metabolic Pattern, Human Toxicol. *7* (1988), 187–189
36. Rettenmeier, A.W., Hennigs, R., Wodarz, R.: Determination of butoxyacetic acid and N-butoxyacetylglutamine in urine of lacquerers exposed to 2-butoxyethanol, Int. Arch. Occup. Environ. Health *65* (1993), 151–153

37. Sakai, T., Araki, T., Masuyama, Y.: Determination of urinary alkoxyacetic acid by a rapid and simple method for biological monitoring of workers exposed to glycol ethers and their acetates, Int. Arch. Occup. Environ. Health *64* (1993), 495–498
38. Sakai, T., Araki, T., Moriata, Y., Masuyama, Y.: Gaschromatographic determination of butoxyacetic acid after hydrolysis of conjugated metabolites in urine from workers exposed to 2-butoxyethanol, Int. Arch. Occup. Environ. Health *66* (1994), 249–254
39. Smallwood, A.W., DeBoid, K.E., Lowry, L.K.: Analyses of Ethylene Glycol Monoalkyl Ethers and Their Proposed Metabolites in Blood and Urine, Environ. Health Perspect. *577* (1984), 249–253
40. Smialowicz, R.J., Williams, W.C., Riddle, M.M., Andrews, D.L., Luebke, R.W., Copeland, C.B.: Comparative Immunosuppression of Various Glycol Ethers Orally, Fundam. Appl. Toxicol. *18* (1992), 621–627
41. Söhnlein, B., Letzl, S., Weltle, D., Rüdiger, H.W., Angerer, J.: Occupational Chronic Exposure To Organic Solvents XIV. Examinations concerning the evaluation of a limit value for 2-ethoxyethanol and 2-ethoxyethyl acetate and the genotoxic effects of these glycol ethers, Int. Arch. Occup. Environ. Health *64* (1993), 479–484
42. Stott, W.T., McKenna, M.J.: Hydrolysis of Several Glycol Ether Acetates and Acrylate Esters by Nasal Mucosal Carboxylesterase in Vitro., Fundam. Appl. Toxicol. *5* (1985), 399–404

Author: J. Angerer
Approved by the Working Group: 23.11.1994

Cobalt

EKA	The correlation between external and internal exposure yields the following data:

Air (µg cobalt/m³)	Whole blood (µg cobalt/l)	Urine (µg cobalt/l)
50	2.5	30
100	5	60
500	25	300

Sampling: no restrictions; with short-term exposure after several shifts

Date of evaluation	1986
Substances	Cobalt metal Cobalt oxides Cobalt salts
MAK [last established: 1971]	Carcinogenic substance: Category III A 2 of the MAK and BAT Values List

1 Metabolism and Kinetics

There are a number of reviews on the uptake, distribution and excretion of cobalt in the human body (16, 34, 45, 55, 60).

According to these reviews the daily intake of cobalt by an adult with food ranges between 40 and 50 µg (27, 53). The body of an adult contains on average approx. 1 mg cobalt. Large amounts are found in the liver, kidneys, heart and muscles. The cobalt taken in with food is only absorbed to a small extent. Between 60 and 95 % are excreted with the faeces (61) the rest with the urine (47, 51). Recent studies indicate that the average cobalt concentration in the urine and also in the blood of normal persons is below 1 µg/l (8, 25).

Cobalt that has been taken in is eliminated from the body in several phases with differing half-lives. After an accidental oral intake of radioactive cobalt 60 successive half-lives of 0.5, 2.7 and 59 days were determined (43).

After inhalational intake, as it usually occurs at the workplace, the cobalt is deposited, depending upon the size of the dust particles, in the various regions of the bronchopulmonary system. From there it is quickly transferred into the blood and is bound to plasma proteins, above all to albumins and globulins (33, 44) and also to

Essential BAT Value Documentations. DFG, Deutsche Forschungsgemeinschaft

ISBN 3-527-31477-6

haemoglobin (56) or erythrocytes (39, 40). Also after inhalational uptake the cobalt is eliminated from the body in several phases, whereby one with a 5 – 10 year duration seems very long (46). With iron and steel workers exposed to cobalt, even after a three-week exposure-free period, considerably increased concentrations of this metal were still found in the blood and urine (17).

Cobalt is also a component of vitamin B_{12}. A deficiency of this vitamin results in macrocytic anaemia. Vitamin B_{12} is taken in above all with animal proteins whereby 3 µg of this vitamin per day is seen as sufficient.

2 Critical Toxicity and Exposure and Effects

There are some reviews which report on the effects on health of cobalt and its compounds (see section 1). With the prevention of occupational illnesses due to cobalt and its compounds in particular its potentially carcinogenic and mutagenic effects, as well as the action of this metal on the bronchopulmonary system, the sensitising effect and the effects on the heart and blood are of interest.

The DFG Commission for the Investigation of Health Hazards of Chemical Compounds in the Work Area has grouped cobalt in the form of inspirable dusts, aerosols of metallic cobalt, as well as practically insoluble cobalt salts in Category III A 2 of the carcinogenic substances which to date have only been shown to be carcinogenic in animal experiments. The Commission bases this classification on results in which rats were given cobalt and sparingly soluble cobalt compounds such as cobalt oxide and cobalt sulphide intramuscularly. With up to 50 % of the treated animals carcinomas occurred at the injection site (18, 20, 21). Inhaled cobalt was not able to produce any carcinomas, however, in animal experiments (65).

Although due to the wide industrial usage of cobalt and its compounds we know a lot about the effects of this metal on health, it has so far not been possible to prove a carcinogenic effect on humans. Recently a mortality study carried out on iron and steel workers exposed to cobalt did show considerable incidences of carcinoma, above all of the lungs and stomach, but these workers were also exposed to arsenic and nickel. Also the smoking of cigarettes could not be excluded as a confounding factor (64).

Similar problems are also encountered in the interpretation of other studies in which an increased cancer risk in cobalt reclaiming plants and nickel refineries is reported (quoted according to NIOSH (45)). These too were mixed exposures to cobalt with other metals such as arsenic and nickel, whose human carcinogenicity is regarded as proven.

A mutagenic effect of some cobalt compounds cannot be excluded. Thus cobalt proved to be an agent which inhibits cell division (11, 26). Cobalt chloride impairs DNA synthesis (58). Mutagenicity tests with *Escherichia coli* and Salmonella proved, however, to be negative (29, 63).

Pulmonary fibrosis after the chronic uptake of hard metal dusts containing cobalt has been recognised as an occupational disease for decades in the Federal Republic of Germany. This disease results in a decrease in the flexibility and elasticity of the lung as the result of a fibrotic change in the tissue which can be objectified radiologically. As a result of the hard metal pneumoconiosis one observes coughing, dyspnoea, restriction of the normal lung function, cor pulmonale etc. Although cobalt occurs at the workplace mostly in mixtures with other metals such as chromium and nickel or metal carbides such as tungsten carbide and titanium carbide one is inclined to the opinion today that the effects described above are mainly to be attributed to the cobalt (36, 62). On the one hand the uptake of these metals or their compounds does not lead to fibrotic changes in the lung (54), on the other hand the hard metal pneumoconiosis is also caused by other cobalt compounds (50).

With tool grinders it was shown that average cobalt concentrations in the air of the workplace between 0.1 and 0.2 mg/m^3 can cause pulmonary fibrosis (41). These results were confirmed over 20 years later (1975) in investigations by Lichtenstein et al. who found impairment of the lung function in hard metal grinders who were exposed to cobalt ambient air concentrations of an average of 0.18 mg/m^3. Swedish studies now indicate that ambient air concentrations of as little as 0.06 mg/m^3 on average can lead to obstructive changes in the lungs (1, 2). Also in animal experiments cobalt ambient air concentrations of 0.1 mg/m^3 lead after a very short time to a decrease in the flexibility of the lung (33). These results led in the USA to the announcement of the reduction of the TLV value of 0.1 to 0.05 mg/m^3 (3). The adherence to the former TLV value of 0.1 mg/m^3 already had the result that inflammations of the skin caused by sensitisation to cobalt no longer occurred.

Cobalt exposures at the levels at which they usually occur at workplaces seem fundamentally also capable of causing damage to the heart muscle. This cardiomyopathy, often with a fatal outcome, was first observed in beer drinkers. Cobalt salt had been added to the beverage to stabilise the foam production. The amounts of cobalt thus taken in came to at least 1.6 and at most 12 mg per day (45). Also with occupational cobalt exposure cardiomyopathy with a fatal outcome has been observed. Kennedy (32) reports such a case which occurred at a cobalt ambient air concentration which exceeded the TLV value of 0.1 mg/m^3. In the urine of this patient a cobalt concentration of 34 μg/l was measured. With hard metal grinders who were exposed to ambient air concentrations of 0.01 mg cobalt/m^3 changes in the electrocardiogram compared to that of a control group occurred. These changes proved, however, to be reversible.

The erythropoietic effects of cobalt were put to use in the treatment of anaemia which was not responsive to other treatment (15, 31). Also with occupational exposure to cobalt, depending on the metal concentration in the ambient air, both an increase in the number of erythrocytes and the haemoglobin content as well as their decrease have been observed (10, 30). There are also indications that cobalt increases the blood coagulation time (59). In 21 persons who were exposed to cobalt concentrations between 0.43 and 1.6 mg/m^3 at their workplaces there was an increase in the erythropoietin level compared to that of normal persons (35). With 35 workers exposed to cobalt increased amounts of immunoproteins and plasma proteins were found in the blood (12). Whether these changes constitute a disease must be left open here.

On taking into consideration the results mentioned above, it is evident that the Technical Exposure Limit (TRK value) of 0.5 mg cobalt/m^3 ambient air valid at the moment in the Federal Republic of Germany for areas of production of cobalt powder, catalysts, hard metals and magnets does not sufficiently guarantee the health of the employees. On the basis of the occupational medical experience available it cannot be excluded that workplace concentrations at this level lead to damage to the lungs and the heart muscle. Also allergic reactions of the lung and skin are to be expected with increased frequency with such concentrations. With the TRK value of 0.1 mg/m^3 valid for workplaces handling other cobalt compounds these risks should be minimal but cannot be completely excluded.

3 Selection of the Indicators

For the estimation of the internal exposure to cobalt and its compounds above all blood and urine seem to be suitable indicator materials.

The cobalt concentrations in the blood and urine show a clear relationship (1, 2, 7, 28). For routine monitoring examinations urine seems suitable. The determination of the cobalt concentration in the blood could then be reserved for confirmation of the findings obtained in the urine.

From the results of investigations of iron and steel workers it can be concluded that the level of the cobalt concentration in the blood and urine is independent of whether metallic cobalt or cobalt salts are handled at the workplace. Also the relation between the cobalt level in the blood and in the urine is apparently independent of the kind of cobalt compound used at the workplace (7). This concept is confirmed on the whole by similar results from the area of hard metal production and processing (1, 2, 28). A possible explanation for this phenomenon is that cobalt, even in metallic form, is quickly dissolved in protein solutions. After binding to plasma proteins, to leucocytes and to erythrocytes (39, 40) the cobalt can be quickly transported away from the place of deposit of the substance, the lung. The binding to these blood components is probably also responsible for the fact that there is a balance between the metal concentration in the blood and in the urine which has proven to be independent of the original form of the cobalt compound.

Serum does not seem to be a suitable indicator material to take the place of whole blood, as it has been observed that individually differing amounts of the cobalt are bound to plasma proteins and to haemoglobin (56). This realisation could on the other hand provide a reason to employ the cobalt content of the erythrocytes as a parameter for monitoring.

4 Methodology

For the determination of the cobalt concentrations in the blood which are increased due to an occupational exposure, the Working Group "Analysen in biologischem Material" ("Analyses of Hazardous Substances in Biological Materials") of the DFG Commission for the Investigation of Health Hazards of Chemical Compounds in the

Work Area has published a tested analytical procedure (5, 9). In this procedure the diluted blood is analysed directly by electrothermal atomic absorption spectrometry (ETAAS). A particularly gentle temperature programme which is suitable for avoiding cobalt losses is used for the mineralisation of the biological matrix. The procedure is characterised by its practicability and its analytical reliability (6). The accuracy was checked in all steps of the procedure with an independent inverse voltammetric method (23). It has been shown that the total cobalt content of the blood is determined independently of the type of cobalt compound. With procedures which allow a deproteinisation of the blood to precede the ETAAS determination, the cobalt concentrations found are systematically too low (24). An ETAAS procedure described by Delves (14) for the determination of cobalt in blood, in which oxygen supports the mineralisation of the biological matrix, seems less suitable for serial analyses as, due to the oxidative attack on the graphite tube, the sensitivity decreases drastically from injection to injection. Sufficiently stable measuring conditions are not provided by this procedure. Other methods are either not sensitive enough to ascertain the increased cobalt content of the blood due to an occupational exposure (38) or seem too troublesome to be used for routine monitoring examinations (37). The physiological cobalt levels of the blood, which amount to about 0.01 µg/l, cannot at present be determined by any of the atomic absorption spectrometric or inverse voltammetric methods described in the literature.

For the determination of cobalt in urine the Working Group "Analysen in biologischem Material" ("Analyses of Hazardous Substances in Biological Materials") of the DFG Commission for the Investigation of Health Hazards of Chemical Compounds in the Work Area has evaluated a sensitive, reliable and very practicable procedure (4). In this procedure the cobalt excreted in the urine is separated from interfering urinary components in a chelation/extraction step, whereby at the same time the metal is concentrated. Thus it is not only possible to determine cobalt concentrations in the urine in the physiological range but, moreover, to carry out the procedure very reliably. The determination of the cobalt in the organic phase is performed by electrothermal atomic absorption spectrometry (57).

5 Evaluation of the Biological Exposure Equivalents for Carcinogenic Substances (EKA)

5.1 Cobalt in Blood

Only the availability of a suitable method for the determination of cobalt in biological material has made it possible in recent years to ascertain the internal cobalt exposure of employees in many and various branches of industry. This is particularly true for the examination of the cobalt concentration in the blood. At present there are four studies available which allow the evaluation of a relationship between the cobalt concentration in the ambient air and the blood. The correspondence between three of these studies has proved to be so good that the results seem sufficient for the evaluation of a provisional relationship between the cobalt concentration in the ambient air and that of blood (1, 2, 7, 28) (c. f. Tab. 1 a/b and 2). The results indicate that an average ambient air concentration of 100 µg/m³ corresponds to a cobalt concentration in the blood between 4.6 and 6.3 µg/l.

Tab. 1 a: Relationships between the cobalt concentrations in the workplace air and in blood; details on the exposure and the group of persons as well as literature references in Tab. 2.

Cobalt Air (µg/m³)	Cobalt Blood (µg/l)	Comments	Study (Reference)
90	5.7	Mean values – ambient air concentration and blood	1
70–8610	2.16	Mean values – blood	2
50–250	0.63	Mean values – blood	3

Tab. 1 b: Correlations between the cobalt concentrations in the workplace air and in blood; details of the exposure and the collective as well as literature references in Tab. 2.

Regression equation $Co_{Blood} = a\ Co_{Air} + b$ Co_{Blood} (µg/l), Co_{Air} (µg/m³)	Correlation coefficient r	Comments	Study
$Co_{Blood} = 0.0425\ Co_{Air} + 0.478$	0.670	Ambient air concentrations (stationary monitoring) compared to blood level	4
$Co_{Blood} = 0.044\ Co_{Air} + 0.23$		Average ambient air concentration (personal air sampling) compared to average blood level	5

The investigations by Christiansen et al. (13) cannot be used for the setting up of such a relationship. For the ambient air concentration only one range is given which, in addition, spans two powers of ten and is thus too inexact to determine a relationship to the blood levels. On the other hand it is known that with the analysis procedure used by this working group, which is based on the deproteinisation of the blood, drastically too low cobalt concentrations are to be expected (24).

Tab. 2: Details on the exposure and the groups of persons in the studies listed in tables 1 a/b and 4 a/b.

Study	Exposure/Occupation	Number of persons examined	Sex	Literature reference
1	Hard metal processing	10	♂	1
2	Porcelain painters	46	♀	13
3	Porcelain painters	15	♀	13
4	Production of cobalt salts, powder, 7 work areas	48	♂	7
5	Hard metal processing, 10 work areas	170 5	♂ ♀	28
6	Hard metal processing	5	♂	1
7	Production of cobalt oxide, processing of cobalt salts	49	♂	42
8	Cobalt powder	6	–	48
9	Hard metal sintering	15	–	48
10	Hard metal processing	7	–	48
11	Hard metal production, 7 work areas	29	–	49
12	Hard metal grinders	153	–	19
13	Hard metal production	26	♂	52

From the studies available it can be concluded that the following values for the external and internal cobalt exposure correspond to each other (Tab. 3).

Tab. 3: Relationships between the cobalt concentration in the workplace air and in the blood

Air (µg Co/m^3)	Blood (µg Co/l)
50	2.5
100	5
500	25

In this evaluation the results by Ichikawa (28) were given greater weight than those of the other two studies, as they are based on the measurement of cobalt in the ambient air through personal air sampling.

5.2 Cobalt in Urine

Three of the studies (c. f. Tab. 4a/b and 2) on the relationship between the cobalt concentration in the ambient air and in urine come to the conclusion that a strict correlation exists between the two parameters (7, 28, 52). Considering the fact that metallic cobalt, cobalt in the form of hard metals and readily soluble cobalt salts were used at the workplaces investigated, the good concurrence of the results is surprising. This seems to indicate that the toxicokinetics of the uptake and excretion of the cobalt are to a large extent independent of its binding state. According to these studies a cobalt concentration of 100 µg/m³ in the ambient air leads to a cobalt excretion in the urine between 54 and 71 µg/l. The urine samples were taken after several days of cobalt exposure at the end of the work period.

Tab. 4a: Relationships between the cobalt concentrations in the workplace air and in urine; details on the exposure and the groups of persons as well as literature references in Tab. 2.

Cobalt Air (µg/m³)	Cobalt Urine (µg/l)	Comments	Study (Reference)
90	60.1	Mean values – cobalt concentration in ambient air and urine	6
520	340	Mean cobalt concentration in the air (personal air sampling) and in urine	7
675–10 000	35.1		8
120–280	9.6		9
180–190	11.7		10
300–15 000	4.6–64[1]		11
70–8 610	8.35[2]	Mean values – urine	2
50–250	0.13[2]	Mean values – urine	3
up to 61	18	Mean values – urine	12

[1] µg/g creatinine; [2] µg/mmol creatinine

Tab. 4b: Correlations between the cobalt concentrations in the workplace air and in urine; details on the exposure and the group of persons as well as literature references in Tab. 2.

Regression equation $Co_{Urine} = a\ Co_{Air} + b$ Co_{Urine} (µg/l), Co_{Air} (µg/m^3)	Correlation coefficient r	Comments	Study (Reference)
$Co_{Urine} = 0.34\ Co_{Air} + 19.9$	0.606	Mean air concentration (stationary monitoring) compared to cobalt concentrations in individual urine	4
$Co_{Urine} = 0.67\ Co_{Air} + 0.9$	0.99	Mean ambient air concentration (personal air sampling) compared to mean cobalt concentrations in urine	5
$Co_{Urine} = 0.29\ Co_{Air} + 0.8$	0.83	Ambient air concentrations (personal air sampling) compared to mean cobalt concentrations in individual urine (Monday)	13
$Co_{Urine} = 0.70\ Co_{Air} + 0.7$	0.81	Ambient air concentrations averaged over the working week (personal air sampling) compared to mean cobalt concentrations in individual urine (Friday)	6

A considerably lower value of approx. 30 µg/l was gained by Scansetti in the comparison between the workplace concentration and the urine samples (52). The sampling took place here at the end of the first day of a working week (52).

Furthermore, these results have been fully confirmed by other studies. A correlation between the external and internal exposure for the concentration range under discussion here is not to be found in these studies, yet the values measured seem so well-founded that an extrapolation to other exposure conditions seems justifiable (1, 2, 42). Also the results reported by Hartung correspond with those described here in their order of magnitude (19). Some further studies do exist but are not usable for the setting up of a relationship between the external cobalt exposure and the excretion of this metal in the urine as they only report the range of the ambient air concentrations measured which varies between extremely wide limits of two powers of ten (13, 48, 49). Also the peak values measured in these studies of 9 and 15 mg/m^3, respectively, do not seem to reflect the external exposure representatively as they correspond to relatively low cobalt concentrations of 64 µg/g creatinine in the urine. A low urine excretion with a high ambient air concentration would mean that there would be a considerable accumulation of cobalt in the body during occupational exposure. This is, however, not supported by what we know of the toxicokinetics.

From the studies discussed it can be concluded that the following values of the external and internal cobalt exposure correspond to one another (c.f. Tab. 5).

Tab. 5: Relationships between the cobalt concentrations in the workplace air and in the urine.

Air (mg Co/m³)	Urine (µg Co/l)
50	30
100	60
500	300

In this relationship those studies in which the ambient air concentrations were measured by personal air sampling have been given more weight (28, 42, 52) than those in which the sampling took place through stationary monitoring (7). That the urine excretion increases linearly with the external exposure is above all supported by the results reported by Morgan, which were measured at an ambient air concentration of around 500 µg/m³ (42).

6 Interpretation of the Data

Taking into consideration the kinetic relationships presented in section 1, the sampling should take place after at least three consecutive work shifts at the end of the work period. Particular attention is drawn to the possibility of contamination during urine sampling.

7 References

1. Alexandersson, R., Lidums, V.: Arbeite och Hälsa *8* (1979), 1–23
2. Alexandersson, R., Swensson, A.: Arh. hig. rada. toksikol. *30* (1979), 355–361
3. American Conference of Governmental Industrial Hygienists: Threshold Limit Values and Biological Exposure Indices for 1985–86. Cincinatti, 1985
4. Angerer, J.: Cobalt. In: D. Henschler (ed.) Analytische Methoden zur Prüfung gesundheitsschädlicher Arbeitsstoffe. Bd. 2: Analysen in biologischem Material. 7. Lfg., VCH Verlagsgesellschaft, Weinheim 1983
5. Angerer, J.: Cobalt. In: D. Henschler (ed.) Analytische Methoden zur Prüfung gesundheitsschädlicher Arbeitsstoffe. Bd. 2: Analysen in biologischem Material. 9. Lfg. VCH Verlagsgesellschaft, Weinheim 1988
6. Angerer, J., Heinrich, R.: Fresenius Z. Anal. Chem. *318* (1984), 37–40
7. Angerer, J., Heinrich, R., Felixberger, F. X., Szadkowski, D., Lehnert, G. in: Verhandlungen der Deutschen Gesellschaft für Arbeitsmedizin. 24. Jahrestagung. Gentner, Stuttgart 1984, pp. 293–296
8. Angerer, J., Heinrich, R., Szadkowski, D., Lehnert, G. in: T. D. Lekkas (ed.) Heavy Metals in the Environment. Vol. 2. CEP Consultants, Edinburgh 1985, pp. 11–13
9. Henschler, D. (ed.) Analyses of Hazardous Substances in Biological Materials. Vol. 2. VCH Verlagsgesellschaft, Weinheim 1988
10. Barborik, M.: Prac. Mk. *19* (1967), 11
11. Bearden, L. J., Cooke, F. W.: J. Biomed. Mat. Res. *14* (1980), 289–309
12. Bencko, V., Wagner, V., Wagnerova, W., Reichertova, R.: J. Hyg. Epidem. Microbiol. Immunol. *27* (1983), 387–394

13. Christensen, J. M., Mikkelsen, S. in: T. D. Lekkas (ed.) Heavy Metals in the Environment. Vol. 2. CEP Consultants, Edinburgh 1985, pp. 86 ff.
14. Delves, H. T., Mensikov, R., Hinks, L. in: Trace Element – Analytical Chemistry in Medicine and Biology. Vol. 2. Walter de Gruyter, Berlin 1983, pp. 1123 ff.
15. Edwards, M. S., Curtis, J. R.: Lancet *I* (1971), 582–583
16. Elinder, C. G., Friberg, L. in: L. Friberg, G. F. Nordberg, V. B. Voux (eds.) Handbook on the Toxicology of Metals. Elsevier, Amsterdam 1979, pp. 399–419
17. Felixberger, F. X., Szadkowski, D., Angerer, J., Ziemsen, B., Lehnert, G. in: Verhandlungen der Deutschen Gesellschaft für Arbeitsmedizin. 24. Jahrestagung. Gentner, Stuttgart 1984, p. 297–300
18. Gilman, J. P. W.: Cancer Res. *22* (1962), 158
19. Hartung, M., Schaller, K. H. in: Verhandlungen der Deutschen Gesellschaft für Arbeitsmedizin. 25. Jahrestagung. Gentner, Stuttgart 1985, pp. 55–63
20. Heath, J. C.: Br. J. Cancer *10* (1956), 668–673
21. Heath, J. C.: Br. J. Cancer *14* (1960), 478
22. Heath, J. C., Webb, M., Caffrey, M.: Br. J. Cancer *23* (1969), 153
23. Heinrich, R., Angerer, J.: Int. J. Environ. Anal. Chem. *16* (1984), 305–314
24. Heinrich, R., Angerer, J.: Fresenius Z. Anal. Chem. *322* (1985), 772–774
25. Heinrich, R., Angerer, J. in: B. Welz (ed.) Fortschritte in der atomabsorptionsspektrometischen Spurenanalytik. Bd. 2. VCH Verlagsgesellschaft, Weinheim 1986, pp. 159–170
26. Herich, R.: Chromosoma *17* (1965), 11
27. Hubbard, D. M., Creech, F. M., Cholak, J.: Arch. Environ. Health *13* (1966), 190
28. Ichikawa, Y., Kusaka, Y., Goto, S.: Int. Arch. Occup. Environ. Health *55* (1985), 269–276
29. Kanematsu, N., Hara, M., Kada, T.: Mutat. Res. *77* (1980), 109
30. Kaplun, Z. S.: Tsvetn. Met. *30* (1957), 42
31. Kato, K.: J. Pediat. *11* (1937), 385
32. Kennedy, A., Dornan, J. D., King, R.: Lancet *I* (1981), 412–414
33. Kerfoot, E. J., Fredrich, W. G., Domeier, E.: Am. Ind. Hyg. Assoc. J. *36* (1975), 17–25
34. Kipling, M. D. in: H. A. Waldron (ed.) Metals in the Environment. Academic, New York 1980, pp. 133–153
35. Klucik, J., Palkovico, M.: Bratisl. Lek. Listy *60* (1973), 445
36. Lahaye, D., Demedts, M., von den Oever, R., Roosels, D.: Lancet *I* (1984), 156–157
37. Lidums, V. V.: Atom Absorpt. Newsl. *18* (1979), 71–72
38. Maessen, F. J. M. J., Posma, F. D., Balke, J.: Anal. Chem. *46* (1974), 1445–1449
39. Merrit, K., Brown, S. A., Sharkey, N. A.: J. Biomed. Mat. Res. *18* (1984), 991–1004
40. Merrit, K., Brown, S. A., Sharkey, N. A.: J. Biomed. Mat. Res. *18* (1984), 1005–1015
41. Miller, C. W., Davis, M. W., Goldman, A., Wyatt, J. P.: Arch. Ind. Hyg. Occup. Med. *8* (1953), 453
42. Morgan, L. G.: J. Soc. Occup. Med. *33* (1983), 181–186
43. Morsy, S. M., El-Assaly, F. M.: Health Phys. *19* (1970), 769
44. Nandetkar, A. K. N., Basu, P. K., Friedberg, F.: Bioinorg. Chem. *2* (1972), 149–157
45. National Institute for Occupational Safety and Health: Occupational Hazard Assessment, Criteria for Controlling Occupational Exposure to Cobalt (82–107). NIOSH, Cincinnati 1981
46. Newton, D., Rundo, J.: Health Phys. *21* (1970), 377
47. Paley, K. R., Sussman, E. S.: Metab. Clin. Exp. *12* (1963), 975
48. Pellet, F., Perdrix, A., Vincent, M., Mallion, J.-M.: Arch. Mal. Prof. *45* (1984), 81–85
49. Posma, F. D., Dijstelberger, S. K. in: T. D. Lekkas (ed.) Heavy Metals in the Environment. CEP Consultants, Edinburgh 1985, pp. 89–91
50. Reinl, W., Schnellbäcker, F., Rahm, G.: Zbl. Arbeitsmed. Arbeitsschutz Prophyl. *29* (1979), 318–325
51. Ripak, E. N.: Vop. Pitan. *20* (1961), 19
52. Scansetti, G., Lamon, S., Talarico, S., Botta, C., Spinelli, P., Sulotto, F., Fantoni, F.: Int. Arch. Occup. Environ. Health *57* (1985), 19–26
53. Schelenz, R.: J. Radioanal. Chem. *37* (1977), 539–548
54. Scherrer, M., Maillard, J.-M.: Schweiz. med. Wschr. *112* (1982), 198–207
55. Sahrauzer, G. N. in: E. Merian (ed.) Metalle in der Umwelt. VCH Verlagsgesellschaft, Weinheim 1984, p. 425–433
56. Schumacher-Wittkopf, E.: Toxicol. Environm. Chem. *8* (1984), 1–9
57. Schumacher-Wittkopf, E., Angerer, J.: Int. Arch. Occup. Environ. Health *49* (1981), 77–81

58. Sirover, M. A., Loeb, L. A.: Science *194* (1976), 1434–1436
59. Smith, A. G, Smith, A. N.: Toxicol. Letters *23* (1984), 349–352
60. Smith, I. C., Carson, B. L.: Trace Metals in the Environment. Vol. 6. Ann Arbor Science, Ann Arbor 1981
61. Smith, T., Edmonds, C. J., Barnaby, C. F.: Health Phys. *22* (1972), 359
62. Sprince, N. L., Chamberlin, R. J., Hales, C. A., Weber, A. L., Kazemi, H.: Chest *86* (1984), 549
63. Tso, W.-W., Fung, W.-P.: Toxicol. Letters *8* (1981), 195–200
64. Wegner, R., Szadkowski, D., Lehnert, G. in: Verhandlungen der Deutschen Gesellschaft für Abeitsmedizin. 25. Jahrestagung. Gentner, Stuttgart 1985, pp. 113–118
65. Wehner, A. P., Bush, R. H., Olson, R. J., Craig, D. U.: Am. Ind. Hyg. Assoc. J. *38* (1977), 338–346

Author: J. Angerer
Approved by the Working Group: 21st February 1986

Cresols (all isomers)

BLW	200 mg total cresol/l urine Sampling time: end of exposure or end of shift	
Date of evaluation	2003	

Chemical name	Synonyms	CAS No.
Isomer mixture		
Methylphenol	Hydroxytoluene	1319-77-3
Individual isomers		
2-Methylphenol	*o*-Cresol, *o*-cresylic acid, 1-hydroxy-2-methylbenzene, 2-hydroxytoluene	95-48-7
3-Methylphenol	*m*-Cresol, *m*-cresylic acid, 1-hydroxy-3-methylbenzene, 3-hydroxytoluene	108-39-4
4-Methylphenol	*p*-Cresol, *p*-cresylic acid, 1-hydroxy-4-methylbenzenel, 4-hydroxytoluene	106-44-5

Formula C_7H_8O

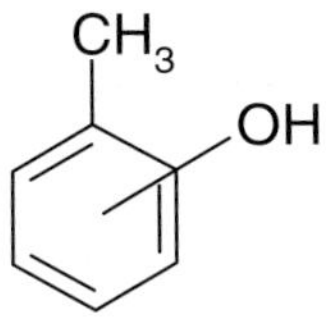

Molecular weight	108.14
Melting point	11.5–34.8°C
Boiling point	191–202.2°C
Vapour pressure at 25°C	0.15–0.39 hPa
Density at 20°C	1.02–1.03 g/cm^3
Odour threshold	0.0012–22 mg/m^3
MAK [last established: 2000]	Carcinogen category 3A

Cresols are colourless to yellowy, oily, poorly water-soluble liquids or crystals with a pungent, tar-like smell, which are of low volatility, are hardly inflammable and burn to produce large amounts of soot. The vapour is much heavier than air. Cresol–air mixtures may explode at high temperatures.

Essential BAT Value Documentations. DFG, Deutsche Forschungsgemeinschaft

ISBN 3-527-31477-6

The isomeric cresols are starting materials for the production of plastics, tanning agents, dyes, disinfectants and perfumes, insecticides and herbicides. In addition, they are used for the production of cresol resins, of solvents for wire coatings, for the production of phosphoric acid esters, hydraulic fluids and of cresyl compounds (ATSDR 1992, Calabrese 1986, Deichmann and Keplinger 1981, Greim 2000a, WHO 1995).

1 Metabolism and Kinetics

1.1 Absorption and distribution

The isomeric cresols are absorbed mainly via the skin and respiratory tract (ATSDR 1992). In analogy to phenol, high levels of absorption are to be expected. As a result of the low volatility and intensive odour (warning signal) of the substance, the danger of acute intoxication from inhalation is, however, small under normal circumstances.

As a result of rapid local anaesthesia and the lack of pain as a warning signal, skin contact often remains unnoticed. Absorption of acutely toxic doses of the substance can therefore take place, and even of lethal doses if large areas of skin are wetted; this is regarded as the main source of danger when handling the substance occupationally (ATSDR 1992).

After ingestion, the substance is quickly absorbed in the gastrointestinal tract, leading rapidly to systemic effects (ACGIH 2001, ATSDR 1992, Deichmann and Keplinger 1981).

1.2 Metabolism and elimination

Percutaneously absorbed and inhaled cresol is rapidly detoxified, mainly by conjugation (sulfate, glucuronide), and excreted by the kidneys. In general, no free cresol can be detected in plasma, even after acute intoxication. Depending on their hydrolysis by intestinal bacteria, conjugates eliminated in the bile enter enterohepatic circulation (ATSDR 1992, Deichmann and Keplinger 1981).

According to the results of animal experiments, for *p*-cresol there is another metabolic pathway that leads via the oxidation of the methyl group to the formation of *p*-hydroxybenzoic acid. A reactive quinone-methide intermediate is formed, which can be bound to glutathione or macromolecules. Such compounds, which are known from the metabolism of benzene (see the chapter on "Phenol" in Volume 1 of this series; Henschler and Lehnert 1994), have been detected to date only for *p*-cresol (DECOS 1998, Thompson *et al.* 1996).

For the other cresol isomers, the extent of ring hydroxylation resulting from the formation of dihydroxytoluenes seems to be small (Deichmann and Keplinger 1981).

Some of the *p*-cresol detected in the urine and faeces is formed during the bacterial breakdown of amino acids in the intestine. Furthermore, all cresol isomers are formed as metabolites of toluene (Greim 2000a, Nise 1992, Sherwood and Carter 1970).

2 Critical Toxicity

2.1 Acute toxicity

The slight differences in the toxicity of the cresol isomers (*p* > *o* > *m*-cresol) are, from a practical point of view, negligible. Their effects, also as a mixture of isomers, are similar to those of phenol; the local effects on the skin and mucous membranes are, however, slightly less pronounced (ATSDR 1992, Greim 2000a).

After direct contact of the eyes with the substance there is the danger of severe damage to the eyes, and even of blindness. Undiluted cresol caused clouding and vascularization in the rabbit eye (ATSDR 1992).

The cresols and their concentrated solutions are caustic to the skin, and if they penetrate deeply also cause damage to the vessels. First of all a burning sensation is felt, which rapidly develops into a local loss of feeling. Finally, white to dark-coloured tissue damage can occur, and even gangrene (ATSDR 1992, Moeschlin 1972).

Diluted solutions cause reddening of the skin and the formation of blisters. In hypersensitive persons inflammation of the skin was induced by solutions with cresol concentrations as low as < 0.1 % (Moeschlin 1972).

The vapour given off when cresol is heated has irritative effects on the respiratory tract, can damage the lungs and can lead, usually with a delay, to pulmonary oedema.

Ingestion of cresol causes painful local effects in the mucous membranes affected; whitish slough is formed, the person has difficulty in swallowing, sometimes oedema of the glottis develops, and nausea and stomach ache are reported. As a result of the local paralysis of the sensitive nerves of the stomach, vomiting is usually not observed even after acute intoxication with cresol (Moeschlin 1972).

The main acute systemic effects, especially after contact with the substance of large areas of skin or ingestion of more than 1 g cresol, are a rapid impairment of the central nervous and cardio-vascular systems. The uptake of more than about 10 g cresol is generally lethal (ATSDR 1992, WHO 1995).

The symptoms observed during the generally slow course of intoxication are: headaches, dizziness, usually a slower pulse and a drop in blood pressure, tinnitus, visual disorders, breathing difficulties, muscle weakness, and sometimes convulsions and impaired consciousness, often leading to unconsciousness. Damage to the blood cells and kidneys has been observed, including the formation of Heinz bodies, methaemoglobinaemia, haemolysis, haematuria, proteinuria, oliguria and sometimes also anuria. The haematological effects were observed mainly in persons with deficient glucose-6-phosphate dehydrogenase (G-6-PDH) activity (Chan *et al.* 1971, Moeschlin 1972, Roots *et al.* 1992).

After some time, further complications, such as bronchopneumonia, damage to the pancreas and liver, and strictures of the oesophagus and intestine can develop. A rapid course of intoxication is possible after the uptake of high doses. Usually a severe state of collapse is observed, which can lead to death as a result of respiratory arrest, sometimes after 10 to 60 minutes, but also immediately (ATSDR 1992, Moeschlin 1972).

As a result of a polymorphism of the isoenzymes of UDP-glucuronosyl transferase (UDPG), around 6 % of Central Europeans can glucuronidize only slowly (see the documentation on "Phenol" in this series; Henschler and Lehnert 1994). In some rare cases this defect is amplified by the lack of phosphoadenosine-phosphosulfate (PAPS) sulfotransferase responsible for sulfation. In these persons, in particular accidental exposure to phenol or cresols generally leads to the increased formation of free phenol and cresols, which can cause massive impairments in kidney function and even acute kidney failure (ATSDR 1992, Calabrese 1986, Lewalter and Neumann 1998, Lewalter *et al.* 1993).

These adverse effects have been extensively investigated in the case of phenol (see the documentation on "Phenol" in this series; Henschler and Lehnert 1994), but there are only case reports available for the cresols.

After the accidental exposure to *m*-cresol of a UDPG-deficient worker, the data for exposure and effects shown in Table 1 were determined during monitoring of the course of intoxication.

Table 1. Case report of intoxication with *m*-cresol of a UDPG-deficient worker (Lewalter, personal communication to the Commission)

Time period after the accident	Urine		Serum
	Free *m*-cresol [μg/l urine]	Total *m*-cresol [mg/l urine]	Creatinine [mg/dl serum]
1 hour	120	226	1.0
12 hours	70	99	2.2
24 hours	30	34	5.0
72 hours	10	6	2.5
3 months (occupational-medical check-up)	< 1.0	0.001	1.0

The slow increase in serum creatinine after acute intoxication with cresol is unusual.

2.2 Chronic toxicity

As seen in man and experimental animals, long-term exposure to cresols affects the same organs which are damaged after short-term exposure, in particular the liver.

In persons who inhaled the substance, headaches, nausea, vomiting, increased blood pressure, renal functional disorders, marked tremor and irritation of the upper airways were observed (ATSDR 1992, Deichmann and Keplinger 1981, Moeschlin 1972). A biochemical change described is the disturbance of the blood–calcium homeostasis. Other possible symptoms are difficulties in swallowing, the increased formation of saliva, diarrhoea, dizziness and impaired consciousness. The prognosis in particular after severe damage to the liver and kidneys is bad; in some cases this can even lead to death.

Cresols can cause discoloration and, in toxic doses, inflammation of the skin.

The genotoxicity studies which have been carried out with the individual cresol isomers *in vivo* have not yielded any evidence of genotoxic effects. A suggestion that the substances could have genotoxic effects in mammalian cells may be deduced from the positive results of some *in vitro* studies, but the relevance of these studies is not always clear (Greim 2000a). It is known that *p*-cresol is converted metabolically to a reactive derivative with a quinoid structure; for *o*-cresol such activation is also theoretically possible. *m*-Cresol, which cannot be activated metabolically in this way, yielded negative results in all genotoxicity studies. The results are thus largely consistent and compatible with a weak genotoxic effect, especially of *p*-cresol (Greim 2000a).

In initiation-promotion studies the cresol isomers reveal a promoting effect like that of phenol. As there is evidence of promoting effects which are independent of the skin irritation, in 1999 the cresol isomers were classified in Carcinogen category 3 Section III of the *List of MAK and BAT Values* (Greim 2000a). In 2000 they were reclassified in the new category 3A (Greim 2000b).

3 Exposure and Effects

3.1 Relationship between external and internal exposure

In the case of the cresol isomers external exposure is any kind of exposure that can lead to inhalation or percutaneous absorption of the substance.

In occupational-medical practice, the excretion of cresols after contact with the substance is often evaluated on the basis of so-called "empirical values" (Lewalter and Neumann 1998). The relationships listed in Table 2 between the external and internal exposure to total cresols are thereby observed (Lewalter, personal communication to the Commission). In the meantime these correlations have been supplemented for the low dose range by a study with coking plant workers (Bieniek 1997).

3.2 Relationship between internal exposure and effects

The internal exposure is the biologically relevant concentration of the cresols above all in the liver and kidneys. Like with phenol, also after increasing exposure to cresols an increase is observed in the free cresols in urine, which in UDPG-deficient workers can be diagnosed even after markedly lower cresol levels (Table 1) (see also the documentation on "Phenol" in this series; Henschler and Lehnert 1994).

The exposure parameters are the concentrations of total cresols and free cresols in body fluids, such as blood and urine, under the specific pharmacokinetic conditions.

Table 2. Data for the relationship between external and internal exposure after occupational contact with cresols

Number of persons [N]	Air Total cresols (mean shift values) [ml/m³]	[mg/m³]	Urine Total cresols [mg/l urine]	References
75	0.05	0.22	19	Bieniek 1997
520	0.91	4	68 (36–103)	Lewalter[1]
340	1.59	7	140 (114–186)	Lewalter[1]
80	2.74	12	250 (201–264)	Lewalter[1]
35	3.41	15	280 (250–315)	Lewalter[1]
./.	5.00	22	450*	

* extrapolation
[1] personal communication to the Commission

Despite extensive case reports of occupational exposure to cresols and studies with significant correlations between the external exposure to cresols and the excretion of cresols in urine, there are to date no studies of the quantitative relationship between exposure to cresols and effect parameters. In view of what is known from exposure to phenol and intoxication with cresols (see Table 1), it can, however, be assumed that the systemic toxic effects of cresol are caused by free cresols (Lewalter and Neumann 1998).

Acute intoxication with cresols, like intoxication with phenol, in some cases caused significantly increased serum creatinine values (see Table 1).

Comparison of the results of the biological monitoring of persons with acute intoxication with cresols showed that even after intensive decontamination of the skin, the serum creatinine level can increase significantly above the normal value of 1.0 (0.55–1.1) mg/dl when, with total cresol levels excreted in the urine of up to 200 mg/l, the proportion of free cresols detected in the urine exceeds a "threshold value" of 150 µg/l (Lewalter, personal communication to the Commission).

Serum creatinine values can be used in occupational medicine for monitoring the course of the intoxication, but are not suitable, however, as effect parameters in accordance with the BAT value concept (Lewalter *et al.* 1993).

4 Selection of the Indicators

The exposure and effect indicators available are not specific, at least for *o*-cresol and *p*-cresol, as a result of the ubiquitous background exposure to these substances. Internal exposure to cresols is best evaluated by determining the amounts of free cresols and total cresols (free cresols and conjugated cresols) excreted in urine.

5 Methods

Differentiation of the excreted cresols according to the free and conjugated forms can be carried out on the basis of hydrolysis with perchloric acid (Baselt 1980, De Smet *et al.* 1998, Teisinger *et al.* 1954) or enzymatically with β-D-glucuronidase (Piotrowski 1971). The often recommended sulfuric acid hydrolyses only some of the cresyl glucuronide (Piotrowski 1971). After cleaning by means of water vapour distillation or with solid-phase cartridges, the cresol is quantified using high-performance liquid chromatography. A reliable and practicable method has been published by the working group "Analyses of Hazardous Substances in Biological Materials" of the DFG Commission for the Investigation of Health Hazards of Chemical Compounds in the Work Area (Angerer and Schaller 1988).

The direct determination of cresyl sulfate and cresyl glucuronide using high-performance liquid chromatography without hydrolysis and concentration also described, is, despite lower sensitivity, also suitable for the determination of the isomeric cresols in urine (Ogata and Yamasaki 1979). The creatinine values are determined enzymatically (Thomas 2000).

6 Background Exposure

o-Cresol and *m*-cresol do not occur in physiological metabolism, *p*-cresol is formed during the bacterial breakdown of amino acids in the intestine (see Section 1.2).

The background exposure to *o*-cresol in urine can be up to 200 µg/g creatinine and is mainly dependent on smoking habits. In non-smokers and the general population not exposed to the substance, *o*-cresol concentrations of about 60 µg/g creatinine were observed, probably as a result of the ubiquitous exposure to toluene. Smokers, however, were found to have concentrations which were three to four times higher (Nise 1992).

The reference value for the physiological excretion of *p*-cresol in urine is 70 mg/g creatinine (Lewalter *et al.* 1993).

7 Evaluation of the BLW Value

In general, inhaled and percutaneously absorbed cresols are rapidly detoxified by glucuronidation. The critical toxic effects of cresol metabolism in the kidneys are caused, however, mainly by free cresols. Normally no free cresols can be detected in plasma, even after exposure to high cresol concentrations.

However, as a result of the polymorphism of the isoenzymes of uridine diphosphate glucuronosyl transferase (UDPG), around 6 % of Central Europeans can glucuronidize only slowly. In rare cases this defect can be amplified by the lack of phosphoadenosine-phosphosulfate (PAPS) sulfotransferase normally responsible for sulfation (Calabrese 1986, Lewalter and Neumann 1998). In these persons high exposure to cresols leads to the increased formation of free cresols, which within a few hours can cause massive renal functional disorders and even acute kidney failure (Lewalter and Neumann 1998). The nephrotoxic effects of exposure to high cresol concentrations, which are evidently based on deficient glucuronidation, can be prevented by limiting the amount of free cresol in the total amount of cresol excreted in urine (Lewalter and Neumann 1998, Lewalter *et al.* 1993, Roots *et al.* 1992).

Increases in the serum creatinine level of over 1 mg/dl are frequently observed when the amount of free cresol detectable in urine exceeds 150 µg/l (Lewalter and Neumann 1998). A threshold value based on free cresols that could be used as a BAT value, has to date not yet been adequately validated. In the light of what is known from industrial contact with the more toxic phenols (see the documentation on "Phenol" in Volume 1 of this series; Henschler and Lehnert 1994), it can be assumed that also for the cresols a value of 150 µg free cresols/l urine in general will not be exceeded by 95 % of persons exposed to cresols with total cresol levels of up to 200 mg/l urine. In view of this, a BLW value has been set of

200 mg total cresol/l urine

Sampling should be carried out at the end of exposure or at the end of the shift.

For 5 % of persons exposed to cresol (UDPG-deficient persons), the determination of total cresol alone is, however, not sufficient. In such cases, additional determination of free cresol is recommended. The BLW value for total cresol is, therefore, to be regarded as provisional.

8 Interpretation of Data

The BLW value does not take into account local effects resulting from the direct contact with cresols of the skin. Even cresol corrosion on small areas of skin should be reported to the physician.

The problem resulting from the excretion of cresol without occupational exposure to cresols or toluene was discussed in the second addendum to the BAT documentation for toluene from 2000.

9 References

ACGIH (American Conference of Governmental Industrial Hygienists) (2001) Cresol. All isomers. TLV® Chemical substances 7th edition, Documentation. Publication # 7DOC-146, ACGIH®, Cincinatti

Angerer J, Schaller KH (1988) Phenole und Aromatische Alkohole. in: Henschler D (Ed.) Analytische Methoden zur Prüfung gesundheitsschädlicher Arbeitsstoffe. Band 2: Analysen in biologischem Material, 9. Lieferung, VCH, Weinheim

ATSDR (Agency for Toxic Substances and Disease Registry) (1992) Toxicological profile for cresols. US Department of Health and Human Services, USA

Baselt RG (1980) Urine Phenol. in: Baselt RC (Ed.) Biological monitoring methods for industrial chemicals, Biomedical Publications, Davis, 41–42

Bieniek G (1997) Urinary excretion of phenols as an indicator of occupational exposure in the coke-plant industry. Int Arch Occup Environ Health 70: 334–340

Calabrese EJ (1986) Ecogenetics: historical foundation and current status. J Occup Med 28: 1096–1102

Chan TK, Mak LW, Ng RP (1971) Methemoglobinemia, Heinz bodies and acute massive intravascular hemolysis in lysol poisoning. Blood 38: 739–744

DECOS (Dutch Expert Committee on Occupational Standards) (1998) Cresols. Health-based recommended occupational exposure limit. Report of the Dutch expert committee on occupational standards, a committee of the Health Council of the Netherlands, to the Minister and State Secretary of Social Affairs and Employment. No. 1998/15WGD, Rijswijk

Deichmann WB, Keplinger ML (1981) Phenols and phenolic compounds. in: Clayton GD, Clayton FE (Eds) Patty's industrial hygiene and toxicology, 3rd revised edition, Vol. 2A Toxicology, John Wiley and Sons, New York–Chichester–Brisbane–Toronto–Singapore, 2567–2627

De Smet R, David F, Sandra P, Van Kaer J, Lesaffer G, Dhondt A, Lameire N, Vanholder R (1998) A sensitive HPLC method for the quantification of free and total *p*-cresol in patients with chronic renal failure. Clin Chim Acta 278: 1–21

Greim H (Ed.) (2000a) Cresols (all isomers). in: Occupational toxicants, Vol. 14, Wiley-VCH, Weinheim

Greim H (Ed.) (2000b) Kresol (alle Isomeren). Gesundheitsschädliche Arbeitsstoffe, Toxikologisch-arbeitsmedizinische Begründungen von MAK-Werten, 30. Lieferung, Wiley-VCH, Weinheim

Henschler D, Lehnert G (Eds) (1994) Phenol. in: Biological exposure values for occupational toxicants and carcinogens – Critical data evaluation for BAT and EKA values, Vol. 1, VCH, Weinheim, pp. 123–128

Lewalter J, Neumann H-G (1998) Biologische Arbeitsstoff-Toleranzwerte (Biomonitoring). Teil XII: Die Bedeutung der individuellen Empfindlichkeit beim Biomonitoring. Arbeitsmed Sozialmed Umweltmed 33: 352–364

Lewalter J, Steffens W, Wimber M (1993) Biomarker der Polymorphismen im Benzol- und Phenol-Stoffwechsel. in: Triebig G, Stelzer O (Eds) Dokumentationsband über die 33. Jahrestagung der Deutschen Gesellschaft für Arbeitsmedizin und Umweltmedizin e.V., Gentner-Verlag, Stuttgart, 209–214

Moeschlin S (1972) Klinik und Therapie der Vergiftungen, G. Thieme Verlag, Stuttgart, 274–275

Nise G (1992) Urinary excretion of *o*-cresol and hippuric acid after toluene exposure in rotogravure printing. Int Arch Occup Environ Health 63: 377–381

Ogata M, Yamasaki Y (1979) High performance liquid chromatography for the quantitative determination of urinary phenylsulfate and phenylglucuronide as indices of benzene and phenol exposure in rats. Int Arch Occup Environ Health 44: 177–184

Piotrowski JK (1971) Evaluation of exposure to phenol: absorption of phenol vapour in the lungs and through the skin and excretion of phenol in urine. Br J Ind Med 28: 172–178

Roots I, Drakoulis N, Brockmöller J (1992) Polymorphic enzymes and cancer risk: concepts, methodology and data review. in: Kalow W (Ed) Pharmacogenetics of drug metabolism, Pergamon Press, New York, 815–841

Sherwood RJ, Carter FWG (1970) The measurement of occupational exposure to benzene vapour. Am Occup Hyg 13: 125–146

Teisinger J, Fiserova-Bergerova V, Kudra J (1954) The metabolism of benzene in man. Prac Lek Ces 82: 175–188

Thompson DC, Perera K, London R (1996) Studies on the mechanism of hepatotoxicity of 4-methylphenol (*p*-cresol) effects of deuterium labeling and ring substitution. Chem Biol Interact 101: 1–11

Thomas L (2000) Creatinin. in: Thomas L (Ed.) Labor und Diagnose, 5. Auflage, TH-Books Verlagsgesellschaft, Frankfurt/Main, 376–384

WHO (World Health Organization) (1995) Cresols. Environmental Health Criteria 168, Geneva

Authors: J. Lewalter, A.W. Rettenmeier, G. Leng

Approved by the Working Group: 05.05.2003

Cyclohexane

BAT	170 mg total 1,2-cyclohexanediol/g creatinine Sampling time: end of exposure or end of shift, with long-term exposure after several previous shifts
Date of evaluation	2001
CAS No.	110-82-7
Synonyms	Hexahydrobenzene Hexamethylene Hexanaphthene
Chemical name (CAS)	Cyclohexane
Formula	C_6H_{12}

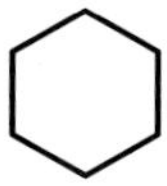

Molecular weight	84.16
Melting point	6.5°C
Boiling point	80.8°C
Density at 25°C	0.78 g/cm^3
Vapour pressure at 20°C	104 hPa
Solubility in water at 20°C	50 mg/l
MAK [last established: 2001]	200 ml/m^3 ≙ 700 mg/m^3

Cyclohexane is a colourless, highly inflammable liquid with a high vapour pressure of 104 hPa at 20°C. It is insoluble in water, but readily soluble in alcohols, hydrocarbons, ethers or chlorinated hydrocarbons.

It is used mainly as an intermediate in the production of nylon. It is used in the production of cyclohexanol and cyclohexanone, and as a solvent for lacquers, resins, glues and for the extraction of ethereal oils. Cyclohexane does not usually occur as the pure product, but is used industrially in accompaniment with other substances. Mainly cyclohexane–toluene mixtures are used. There are therefore only few data available from field studies for pure cyclohexane at the workplace.

Essential BAT Value Documentations. DFG, Deutsche Forschungsgemeinschaft

ISBN 3-527-31477-6

1 Toxicokinetics

1.1 Absorption and distribution

Cyclohexane is absorbed mainly by inhalation; a large proportion is exhaled unchanged (Sandmeyer 1981). Pulmonary retention of the substance was given as 18.4 % (resting conditions) and 34 % (workplace conditions) (Mutti *et al.* 1981). Cyclohexanol in urine, however, represents only about 1 % of the absorbed dose.

Wetting an area of skin of 360 cm^2 (about 2 % of the body surface) with a saturated solution of cyclohexane in water did not lead to any significant increase in the internal exposure to the substance (Fiserova-Bergerova *et al.* 1990).

In persons exposed to cyclohexane in concentrations of 350 mg/m^3 and up to 2500 mg/m^3, respectively, the cyclohexane concentrations in the ambient air and those in alveolar air correlated linearly (Mutti *et al.* 1981, Perbellini *et al.* 1980).

Oil/air and blood/air distribution coefficients in man were given as 293 and 1.3 (Perbellini *et al.* 1985). The corresponding tissue/air coefficients were found to be 11 in the liver, 7 in the kidneys, 10 in the brain, 11 in muscle, 6 in the heart, 3 in the lung and 260 in body fat. These data indicate that after cyclohexane has been incorporated it is distributed mainly in adipose tissue.

1.2 Metabolism

The metabolism of cyclohexane to cyclohexanone has been described (Elliott *et al.* 1959, Mráz *et al.* 1994, Perbellini and Brugnone 1980, Yasugi *et al.* 1994) and is shown in Figure 1. Data for the biotransformation of cyclohexane in man are to date inadequate. After volunteers were exposed to cyclohexane concentrations of 1050 mg/m^3 for 8 hours, over a period of 72 hours 0.5 % was excreted in the urine as cyclohexanol, 23.4 % as 1,2-cyclohexanediol and 11.3 % as 1,4-cyclohexanediol, determined as the sum of the free and conjugated compounds.

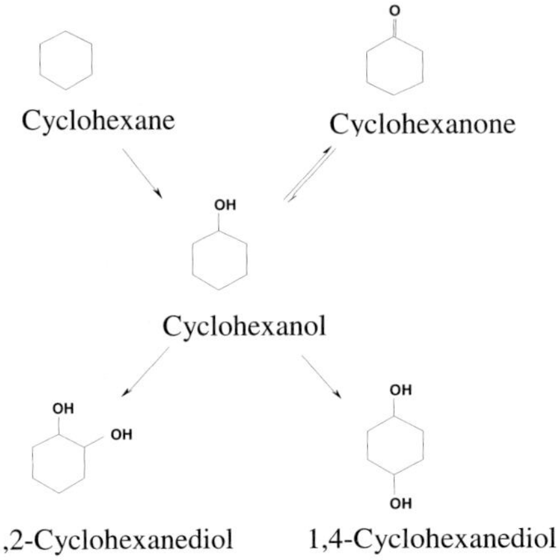

Figure 1. The metabolism of cyclohexane in man

1.3 Elimination

According to data from the literature, alveolar exhalation of the substance nine hours after exposure does not exceed 10 % of the total amount absorbed (Mutti *et al.* 1981). In animal experiments cyclohexane is excreted with the urine partly in unchanged form and after biotransformation in the liver and in the kidneys in the form of its metabolites. Renal excretion of the three cyclohexane metabolites, cyclohexanol, 1,2-cyclohexanediol and 1,4-cyclohexanediol, was found to be 0.5 %, 23.4 % and 11.3 %, respectively, of the total dose of cyclohexane absorbed (Mráz *et al.* 1994). Cyclohexanol and the two diols are excreted in man both in glucuronidized and also in free, non-conjugated form (Trabs 1999). As a result of further oxidative biotransformation the amount of cyclohexanol renally excreted is small; only about 10 % of the amount of 1,2-cyclohexanediol excreted (Mráz *et al.* 1998, Trabs 1999, Walter *et al.* 1999). The resulting elimination half-times for 1,2-cyclohexanediol were found to be on average 17.0 ± 5.2 hours (Mráz *et al.* 1998) and 15.8 ± 1.9 hours (Trabs 1999, Walter *et al.* 1999). The half-time for 1,4-cyclohexanediol determined by Mráz *et al.* 1998 is of a comparable order of magnitude, while Trabs determined a half-time that was around twice as high, with an average value of 31.5 hours (Trabs 1999). This indicates that both metabolites accumulate. Cyclohexanol, however, was found to be eliminated with mean half-times of 4.6 hours (Trabs 1999, Walter *et al.* 1999) and 1.5 hours (Mráz *et al.* 1998). For the monitoring of occupationally exposed persons, the cyclohexane metabolites 1,2-cyclohexanediol and 1,4-cyclohexanediol should therefore be determined at the end of the shift after several previous shifts.

2 Critical Toxicity

2.1 Acute toxicity

Cyclohexanol is of low acute toxicity (Sandmeyer 1981). It has depressive effects on the central nervous system and is narcotic in high concentrations.

2.2 Chronic toxicity

High vapour concentrations are reported to cause irritation of the mucous membranes of the eyes and the respiratory tract, which produce drowsiness, dizziness, nausea, coughing and vomiting, and at extremely high concentrations can provoke respiratory arrest, unconsciousness and collapse. Further details are at present not available. The cyclohexanol metabolite cyclohexanone was classified as carcinogenic in Category 3 (now Carcinogen category 3B) in 1994 and the MAK value of 50 ml/m^3 was withdrawn (Greim 1994).

In a field study, in which 33 female workers from the glue industry were subdivided into a group of 17 women with low exposure (5 to 13 mg/m^3) and a group of 16 women with high exposure (15 to 274 mg/m^3), in neither subgroup were symptoms described. Laboratory analysis did not yield any unusual findings (Yasugi *et al.* 1994).

3 Exposure and Effects

Field studies and the results of laboratory analyses are available for the external and internal exposure to cyclohexane (e.g. Mráz *et al.* 1994, 1998, Mutti *et al.* 1981, Ong *et al.* 1991, Perbellini *et al.* 1980, Perbellini and Brugnone 1980, Perico *et al.* 1999, Trabs 1999, Walter *et al.* 1999, Yasugi *et al.* 1994). In particular the field study of Perico *et al.* (1999), a simulation model of the same author based on data of Perbellini *et al.* (1988, 1990) and Mráz *et al.* (1994), and laboratory studies of Mráz *et al.* (1998), Trabs (1999) and Walter *et al.* (1999) can be used as the basis for the evaluation of a BAT value for cyclohexane. Table 1 compares the results of the studies. The cyclohexane metabolites cyclohexanol and in particular 1,2-cyclohexanediol and 1,4-cyclohexanediol are suggested in all of the studies as possible exposure parameters after exposure to cyclohexane. Similar metabolite ratios were found in all.

4 Selection of the Indicators

In principle, the solvent itself and all the metabolites formed that are detectable in urine, but in particular the parameters named below, are suitable for the biological monitoring of workers exposed to cyclohexane:

- the cyclohexane concentration in alveolar air
- the cyclohexane concentration in blood
- the cyclohexanol concentration in urine
- the 1,2-cyclohexanediol and 1,4-cyclohexanediol concentration in urine

Cyclohexanol and the two isomeric diols are excreted in free and in glucuronidized form. As the critical toxicity is based on cyclohexanol, this metabolite is of particular importance. Parameters for monitoring the effects are at present unknown.

Table 1. Field studies, PBPK modelling and experiments in man to determine the correlation between external exposure to cyclohexane and the internal exposure on the basis of the cyclohexane metabolites excreted

References	Study, exposure conditions	Air cyclohexane (mg/m^3)	Urine cyclohexane metabolites (mg/g creatinine) 1,2-cyclo-hexanediol	1,4-cyclo-hexanediol	cyclo-hexanol	Comments
Perico *et al.* 1999	**field study in a shoe factory** (N = 156 workers) 5 workdays (8 h/day)	102 ± 115 (7–617)				exposure to a mixture of solvents
		120 ± 128 (Monday)	13.7	8.4		y(1,2-diol) = 0.081x (CH_{Air}) + 3.9
		80 ± 92 (Thursday)	27.8	14.1		y(1,4-diol) = 0.049x (CH_{Air}) + 2.5
		700	*60.6*	*36.8*		*extrapolated to the MAK value of 700 mg/m³*
Perico *et al.* 1999 (with data from Perbellini *et al.* 1988, 1990 and Mráz *et al.* 1994)	**simulation model (PBPK)** 5 days (8 h/day), physical activity:	1030	day 1:	day 5:		PBPK calculated for normal and increased physical activity (expressed as AV and Q)
	AV = 15 l/min, Q = 6 l/min		200	350		
	AV = 10 l/min, Q = 10 l/min		150	250		
		700	day 1:	day 5:		*extrapolated to the MAK value of 700 mg/m³*
	AV = 15 l/min, Q = 6 l/min		136	238		
	AV = 10 l/min, Q = 10 l/min		102	170		
Mráz *et al.* 1998	**laboratory study** (N = 8 persons) 8 hours, at rest	1010	136.9	71.4	12.9	excretion of the metabolites determined 6–8 hours after the beginning of exposure; urinary excretion increased on days 2 and 3 of exposure by about 40 % and 60 %
		700	*95*	*50*	*9*	*extrapolated to the MAK value of 700 mg/m³*
Trabs 1999, Walter *et al.* 1999	**laboratory study** (N = 17 persons) 8 hours, physical activity of 75 watts, 10 min/h	1015 ± 77	191.4 ± 107.4	88.5 ± 56.5	16.5 ± 9.2	excretion of the metabolites determined 8–10 hours after the beginning of exposure
		700	*132.0 (170)*	*61.0 (85)*	*11.4 (20)*	*extrapolated to the MAK value of 700 mg/m³ (95th percentile)*

AV = alveolar ventilation; Q = flow rate of the blood; 1,2-diol = 1,2-cyclohexanediol; CH = cyclohexane; 1,4-diol = 1,4-cyclohexanediol

4.1 Cyclohexane in alveolar air

The available data do not allow any statement to be made about the extent to which alveolar air is a diagnostically valid parameter for detecting exposure to cyclohexane. In addition, there is no standardized sampling procedure available for routine practice (Lauwerys and Hoet 1993, Mutti *et al.* 1981, Perbellini *et al.* 1979, 1980, Rosenberg *et al.* 1989).

4.2 Cyclohexane in blood

In the standardized test procedures of the studies of Trabs (1994) and Walter *et al.* (1999), defined sampling times were set to determine the concentrations and kinetics of cyclohexane in blood during the invasion, equilibrium and elimination phases (Trabs 1999, Walter *et al.* 1999). The data collected yielded differentiated information e.g. about differences in the invasion and evasion kinetics, the steady state and the calculation of biological half-times. The invasion of cyclohexane in the blood increases linearly in the first half hour with a correlation coefficient of $r = 0.90$. During the exposure period, the cyclohexane concentration reaches a plateau one hour after the beginning of exposure with a more or less constant concentration during the determination period. The mean cyclohexane concentration during this steady state is 1.23 ± 0.32 mg/l.

On the other hand, in another field study with external exposure to cyclohexane concentrations of 300 ml/m^3 with a fluctuation range of 17 to 2484 mg/m^3, a cyclohexane concentration in blood of about 0.50 mg/l was found (Perbellini and Brugnone 1980). With the support of another field study, the authors recommended a cyclohexane value of 0.44 mg/l blood as the parameter in biological material, which correlates with a cyclohexane concentration of 300 ml/m^3 (Brugnone and Perbellini 1985). The concentrations determined after occupational and experimental exposure to cyclohexane therefore differ by a factor of about 2.5. Experimentally determined half-times for the elimination of cyclohexane from the blood show that a biphasic course of elimination must be taken into account (Trabs 1999). In the first hour after the end of the standardized exposure, cyclohexane is eliminated from the blood with a half-time of 0.39 ± 0.09 hours. After this period elimination takes place with a half-time of 1.24 ± 0.36 hours. In individual cases the determination of the blood cyclohexane concentration can provide valuable evidence of incorporation, as it reflects, as a result of the short invasion and elimination times, the current external exposure situation. This parameter is less suitable for routine investigations and in particular as the basis for the evaluation of a threshold limit value.

4.3 Cyclohexane metabolites in urine

The metabolites cyclohexanol, 1,2-cyclohexanediol and 1,4-cyclohexanediol can be determined simultaneously. The main advantages of the determination of the metabolites in urine are that

- cyclohexanol and the isomeric diols are not detectable in the urine of persons not occupationally exposed to cyclohexane
- the concentrations of the cyclohexane metabolites, in particular those of the diols, are comparatively high
- the metabolite concentrations in urine are proportional to the external exposure
- these metabolites can also be used as biological parameters for occupational exposure to cyclohexanone and cyclohexanol.

5 Methods

The gas chromatographic head space method is a suitable and tested procedure for the determination of cyclohexane in alveolar air and blood. It is carried out in analogy to the quantification of cyclohexanone in blood (Angerer and Schaller 1983). Gas chromatographic methods of analysis are particularly suitable for the determination of the cyclohexane metabolites in urine. The working group "Analyses of Hazardous Substances in Biological Materials" of the DFG Commission for the Investigation of Health Hazards of Chemical Compounds in the Work Area has tested and approved a capillary gas chromatographic procedure with flame ionization detector for the determination of cyclohexanol and of 1,2-cyclohexanediol and 1,4-cyclohexanediol in urine.

After acid hydrolysis and the addition of an internal standard, the cyclohexane metabolites are extracted with ethyl acetate. The analytical detection limit is around 1 mg of each component per l urine. Analytical determination of the metabolites includes both the conjugated fraction in the urine and also that in unbound form. The above procedure does not allow the separation of the metabolically formed cis/trans isomers 1,2-cyclohexanediol and 1,4-cyclohexanediol, or only in negligible amounts, so that the determination also takes into account the total amount of both components.

6 Background Exposure

Cyclohexane is a component of some glues and resins. The indoor survey 1985/86 of the German Federal Environmental Agency yielded on the basis of 479 indoor determinations a median value of 6 $\mu g/m^3$ and a 95th percentile of 18 $\mu g/m^3$ (Krause *et al.* 1987). The highest value determined was 590 $\mu g/m^3$. In urine samples of the general population cyclohexane metabolites were not detected with the usual analytical methods. Using a sensitive method, Perico *et al.* (1999) determined mean amounts of 1,2-cyclohexanediol excreted in the urine of 31 workers not exposed to the substance of 0.5 mg/g creatinine, with a median of 0.3 mg/g creatinine.

7 Evaluation of the BAT Value

The studies shown in Table 1 were used to evaluate a BAT value for cyclohexane. In these studies the parameters used are the excretion of the metabolites 1,2-cyclohexanediol and 1,4-cyclohexanediol. In addition in Table 1 the amounts of cyclohexanol excreted in urine are given. From the study of Perico *et al.* (1999) relationships between external and internal exposure can be deduced. A cyclohexane concentration in air of 300 ml/m^3 corresponds to metabolite concentrations in urine of about 61 mg 1,2-cyclohexanediol/g creatinine and 37 mg 1,4-cyclohexanediol/g creatinine (Perico *et al.* 1999).

The results of biomonitoring demonstrate the cumulative properties of both metabolites. In a simulation model also described by Perico *et al.* (1999), which includes the laboratory studies of Mráz *et al.* (1994) and Perbellini *et al.* (1988, 1990), at the end of days 1 and 5 of exposure, with alveolar ventilation of 15 l/min and after extrapolation to 300 ml/m^3, 1,2-cyclohexanediol concentrations were calculated of 136 mg and 238 mg/g creatinine.

The two experimental studies in man of Mráz *et al.* (1998), and Trabs (1999) and Walter *et al.* (1999), were carried out with comparable external exposure to cyclohexane of about 300 ml/m^3. The results of the two studies are of a similar order of magnitude.

In the study of Trabs (1999) there are data available for the 95th percentile of the metabolite concentrations which can be used in the evaluation of a BAT value. On this basis the BAT value has been set at

170 mg total 1,2-cyclohexanediol/g creatinine

Sampling of the urine should be carried out at the end of the shift after several previous shifts.

8 References

Angerer J, Schaller KH (1983) Head-Space-Technik, Sammelmethode. in: Henschler D (Ed.) Analytische Methoden zur Prüfung gesundheitsschädlicher Arbeitsstoffe, Band 2: Analysen in biologischem Material, 5. Lieferung, VCH, Weinheim

Brugnone F, Perbellini L (1985) Biological monitoring of occupational exposure to solvents by analysis of alveolar air and blood. in: WHO Regional office for Europe, Nordic Council of ministers (Ed.) Chronic effects of organic solvents on the central nervous system and diagnostic criteria, Report on a joint WHO/Nordic Council of Ministers working group, Copenhagen, 56–89

Elliott TH, Parke DV, Williams RT (1959) Studies in detoxication: the metabolism of cyclo[^{14}C]hexane and its derivatives. Biochem J 72: 193–200

Fiserova-Bergerova V, Pierce JT, Droz PO (1990) Dermal absorption potential of industrial chemicals: criteria for skin notation. Am J Ind Med 17: 617–635

Greim H (Ed.) (1998) Cyclohexanone. in: Occupational toxicants, Vol. 10, Wiley-VCH, Weinheim

Krause C, Mailahn W, Nagel R, Schulz C, Seifert B, Ullrich D (1987) Occurrence of volatile organic compounds in the air of 500 homes in the Federal Republic of Germany. in: Indoor air '87: Proceedings of the 4th international conference on indoor air quality and climate, Volume 1, Institute for Soil, Water and Air Hygiene, Berlin, 102–106

Lauwerys RR, Hoet P (1993) Industrial chemical exposure: guidelines for biological monitoring. Biological monitoring of exposure to organic substances. Lewis Publishers, Boca Raton–Ann Arbor–London–Tokyo, 105–108

Mráz J, Gálová E, Nohová H, Vitková D (1994) Markers of exposure to cyclohexanone, cyclohexane and cyclohexanol: 1,2- and 1,4-cyclohexanediol. Clin Chem 40: 1466–1468

Mráz J, Gálová E, Nohová H, Vitková D (1998) 1,2- and 1,4-cyclohexanediol: major urinary metabolites and biomarkers of exposure to cyclohexane, cyclohexanone and cyclohexanol in humans. Int Arch Occup Environ Health 71: 560–565

Mutti A, Falzoi M, Lucertini S, Cavatorta A, Franchini I, Pedroni C (1981) Absorption and alveolar excretion of cyclohexane in workers in a shoe factory. J Appl Toxicol 1: 220–223

Ong CN, Sia GL, Chia SE, Phoon WH, Tan KT (1991) Determination of cyclohexanol in urine and its use in environmental monitoring of cyclohexanone exposure. J Anal Toxicol 15: 13–16

Perbellini L, Brugnone F, Fracasso ME, Leone R (1979) Studio sulla biotransformazione del cicloesano in ratti e nell' uomo. Il Convegno sulla Patologia indotta dai tossici ambientali ed occupazionali Turin: 21–22

Perbellini L, Brugnone F (1980) Lung uptake and metabolism of cyclohexane in shoe factory workers. Int Arch Occup Environ Health 45: 261–269

Perbellini L, Brugnone F, Pavan I (1980) Identification of the metabolites of *n*-hexane, cyclohexane, and their isomers in men's urine. Toxicol Appl Pharmacol 53: 220–229

Perbellini L, Brugnone F, Caretta D, Maranelli G (1985) Partition coefficients of some industrial aliphatic hydrocarbons (C5–C7) in blood and human tissues. Br J Ind Med 42: 162–167

Perbellini L, Mozzo P, Turri PV, Zedde A, Brugnone F (1988) Biological exposure index of styrene suggested by a physiologico-mathematical model. Int Arch Occup Environ Health 60: 187–193

Perbellini L, Mozzo P, Olivato D, Brugnone F (1990) "Dynamic" biological exposure indexes for *n*-hexane and 2,5-hexanedione suggested by a physiologically based pharmacokinetic model. Am Ind Hyg Assoc J 51: 356–362

Perico A, Cassinelli C, Brugnone F, Bavazzano P, Perbellini L (1999) Biological monitoring of occupational exposure to cyclohexane by urinary 1,2- and 1,4-cyclohexanediol determination. Int Arch Occup Environ Health 72: 115–120

Rosenberg J, Fiserova-Bergerova V, Lowry LK (1989) Biological Monitoring IV: measurements in urine. Appl Ind Hyg 4: 16–21

Sandmeyer EE (1981) Alicyclic hydrocarbons. in: Clayton GD, Clayton EE (Eds) Patty's industrial hygiene and toxicology, 3rd ed., Wiley-Interscience, New York, 3221–3250

Trabs A (1999) Biologisches Monitoring nach standardisierter Cyclohexan-Einwirkung. Inaugural-Dissertation des Fachbereichs Humanmedizin der Justus-Liebig-Universität Gießen

Walter D, Trabs A, Knecht U, Woitowitz HJ (1999) Toxikokinetische Daten zur Evaluierung eines BAT-Wertes für Cyclohexan. in: Rettenmeier A, Feldhaus Ch (Eds) Dokumentationsband über die 39. Jahrestagung der Deutschen Gesellschaft für Arbeitsmedizin und Umweltmedizin e.V., Rindt-Druck, Fulda, 265–268

Yasugi T, Kawai T, Mizunuma K, Kishi R, Harabuchi I, Yuasa J, Eguchi T, Sugimoto R, Seiji K, Ikeda M (1994) Exposure monitoring and health effect studies of workers occupationally exposed to cyclohexane vapor. Int Arch Occup Environ Health 65: 343–350

Authors: U. Knecht, K.H. Schaller

Approved by the Working Group: 20.02.2001

4,4′-Diaminodiphenylmethane

Synonyms	p,p′-Diaminodiphenylmethane 4,4′-Methylenedianiline MDA
Formula	$C_{13}H_{14}N_2$

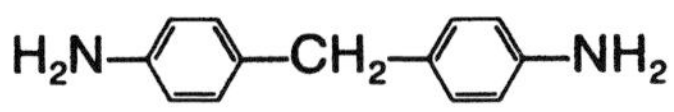

Molecular weight	198.27
Melting point	92 °C
Boiling point	398.5 °C
Vapour pressure at 20 °C	0.06 hPa
MAK [last established: 1987]	Carcinogenic substance: category IIIA2 of the List of MAK and BAT Values
TRK Value [1993]	0.1 mg/m^3

4,4′-Methylenedianiline (MDA) has been produced industrially from aniline and formaldehyde since 1920. Pure MDA consists of pale yellow crystals with a slight amine-like smell. Technical grade MDA contains up to 5 % of the 2,2′-isomer and 2,4′-isomer of the diamine. In general MDA is processed to MDI (4,4′-methylenediphenyl-diisocyanate). Up to 10 % of the MDA is used directly as a cross-linker in epoxy resins, polyurethanes and other polymers as well as in the production of rubber chemicals (4, 12, 15, 19).

1 Metabolism and Kinetics

Details of the metabolism and toxicology of MDA have already been published by the DFG Commission for the Investigation of Health Hazards of Chemical Compounds in the Work Area (22).

Like other aminoaromatics (see 4-aminodiphenyl, aniline, 2-naphthylamine, benzidine) 4,4′-diaminodiphenylmethane is transformed into metabolites which form haemoglobin adducts in erythrocytes (see Tab. 1).

Essential BAT Value Documentations. DFG, Deutsche Forschungsgemeinschaft
Copyright © 2006 WILEY-VCH Verlag GmbH & Co. KGaA, Weinheim
ISBN 3-527-31477-6

Tab. 1: Haemoglobin adduct level (µg/l) in persons occupationally exposed to high levels of MDA (E. Bailey, unpublished results 1992 (2))

Person	Haemoglobin adduct level (µg/l blood) MDA	N-Acetyl-MDA	Relationship between N-acetyl-MDA and free MDA (mol/mol)	Acetylator phenotype
A	1807	3637	1.7	i
B	414	N	./.	s
C	409	1246	2.5	f
D	536	697	1.1	s
E	639	N	./.	s
F	191	869	5.9	f
G	356	1003	2.3	f
H	242	404	1.4	s
I	639	1064	1.4	s
J	261	1466	4.6	f
K	955	1780	1.5	i
L	463	1785	3.2	f
N = not detectable			Average: 2.6	f : s : i = 42 : 42 : 16 f: fast, s: slow, i: indifferent

2 Critical Toxicity

2.1 Liver Toxicity

MDA feeding experiments with male beagle dogs led, in addition to weight loss, to disturbances in liver metabolism with significantly increased activity of the liver enzymes (13, 42). Oral or dermal exposure or inhalation of MDA on one or a few occasions has also led in humans to disturbances in liver metabolism. In the accident known as "Epping Jaundice" 84 persons contracted hepatitis with markedly increased SGOT, SGPT and bilirubin values after eating bread contaminated with MDA; the bread contained up to 3 mg MDA/kg flour. In one patient haematuria was also observed (25, 26, 39).

Further cases of hepatitis-like diseases have been reported in persons after contact with epoxide resins containing MDA (3, 4, 27, 32).

2.2 Genotoxicity and Carcinogenicity

4,4′-Diaminodiphenylmethane has been classified by the DFG Commission for the Investigation of Health Hazards of Chemical Compounds in the Work Area in category IIIA2. Details can be found in the appropriate documentation (22).

In the Ames test MDA was mutagenic after metabolic activation (36, 37, 43, 44, 52).

In an epidemiological study of 179 MDA workers, three tumours of the efferent urinary passages were observed instead of the expected 0.88 cases (15, 16). This could not be confirmed in two further studies on employees exposed to MDA in a chemical factory and power plant (34, 40, 51).

2.3 Other Effects

The ability of MDA to induce skin sensitisation in humans has been repeatedly reported. The allergen ultimately responsible is unknown. It is possibly a photo-allergen (28, 31). In individual cases impairment of the visual ability has also been described after exposure to MDA. In all cases there was massive exposure to MDA which, however, was not quantified (11, 18, 27, 28).

3 Exposure and Effects

In the case of MDA every exposure is to be regarded as external exposure which can lead to inhalation or percutaneous absorption. The internal exposure is the biologically relevant concentration of the reactive metabolite in the target organ, above all in the liver and in the efferent urinary passages (5, 6, 18). The internal exposure parameters are the MDA concentrations in body fluids such as blood, plasma and urine which correlate with the internal exposure under the specific pharmacokinetic conditions. MDA adducts in erythrocytes (Hb adducts) or leucocytes (DNA adducts) as well as changed activities of liver enzymes are understood as parameters of effect for MDA.

4 Selection of the Indicators

The possible internal exposure and effect after contact with MDA can be determined via analysis of the substances in urine, blood and plasma, as well as via protein and DNA adducts in the blood cells (7, 20).

4.1 MDA in Urine

For some time now, MDA exposure has been measured via the excretion of free and conjugated MDA in urine. Despite extensive studies, exact correlations between inhaled MDA concentrations and the urinary excretion of MDA are not yet available (5, 11, 27, 28). This is not least due to the often predominant percutaneous absorption which cannot be quantitatively determined in the total exposure to MDA. In occupational-medical practice the excretion of MDA after contact with MDA is often judged on the basis of so-called "empirical values" (23, 29, 47).

4.2 MDA Protein Adducts

According to investigations by various research groups, a metabolite of MDA in which an amino group was oxidised to the nitroso group reacts with the sulphhydryl groups of glutathione (GSH) and of proteins. In particular MDA adducts with serum albumin (HSA) and haemoglobin can be used for biological monitoring (7, 56).

For the reasons mentioned in section 4.1, published investigations on the correlation between defined Hb-adducts and the level of external exposure to MDA are not yet available.

4.3 DNA Adducts

In DNA, metabolites of MDA react mostly with the C8 position in desoxyguanosine. *N*-(Desoxyguanosine-8-yl)-MDA is formed in the reaction with *N*-hydroxy-MDA (24).

Biological monitoring via the MDA-DNA adducts in leucocytes is possible in principle (4a). To what extent the detection of DNA adducts can be correlated with a DNA effect in other tissues or with the genotoxicity of MDA requires further investigation. A genotoxic effect can in certain cases also be determined non-specifically by investigating the incidence of DNA strand breaks in leucocytes (41).

5 Methodology

Analysis of MDA in urine or of HSA or Hb adducts takes place by high-pressure liquid chromatography with an LC-UV detector (1, 6, 14, 17, 33, 35, 46, 53) or an LC-ECD detector (30, 48, 49, 50) or, after derivatisation, by capillary gas chromatography with a GC-ECD detector or by GC-MS (2, 8, 9, 10, 38). DNA adducts in the leucocytes are analysed, after being cleaved hydrolytically, by GC-MS (6, 43, 54, 55) or directly using the ^{32}P-postlabelling technique (4a, 45). Using the alkaline elution method, the incidence of DNA strand breaks in the leucocytes can be determined (41).

5.1 Calculation of the MDA Content of Haemoglobin (Hb) and DNA Adducts

During preparation the erythrocytes and leucocytes are isolated from whole blood, washed and then suspended in a volume of physiological saline corresponding to the original volume of blood.

The MDA content of the Hb adduct (ng MDA_{Hb}) and the DNA adducts of the leucocytes (ng MDA_{DNA}), is calculated, allowing for possible preparation losses, by use of the packed cell volumes (PCV), relating the PCV of the erythrocyte or leucocyte suspension to that of the whole blood, according to the equation:

$$C_{\text{Hb or DNA}}(\text{MDA/l blood}) = \frac{PCV_{\text{Blood}}}{PCV_{\text{Suspension}}} \times C_{\text{Suspension}}\ (\text{MDA/l Suspension})$$

$C_{\text{Hb or DNA}}$	= Amount of MDA bound to haemoglobin (erythrocytes) or to DNA (leucocytes) per blood volume in ng MDA per l blood
$C_{\text{Suspension}}$	= MDA level measured in the erythrocyte or leucocyte suspension in ng MDA per l suspension
PCV_{Blood}	= Packed cell volume of the whole blood
$PCV_{\text{Suspension}}$	= Packed cell volume of the erythrocyte or leucocyte suspension

6 Evaluation of the Biological Exposure Equivalents for Carcinogenic Substances (EKA)

The current concentration of MDA intermediates after inhalation and percutaneous MDA absorption cannot be directly determined in the human organism, in particular in the liver or in bladder tissue. Conclusions as to individual biologically effective MDA exposure in these target tissues can be deduced, however, from the level of MDA conjugates in erythrocytes (Hb) and also in leucocytes (DNA).

6.1 MDA in Urine

Despite many years of monitoring MDA excretion in urine after industrial exposure to MDA, detailed investigations of its dependence on the inhaled MDA concentration are not available in the literature. Only the British Health and Safety Executive (HSE) recommends in its guidance note on MDA a so-called "yardstick value" of 88 µg MDA/g creatinine which surprisingly was correlated with an 8-hour exposure to only 0.01 ppm (80 µg/m^3) MDA (23). In German occupational-medical practice the value of 100 µg MDA/l urine named earlier in the specific effect definitions has been used to monitor occupational exposure to MDA (29, 47). This value was, however, not scientifically founded. It therefore corresponds to the HSE recommendation. It could not be clarified to what extent the two reference value recommendations take into consideration the percutaneous absorption characteristic of exposure to MDA.

6.2 MDA in Blood Cells

In the literature, adduct data are only described from a few sub-areas, e.g. from isolated Hb samples from persons involved in accidents. After low MDA exposures no significant correlation between the MDA values in the exposure air and those in the adducts in the erythrocytes could be observed (54). The Commission, however, has access to extensive data from chemical plants. The most important results are quoted below. Using current analytical methods no MDA-Hb conjugates are found in persons not exposed to MDA (21, 30).

The typical forms of industrial exposure to MDA are listed in table 2.

Tab. 2: Results of biological monitoring after industrial contact with MDA and various forms of exposure (average values, J. Lewalter, unpublished investigations, 1989–1992)

Air µg MDA/m³	Urine ng MDA/l	Hb adducts ng MDA/l blood	Persons N
1. Continual exposure (routine operation):			
10	270	10	24
20	780	30	12
33	2500	90	6
50	20000	850	3
			→45 persons
2. Intermittent exposure			
	≤50	10	15
	≤100	40	38
	≤1000	170	74
	≤10000	500	137
	≤50000	2300	21
	≤100000	9500	8
			→293 persons
3. Single exposure (intoxication)			
	≤1000	≤50	5
	≤10000	200	29
	≤50000	700	68
	≤100000	2000	43
			→145 persons

Among the persons investigated intermittent contact with MDA with occasional, sometimes very high-level peak exposures, dominated. This can lead to a significant accumulation of the MDA-Hb adducts.

6.3 Conclusions

After occupational contact with MDA concentrations below the currently valid TRK value (100 µg MDA/m³) there is a dose-dependent increase of MDA in urine and the erythrocytic Hb adduct. The data available so far are incomplete. There appear to be difficulties in evaluation due to the high levels of skin absorption. The data in table 2 show a good correlation between the MDA excretion in urine and the Hb adducts in erythrocytes. This indicates the validity of the methods used and their fundamental usefulness for biological monitoring. On the other hand there is no linear correlation between the air values and the biological values. Apparently at workplaces with higher MDA air exposure there is an increased opportunity for immediate skin contact. In table 3 pairs of values are listed which have been assembled, with all necessary reservations, from the values in table 2.

Tab. 3: Concentrations of MDA in air and the associated biological parameters (data taken from table 2)

Air µg MDA/m³	Urine ng MDA/l	Hb adducts ng MDA/l blood
–	50	10
–	100	40
10	270	–
20	780	–
–	1000	170
33	2500	–
–	10000	500
50	20000	–
–	50000	2300
–	100000	9500

Due to the extreme non-linearity of the relationship between the air concentrations and the biological values in table 3 the DFG Commission for the Investigation of Health Hazards of Chemical Compounds in the Work Area was not prepared to set EKA values for MDA at present. In biological monitoring practice the values in tables 2 and 3 can serve for orientation. MDA will be listed for the time being under the rubric IX/2 (until 1992 VIII/2) of the List of MAK and BAT Values until there are further data or concepts for evaluation.

7 Interpretation of the Data

The MDA excretion determined in urine is not of equal value to the cellular effect of MDA measured in Hb adducts. The cellular effects are the result of individual, metabolic activation determined among other things by the individual acetylation (detoxification) potential and N-oxidation (toxification) potential of the organism. These many and various levels of performance of individual metabolism can only be evaluated at present in the MDA adduct formation with haemoglobin as a marker for reactions with other macromolecules.

In practice, e.g. during occupational medical health surveillance, the routine determination of erythrocytic MDA-Hb adducts is to be recommended. In this way not only the current exposure but also MDA exposures during the previous three months are determined.

Investigations in erythrocytes are not bound to any particular sampling time. On the other hand urine investigations only yield reliable results if sampling takes place immediately after exposure.

8 References

1. Avery, M. J.: Determination of aromatic amines in urine and serum. J. Chromatogr. *488* (1989), 470–475
2. Bailey, E., Brooks, A. G., Bird, I., Farmer, P. B., Street, B.: Monitoring exposure to 4,4′-methylenedianiline by the gas chromatography-mass spectrometry determination of adducts to hemoglobin. Anal. Biochem. *190* (1990), 175–181
3. Bastien, P. G.: Medic: Occupational hepatitis caused by methylenedianiline. Med. J. Australia (1984) 533–535
4. Beard, R. R., Noe, J. T.: Aromatic nitro and amino compounds. In: Patty, F. A. (ed.): Industrial Hygiene and Toxicology, 3rd ed., Vol. 2A. Wiley and Sons, New York 1981, pp. 2413–2489

4a. Beach, A. C., Gupta, R. C.: Human biomonitoring and the ^{32}P-postlabelling assay. Carcinogenesis *13* (7) (1992), 1053–1074

5. Kusters, E.: Biological monitoring of MDA (a letter). Br. Ind. Med. *49* (1992), 72
6. Brunmark, P., Persson, P., Skarping, G.: Determination of 4,4′-methylenedianiline in hydrolysed human urine by micro liquid chromatography with ultraviolet detection. J. Chromatogr. *7* (1992), 1–5
7. Bryant, M. S., Osterman-Golkar, S. M.: Hemoglobin adducts as dosimeters of exposure to DNA-reactive chemicals. CIIT Activities *11* (1991), 1–12
8. Cocker, J., Gristwood, W., Wilson, H. K.: Assessment of occupational exposure to 4,4′-diaminodiphenylmethane (methylenedianiline) by gaschromatography-mass spectrometry analysis of urine. Br. J. Ind. Med. *43* (1986), 620–625
9. Cocker, J., Brown, L. C., Wilson, H. K.: A GC/MS method for the determination of 4,4′-diaminodiphenylmethane and substituted analogues in urine. J. Anal. Toxicol. *12* (1988), 9–14
10. Cocker, J., Boobis, A. R., Davies, D. S.: Determination of the N-acetyl-metabolites of 4,4′-methylenedianiline and 4,4′-methylene-bis-(2-chloro-aniline) in urine. Biomed. Env. Mass Spectro. *17* (1988), 161–167
11. Cohen, S. R.: Yellow staining caused by 4,4′-methylenedianiline exposure. Arch. Dermatol. *121* (1985), 1022–1027
12. Darby, T. D., Johnson, H. J., Northup, S. J.: An evaluation of a polyurethane for use as a medical grade plastic. Toxicol. Appl. Pharmacol. *46* (1978), 449–453
13. Deichmann, B., MacDonald, W. E., Coplan, M., Woods, F., Blum, E.: Di-(4-aminophenyl)-methane(MDA): 4-year dose feeding study. Toxicology *11* (1978), 185–188
14. Ernes, D. A., Hanshumaker, D. T.: Determination of extractable methylene-bis(aniline) in polyurethane films by liquid chromatography. Anal. Chem. *55* (1983), 408–409
15. International Agency for Research on Cancer (IARC): 4,4′-Methylenedianiline and its dihydrochloride. In: The evaluation of the carcinogenic risk of chemicals to humans. IARC Monograph No. 39. IARC, Lyon 1986, pp. 347–365
16. International Agency for Research on Cancer (IARC): 4,4′-Methylenediphenyl diisocyanate and polymethylene polyphenyl isocyanate. In: The evaluation of the carcinogenic risk of chemicals to humans. IARC Monograph No. 19. IARC, Lyon 1974, pp. 314 ff.
17. Frei, R. W., Nielen, M. W. F., Brinkman, U. A. T. H.: Handling of Environmental and biological samples via precolumn technologies. Inter. J. Environ. Chem. *25* (1986), 3–35
18. Fukushima, S., Shibata, M., Hibino, T., Yoshimura, T., Hirose, M., Ito, N.: Intrahepatic bile duct proliferation induced by 4,4′-diaminodiphenylmethane in rats. Toxicol. Appl. Pharmacol. *48* (1979), 145–155
19. Grayson, M. (ed.): Methylenedianiline. Kirk-Othmer-Encyclopedia of chemical technology, Vol. 2. Wiley and Sons, New York 1978, pp. 338 ff.
20. Henderson, R. F., Bechtold, W. E., Bond, J. A., Sun, J. D.: The Use of Biological Markers in Toxicology. Toxicology *20* (1989), 65–82
21. Schütze, D., Sepai, D., Lewalter, J., Miske, L., Henschler, D., Sabbioni, G.: Biomonitoring of workers exposed to 4,4′-methylenedianiline (MDA) or 4,4′-methylenediphenyldiisocyanate (MDA). Carcinogenesis, (1995) in press
22. Henschler, D. (ed.): Gesundheitsschädliche Arbeitsstoffe. Toxikologisch-arbeitsmedizinische Begründung von MAK-Werten: 4,4′-Diaminodiphenylmethan und -Dihydrochlorid. 12. Lfg. VCH-Verlagsgesellschaft, Weinheim 1987

23. Fairhurst, S., South, D., Williams, C., Cocker, J., Brown, R.: 4,4′-Methylenedianiline. Criteria document for an occupational exposure limit. Health and Safety Executive, HMSO, London 1993
24. Kadlubar, F. F., Miller, J. A., Miller, E. C.: Hepatic microsomal N-glucuronidation and nucleic acid binding of N-hydroxyarylamines in relation to urinary bladder carcinogenesis. Cancer Res. *37* (1977), 805–814
25. Koppelmann, H., Scheuer, P. J., Williams, R.: The liver lesion of the Epping jaundice. Quart. J. Med. *35* (1966), 553–564
26. Koppelmann, H., Robertson, M. H., Sanders, P. G., Ash, I.: The Epping jaundice. Br. Med. J. *1* (1966), 514–516
27. Larroque, M., Vian, L., Blaise, A., Brun, S.: Méthodes de dosage des monomères résiduels des résines époxydiques dans des simultans du vin. J. Chromatogr. *445* (1988), 107–117
28. LeVine, M. J.: Occupational photosensitivity to diaminodiphenylmethane. Cont. Derma. *9* (1983), 488–490
29. Lewalter, J.: Auswertung der arbeitsmedizinischen Vorsorge- und Biomonitoringuntersuchungen von MDA-Belasteten (1980 bis 1992). III MDA review meeting, Straßburg 1993
30. Lewalter, J., Bussmann, R.: Simultanbestimmung von Aminoaromaten in Harn, Plasma und Hämoglobin mit HPLC-ECD. In: Henschler, D. (ed.): Analytische Methoden zur Prüfung gesundheitsschädlicher Arbeitsstoffe. Bd. 2: Analysen in biologischem Material, 11. Lfg., Deutsche Forschungsgemeinschaft, VCH Verlagsgesellschaft, Weinheim 1993
31. McCarthy, D. J., Struck, R. F., Shih, T.-W., Suling, W. J., Hill, D., Enke, S. E.: Disposition and metabolism of the carcinogen reduced Michler's ketone in rats. Cancer Res. *42* (1982), 3475–3479
32. McGill, D. B., Motto, J. D.: An industrial outbreak of toxic hepatitis due to methylene-dianiline. N. Engl. J. Med. *291* (1974), 278–282
33. National Institute for Occupational Safety and Health (NIOSH): 4,4′-methylene-bis-(phenylisocyanate) (MDI). NIOSH Manual of Analytical Methods, Vol. 7, Method No. 347. U. S. Government Printing Office, Washington DC. 1981, pp. 1–13
34. National Institute for Occupational Safety and Health (NIOSH): NIOSH Health hazard evaluation report Boeing Verol Co., HETA 82-146-1388, Philadelphia, PA. Cincinnati, OH., 1983
35. Neumeister, C.E.: Analysis of urine to monitor exposures to benzidine, *o*-Dianisidine, *o*-Toluidine and 4,4′-Methylenedianiline. Appl. Occup. Environ. Hyg. *6* (1991), 953–958
36. Parodi, S., Taningher, M., Russo, P., Pala, M., Tamaro, M., Monti-Bragadin, C.: DNA-damaging activity in vivo and bacterial mutagenicity of sixteen aromatic amines and azo-derivatives, as related quantitatively to their carcinogenicity. Carcinogenicity *2* (1981), 1317–1326
37. Pludre, G., Karlowski, K., Mankowska, M., Woggon, H., Uhde, W.-J.: Toxicological and chemical studies of some epoxy resins and hardeners. I.: Determination of acute and subacute toxicity of phthalic acid anhydride, 4,4′-diaminodiphenylmethane and of the epoxy resin: Epilox EG-34. Acta. Pol. Pharm. *26* (1969), 352–364
38. Rosenberg, C., Savolainen, H.: Mass fragmentographic determination of urinary amine metabolites in rats exposed to degradation products from heated rigid polyurethane. J. Chromatogr. *358* (1986), 385–392
39. Roy, C. W., McSorley, P. D., Syme, I. G.: Methylene dianiline: a new toxic cause of visual failure with hepatitis. Hum. Toxic. *4* (1985), 61–66
40. Seldén, A., Berg, P., Jakobsson, R., Lavel de, J.: Methylene dianiline: assessment of exposure and cancer morbidity in power generator workers. Int. Arch. Occup. Environ. Health *63* (1992), 403–408
41. Skare, N., Schretel, K.R.: Alkaline elution of rat testicular DNA: Detection of DNA strand breaks after in vivo treatment with chemical mutagens. Mutat. Res. *130* (1984), 283–294
42. Steinhoff, D., Grundmann, E.: Zur kanzerogenen Wirkung von 4,4′-Diaminodiphenylmethan und 2,4-Diaminodiphenylmethan. Naturwissenschaften *57* (1970), 247–248
43. Tamura, N., King, Ch.M.: Comparative survival of aminobiphenyl- and aminofluorene-substituted plasmid DNA in *Escherichia coli* Uvrendonuclease deficient strains. Carcinogenesis *11* (1990), 535–540
44. Tanaka, K., Ino, T., Sawahata, T., Marui, S., Igaki, H., Yashima, H.: Mutagenicity of N-acetyl and N,N′-diacetyl derivatives of 3 aromatic amines used as epoxy-resin hardeners. Mutat. Res. *143* (1985), 11–15
45. Talaska, G., Dooley, K.L., Kadlubar, F.F.: Detection and characterization of carcinogen-DNA adducts in exfoliated urothelial cells from 4-aminobiphenyl-treated dogs by 32P-postlabelling and subsequent thin-layer and high-pressure liquid chromatography. Carcinogenesis *11* (1990), 639–646

46. Tiljander, A., Skarping, G.: Determination of 4,4′-methylenedianiline in hydrolysed human urine using liquid chromatography with UV detection and peak identification by absorbance ratio. J. Chromatogr. *511* (1990), 185–194
47. Spezifische Einwirkungsdefinitionen, ZH1/600. Hauptverband der gewerblichen Berufsgenossenschaften, Bonn 1979, pp. 75–78
48. Tiljander, A.: Chromatographic determination of 4,4′-methylenedianiline in biological fluids. Dissertation, Department of Occupational and Environmental Medicine, Lund 1989
49. Tortoreto, M., Catalani, P., Bianchi, M., Blonda, C., Pantarotta, C., Paglialunga, S.: Determination of 4,4′-diaminodiphenylmethane in blood by gasliquid chromatography with electron-capture detection. J. Chromatogr. *262* (1983), 367–372
50. Trippel-Schulte, P., Zeiske, J., Kettrup, A.: Trace analysis of selected benzidine and diaminodiphenylmethane derivates in urine by means of liquid chromatography using precolumn sample preconcentration, UV and electrochemical detection. Chromatogr. *22* (1986), 138–146
51. Vaudaine, Lery, N., Diter, J. N., Droin, M., Chamaillard, C.: Le diamino diphenyl methane: un example de toxicolovigilance dans les ateliers de fabrication de rhone-poulenc-industrie. Journal de Toxicologie Medicale *2* (1982), 207–214
52. Weisburger, E. K., Murthy, A. S. K., Lilja, H. S., Lamb, J. C.: IV: Neoplastic response of F344 rats and B6C3F1 mice to the polymer and dyestuff intermediates 4,4′-methylene bis-(N,N-dimethyl)-benzeneamine, 4,4′-oxydianiline, and 4,4′-methylenedianiline. J. Natl. Cancer Inst. *72* (1984), 1457–1463
53. Winkler, E., Hohaus, E., Felber, E.: High-performance liquid chromatographic separation of ethylenediamine and triethylenetetramine after derivatization with salicylaldehyde-diphenylboron chelate and separation of 4,4′-diaminodiphenylmethane by high-performance liquid chromatography. J. Chromatogr. *436* (1988), 447–454
54. Schütze, D.: Methoden und Grundlagen zum Expositionsnachweis und zur Risikoermittlung von Bis-(4-Aminophenyl)-methan und davon abgeleiteten Industriechemikalien. Dissertation, Universität Würzburg (1993)
55. Bakthavachalam, J., Abdel-Baky, S., Giese, R. W.: Release of 2-aminofluorene from N-(desoxyguanosin-8-yl)-2-aminofluorene by hydrazinolysis. J. Chromatogr. *538* (1991), 447–451
56. Neumann, H. G., Birner, G., Kowallik, P., Schütze, D., Zwirner-Baier, I.: Hemoglobin adducts of N-substituted aryl compounds in exposure control and risk assessment. Environ. Health Perspect. *99* (1993), 65–69

Author: J. Lewalter

Approved by the Working Group: 27th May 1993

Dimethyl sulfate

EKA The correlation between external and internal exposure yields the following data:

Air Dimethyl sulfate ml/m³	mg/m³	Globin N-Methyl valine µg/l blood
0.002	0.010	10
0.006	0.030	13
0.01	0.050	17
0.04	0.200	[40]*

* obtained by extrapolation of the linear regression equation

Sampling: not restricted

Date of evaluation 1996

CAS No. 77-78-1

Synonyms DMS,
Sulfuric acid dimethyl ester
Methyl sulfate

Formula $C_2H_6SO_4$

$(CH_3)_2\ SO_4$

Molecular weight 126.13

Melting point –32 °C

Boiling point 188 °C

Vapour pressure at 20 °C < 1 torr

MAK [last established: 1971] Carcinogenic substance: Section III Category 2 of the List of MAK and BAT Values

TRK value [1998]

	ml/m³	mg/m³
Production	0.02	0.1
Use	0.04	0.2

Essential BAT Value Documentations. DFG, Deutsche Forschungsgemeinschaft

ISBN 3-527-31477-6

1 Metabolism and Kinetics

Dimethyl sulfate is absorbed rapidly after inhalation. According to animal experiments carried out by Mathison *et al.* (11) with rats, the substance has a marked sensory irritative effect on the mucous membranes of the upper respiratory tract, which is obvious at concentrations of about 8 ppm. DNA methylation is detected in the mucous membranes of the nasal cavity, most pronounced in the respiratory mucosa, weaker in the olfactory mucosa and markedly weaker in that of the lungs. Dimethyl sulfate is therefore to be regarded as a powerful methylating agent with particular local effects on the mucosa of the upper respiratory tract.

Five minutes after intravenous administration of dimethyl sulfate doses of 75 mg/kg to rats, the substance was no longer detectable in the blood of the animals (15). According to a metabolism diagram drawn up by Mathison *et al.* (11), dimethyl sulfate is hydrolysed to sulfate and methanol, which in turn via formaldehyde and formiate enters C_1 metabolism or is excreted as formiate. After administration of dimethyl sulfate to rats, urinary excretion of methylated purines was also found (10).

Figure 1 represents a schematic diagram of the known metabolic steps.

2 Critical Toxicity

The reactivity of dimethyl sulfate is the cause of the local irritative effects on the respiratory tract observed in animal experiments (see above) and also the reason for its genotoxic and carcinogenic effects (14). In numerous genotoxicity tests *in vitro* (4) positive results have been found. After inhalation of dimethyl sulfate, tumours of the nasal area and the lungs were found in rats (13). The carcinogenic effects of the substance were also confirmed by Druckrey *et al.* (3).

Druckrey *et al.* (2) reported the occurrence of a bronchial carcinoma in a 47-year-old; the tumour occurred 11 years after industrial exposure to dimethyl sulfate. There are no other reports available of carcinogenic effects of dimethyl sulfate in man. The current database for carcinogenic effects of dimethyl sulfate in man was described by the IARC as "inadequate" (5, 6). In view of the directly alkylating effect of dimethyl sulfate and the very clear results from animal experiments it should, however, be assumed, that dimethyl sulfate can also have carcinogenic effects in man.

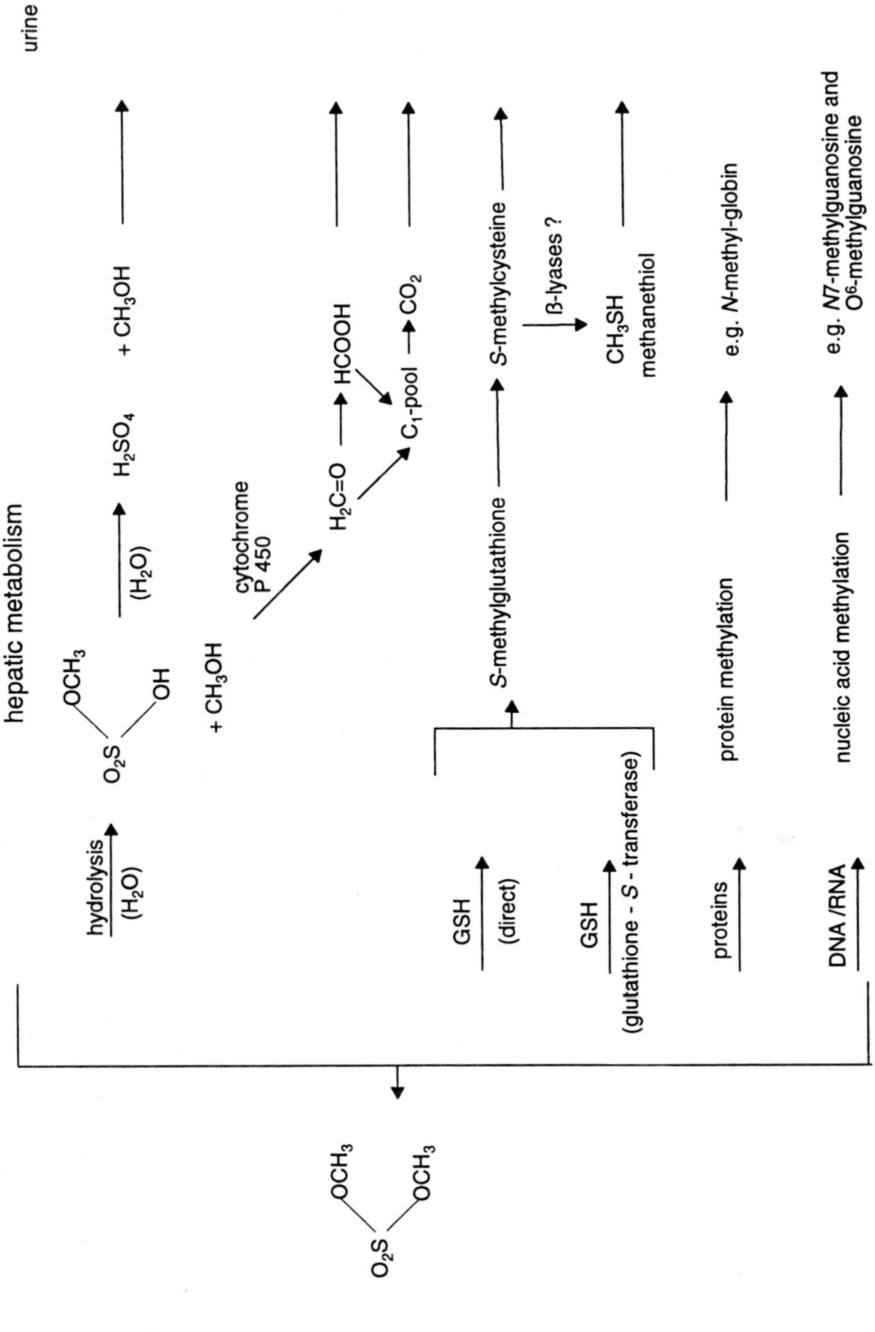

Fig. 1: Metabolism of dimethyl sulfate

3 Exposure and Effects

According to the above, the critical effect of exposure to dimethyl sulfate is to be seen in its ability to alkylate macromolecules of the organism, both locally (epithelia of the respiratory tract) and also systemically. One way of quantifying the systemic effects is to analyse the methylation products of haemoglobin (16–18).

4 Selection of the Indicators

In accordance with the exposure–effect concept, those bio-indicators should be used which allow the effects on the organism to be evaluated. It is known that protein methylation correlates closely with the methylation of DNA.

The determination of *N*-methyl-valine in haemoglobin can be used as a parameter of the methylating potency on the organism exposed to dimethyl sulfate. Investigations with non-exposed persons have shown that also without occupational exposure even in non-smokers there is a detectable background level of *N*-methyl-valine of up to 10.4 µg/l blood, determined after release from the globin of the erythrocytes (7, 8).

5 Methodology

The analysis of *N*-methyl-valine in the erythrocytes is carried out (after Edman degradation of the globin) by GC-MS quantification of the separated hydantoin derivative (1, 7, 8). An analytically tested, practicable method has been published by the working group Analyses of Hazardous Substance in Biological Materials of the DFG Commission for the Investigation of Health Hazards of Chemical Compounds in the Work Area (12). 10 ml venous blood stabilised with EDTA is needed for analysis; the sampling time is not restricted. After sampling, the matrix must be centrifuged and the plasma removed. The isolated erythrocytes can be stored in the refrigerator for 3 days or deep-frozen at –20 °C.

6 Background Exposure

According to Lewalter and Neumann (9) the average background exposure for non-smokers is 7.0 μg *N*-methyl-valine (matrix globin), for smokers 8.5 μg *N*-methyl-valine per litre blood.

7 Evaluation of the Biological Exposure Equivalents for Carcinogenic Substances (EKA)

As a carcinogenic substance, dimethyl sulfate is not given a BAT value. To date no biological value can be given which can be regarded as safe.

A TRK value of 0.1 mg/m^3, valid for the production of dimethyl sulfate, corresponds with about 25 μg *N*-methyl-valine per litre blood. An *N*-methyl-valine concentration of about 40 μg per litre blood corresponds with a TRK value of 0.2 mg/m^3 (use of dimethyl sulfate). Data on the biological monitoring of persons exposed to dimethyl sulfate have only recently been published (8). Further investigations with exposed workers are necessary. The data available to the Commission are represented in Figure 2 (8).

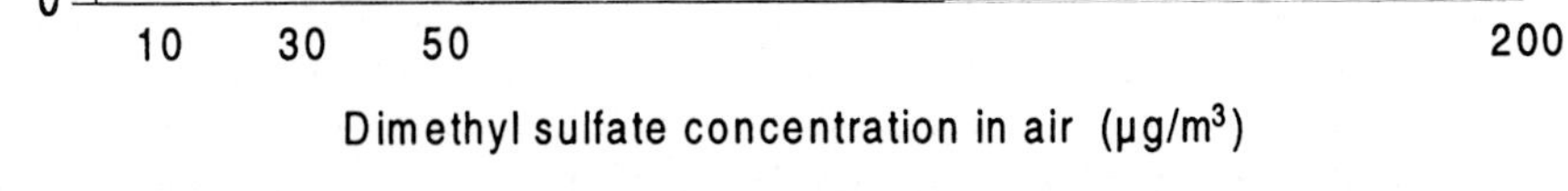

μg DMS/m^3 air	10 (7–15)	30 (19–41)	50 (38–74)	[200] (extrapolated by linear regression)
μg *N*-methylvaline/l blood* {number of persons exposed}	9.7 (4.2–15.8) {24}	13.1 (6.8–19.1) {19}	16.5 (8.2–22.7) {7}	[42]

* Calibration with the *N*-methyl-Val-Leu-anilide standard

Fig. 2: Relationship between external exposure to dimethyl sulfate (DMS) and the formation of adducts with the *N*-terminal valine in globin

8 Interpretation of the Data

When interpreting the data on internal exposure to dimethyl sulfate the influence of smoking habits on the results must be taken into consideration with low values.

By evaluating the *N*-methyl-valine adducts in the erythrocytes, not only the current exposure to dimethyl sulfate, but also exposure up to 3 months previously is recognised.

9 References

1. Bader, M., Lewalter, J., Angerer, J.: Analysis of N-alkylated amino acids in human hemoglobin: evidence for elevated N-methyl-valine levels in smokers, Int. Arch. Occup. Health *67* (1995) 237–242
2. Druckrey, H., Preussmann, R., Nashed, N., Ivankovic, S.: Carcinogene alkylierende Substanzen. I. Dimethylsulfat, carcinogene Wirkung an Ratten und wahrscheinliche Ursache von Berufskrebs, Z. Krebsforsch. *68* (1966) 103–111
3. Druckrey, H., Kruse, H., Preussman, R., Ivankovic, R., Landschütz, C.: Carcinogene alkylierende Substanzen. II. Dimethylsulfat, carcinogene Wirkung an Ratten und wahrscheinliche Ursache von Berufskrebs, Z. Krebsforsch. *74* (1970) 241–273
4. Hoffmann, G.R.: Genetic effects of dimethyl sulfate, diethyl sulfate, and related compounds. Mutat. Res. *75* (1980) 63–129
5. International Agency for Research on Cancer. IARC Monographs on the Evaluation of the Carcinogenic Risk of Chemicals to Man. Vol. 4, Some Aromatic Amines, Hydrazine and Related Substances, N-Nitroso Compounds and Miscellaneous Alkylating Agents (1974) pp. 271–276
6. International Agency for Research on Cancer. IARC Monographs on the Evaluation of the Carcinogenic Risk of Humans – Overall Evaluations of Carcinogenicity: An Updating of IARC Monographs, Vol. 1 - 42, Suppl. 7, (1987) 271–276
7. Lewalter, J.: Monitoring and immunologische Bedeutung von Schadstoffaddukten, Bericht der Österreichischen Gesellschaft für Klinische Chemie (ÖGKC) *17* (1994) 9–18
8. Lewalter, J.: N-Alkylvaline levels in globin as a new type of biomarker in risk assessment of alkylating agents. Int. Arch. Occup. Environ. Health *68* (1996) 519–530
9. Lewalter, J., Neumann, H.G.: Biologische Arbeitsstoff-Toleranzwerte (Biomonitoring), Teil VIII; Bewertung der Hintergrundbelastungen bei beruflich nicht-exponierten Personen, Arbeitsmed. Sozialmed. Umweltmed. *31, 10* (1996) 418–432
10. Löfroth, G., Osterman-Golkar, S., Wennerberg, R.: Urinary excretion of methylated purines following inhalation of dimethyl sulphate. Experientia *30* (1974) 641–642
11. Mathison, B.H., Tylor, M.L., Bogdanffy, S.: Dimethyl sulfate uptake and methylation of DNA in rat respiratory tissues following acute inhalation. Fundamental and Applied Toxicology *28* (1995) 255–263
12. Van Sittert, N.J.: N-2-Cyanoethyl-Valin, N-2-Hydroxyethyl-Valin, N-Methyl-Valin (zum Nachweis einer Belastung/Beanspruchung durch Acrylnitril, Ethylenoxid sowie methylierende Substanzen) in: Angerer, J., Schaller, K.H. (Eds.): Analysen in biologischem Material, Deutsche Forschungsgemeinschaft, Bd 2, 12. Lieferung (1996) and in English translation
13. Schlögel, F., Bannasch, P.: Toxicity and carcinogenic properties of inhaled dimethyl sulfate. Naunyn-Schmiedeberg's Arch. Pharmacol. *266* (1970) 441

14. Swann, P. F., Magee, P.N.: Nitrosamine-induced carcinogenesis. The alkylation of nucleic acids of the rat by N-methyl-N-nitrosourea, dimethylnitrosamine, dimethyl sulphate und methyl methane sulphonate, Biochem. J. *110* (1968) 37–47
15. Swann, P.F.: The rate of breakdown of methyl methane sulphonate, dimethyl sulphate and N-methyl-N-nitrosourea in the rat. Biochem. J. *110* (1968) 49–52
16. Törnqvist, M., Osterman-Golkar, S., Klutiainen, A., Harms-Ringdahl, M., Granath, F., Ehrenberg, L.: Methylations in human haemoglobin, Mutation Research *204* (1988) 521–529
17. Törnqvist, M., Svertengren, M., Ericsson, C.H.: Methylation in hemoglobin from monzygotic twins discordant for cigarette smoking: hereditary and tobacco-related factors. Chem.-Biol. Interact. *82* (1992) 92–98
18. Törnqvist, M., Landing, H.H.: Hemoglobin adducts for in vivo dose monitoring and cancer risk estimation. JOEM *37* (1995) 1077–1085

Authors: J. Lewalter, H.M. Bolt
Approved by the Working Group: November 1996

Ethylene oxide

EKA The correlation between external and internal exposure yields the following data:

Air ethylene oxide (ml/m³)	Air ethylene oxide (mg/m³)	Whole blood hydroxy-ethylvaline (µg/l)
0.5	0.92	45
1	1.83	90
2	3.66	180
3	5.49	260
4	7.32	350
5	9.15	440

Sampling: no restrictions

Date of evaluation 1993

MAK [last established: 1984] Carcinogenic substance: category IIIA2 of the List of MAK and BAT Values

1 Haemoglobin Adducts

Due to its electrophilic properties ethylene oxide reacts directly with cellular macromolecules (10, 4, 34, 39, 38). In addition to DNA adduct formation, in particular hydroxyethyl adducts of cysteine, histidine and the N-terminal valine in haemoglobin are described. The last have been suggested for biological monitoring of persons exposed to ethylene oxide (30, 11). These alkylation products are enriched by use of a modified Edman degradation of the haemoglobin (37).

2 Evaluation of Exposure Equivalents

Exposure equivalents for the formation of hydroxyethylvaline in human haemoglobin can be calculated with the formula given by Denk (5)

Essential BAT Value Documentations. DFG, Deutsche Forschungsgemeinschaft

ISBN 3-527-31477-6

$$\text{HOEtVal [nmol/g Hb]} = \frac{P_{EO} \cdot t_{1/2}\,ery \cdot RC_{EO} \cdot 10^9}{\dfrac{\ln 2}{t_{1/2_{EO}}}}$$

where

P_{EO} is the uptake of ethylene oxide into the organism per kg body weight and day [mol/(kg · d)]
$t_{1/2}ery$ is the half-life of the erythrocytes [d] = 63
RC_{EO} is the reaction constant of the reaction of ethylene oxide with the N-terminal valine of haemoglobin [kg/(g · h)] = $5 \cdot 10^{-5}$
$t_{1/2_{EO}}$ is the half-life of ethylene oxide in the organism [h] = 42/60

A detailed calculation can be found in Filser et al. (13).

Denk (5) calculates a value of 42 minutes for the half-life of ethylene oxide in humans from the results of measurements which Brugnone et al. (3) carried out in employees exposed to ethylene oxide. Hattis (19) estimated a half-life of 41 minutes using the same data and a physiological pharmacokinetic model. Filser and Bolt (12) obtained a similar value of 39 minutes for humans using an allometric extrapolation of the half-life of 6 minutes determined in the rat. In rats, Filser and Bolt (12) found that 40 % of the substance inhaled per respiratory minute volume was cleared from the lung per minute. Observations with other readily water-soluble gases (5) indicate that this value can be applied to humans which means that 40 % of the ethylene oxide inhaled per unit of time is absorbed by the organism. Under these conditions and on the assumption of a half-life of 42 minutes (5), a steady state constant of 2.7 can be calculated for the accumulation of ethylene oxide in the organism. Correspondingly, Brugnone et al. (3) measured a 2.5-fold accumulation of ethylene oxide in the blood compared to the concentration in the ambient air.

From this data, exposure equivalents for hydroxyethylvaline in the haemoglobin of 1.8–18.1 nmol/g or 45–440 µg/l blood could be calculated using the formula given by Törnqvist et al. (37) for an air concentration of 0.5–5 ml/m^3 and an alveolar air concentration of 0.12–1.2 ml/m^3, assuming that 1 litre blood contains approx. 150 g haemoglobin (Tab. 1).

Tab. 1: EKA values for ethylene oxide

Air Ethylene oxide (ml/m^3)	Air Ethylene oxide (mg/m^3)	Alveolar air Ethylene oxide (ml/m^3)	Alveolar air Ethylene oxide (mg/m^3)	Blood HOEtVAL (nmol/g haemoglobin)	Blood HOEtVAL (µg/l)
0.5	0.92	0.12	0.22	1.8	45
1	1.83	0.24	0.44	3.6	90
2	3.66	0.48	0.88	7.2	180
3	5.49	0.72	1.32	10.9	260
4	7.32	0.96	1.76	14.5	350
5	9.15	1.2	2.2	18.1	440

For P_{EO} the formula $P_{EO} = C \cdot Q_{alv} \cdot 40\ \%$ was used where C_{alv} represents the concentration of ethylene oxide in the alveolar air. Q_{alv} was assumed to be 288 l kg^{-1} · d^{-1} and an exposure of 40 hours/week was taken as a basis.

Prerequisite for the theoretical derivation of these exposure equivalents is the notion of a linear function between the internal ethylene oxide dose and the external ethylene oxide exposure concentration. This has been demonstrated for the rat up to concentrations of 100 ppm (12, 19), and for humans up to at least 8 ppm by the investigations of Brugnone et al. (3). In inhalation studies with rats a linear relationship between exposure concentrations (0–110 ppm) and the level of haemoglobin adducts was also found (35, 31). The hydroxyethylation of haemoglobin bears a direct relationship to the hydroxyethylation of DNA (9, 31, 11, 29, 33). After short-term exposure in the concentration range between 1 and 33 ppm the hydroxyethylation of haemoglobin and of the liver DNA of the rat was directly proportional to the air concentration (33). With constant exposure concentration a direct proportionality between exposure duration and hydroxyethylation of the guanine was found (14).

More recent findings by Föst et al. (15), which suggest an enzyme dimorphism of the glutathione-S-transferase in human erythrocytes, call into question the validity of extrapolation to humans of functions deduced in animal experiments for the haemoglobin binding of ethylene oxide. Whether the level of internal exposure in individuals with slow adduct formation may be underestimated has yet to be clarified.

3 Relationships to Carcinogenic Risk

The linear relationship given also corresponds to linear relationships in the given concentration range between external exposure and carcinogenic risk. Estimation of this risk was carried out for the mutagenic effects of ethylene oxide by Latarjet et al. (25), by Ehrenberg et al. (9) and by Kolman et al. (24) by means of a so-called rad-equivalent approach. More recent estimations use a rad-equivalence factor deduced from empirical data from Denk (5) and from Denk and Filser (6). The authors also calculate the cancer risk allometrically by transfer of observations in rats to humans. For exposure of humans to 1 ppm ethylene oxide 40 hours per week for 45 years the cancer risk was estimated allometrically as 1.04 per 100 exposed persons. Using the rad-equivalence factor the risk for this exposure was estimated as being between 1.7 and 8.5 per 100 exposed persons. Corresponding to the notion of a linear dependence between risk and air concentration there is for an airborne concentration of 3 ppm a 3-fold higher cancer risk. The cancer risk from ethylene oxide in humans was also determined using a rad-equivalence factor by the research group associated with Ehrenberg (38). The risk estimation yielded a 20-fold higher value than that calculated by Denk (5) and Denk and Filser (6). The differing values are due to different assumptions for the rad-equivalence factors and for the half-life of ethylene oxide in the body. Not only the well-founded derivation of the factors used by Denk (5) and Denk and Filser (6) but also epidemiological observations by Hogstedt et al. (23) and Gardner et al. (16), which suggest an even lower cancer risk, speak for the somewhat greater plausibility of the risk assessment by Denk (5) and Denk and Filser (6). Four smaller epidemiological studies carried out predominantly with persons exposed to mixtures (21, 36, 22, 23) indicate that ethylene oxide induces malignant diseases of the lymphatic and haemotopoietic systems (1) and stomach carcinoma. These observations stand in contrast with the negative epidemiological findings of Morgan et al. (27), Gardner et al. (16), Hagmar et al. (20) and Wong et al. (40). The carcinogenic effect of ethylene oxide has been proved without doubt in animal experiments (7, 8, 35, 26, 17, 18, 28).

4 Methodology

The pentafluorophenylhydantoin derivative of hydroxyethylvaline produced in the modified Edman degradation according to Törnqvist et al. (37) is transformed into the trimethylsilyl ether derivative (32) and then determined selectively with the GC/MS technique on the mass m/z 440 (molecule-ion). The deuterated analogous compound serves as an internal standard.

5 Interpretation of the Data

N-Hydroxyethylvaline can also regularly be found as a haemoglobin adduct in persons not occupationally exposed. As the proved endogenous ethylene production in the organism does not fully explain the measured value (5), it must be assumed that ethylene is taken up from the environment in regionally greatly differing amounts. This has been analytically proved for industrialised regions (review in 5). Further uptake of ethylene has been demonstrated in cigarette smokers (37, 11, 32). Törnqvist et al. give 57 ± 25 pmol/g as the median value for non-smokers and 289 ± 138 pmol/g as the median value for smokers. Passingham et al. (32) describe a correlation between the formation of the hydroxyethylvaline adduct in haemoglobin and the number of cigarettes smoked daily. The highest value determined for 30 cigarettes/day was below the lowest given exposure level of 0.5 ml/m^3 ethylene oxide which led to an adduct level of 1.8 nmol/g Hb. It should nevertheless be taken into account in the interpretation of the data.

The correlation given does not apply for short-term exposures of a few hours or single days but to long-term activities with regularly recurring exposures. Greatly fluctuating exposures on different days can also be determined as the effect is cumulative. A definite sampling time is not necessary.

6 Conclusions

The applicability of the given exposure equivalents for biological monitoring has not been deduced directly from observations in humans but theoretically from experimental data in rats and humans. They correspond well, however, with data obtained experimentally in humans (20). Thus Bryant and Osterman-Golkar (2) give for an ethylene exposure level of 1 ppm a HOEtVal concentration of 2.4 nmol/g Hb. The exposure equivalents seem, however, as provisional equivalents to be sufficiently well-founded. They correlate roughly with the carcinogenic risk caused by exposure. They can only be used strictly with non-smokers as above all the uptake of ethylene in cigarette smoke leads to a higher internal exposure of the smoker to ethylene oxide. In small amounts ethylene is also formed endogenously and taken up from the environment. The determination of hydroxyethylvaline makes it possible to check exposure conditions at longer intervals of weeks or months. Whether a dimorphism of the erythrocytic glutathione transferase can result in underestimation of the internal exposure to ethylene oxide in individuals with slow adduct formation is at present awaiting clarification.

7 References

1. Bisanti, L., Maggini, M., Raschetti, R., Spila Alegiani, S., Menniti Ippolito, F., Caffari, B., Segnan, N., Ponti, A.: Cancer mortality in ethylene oxide workers. B. J. Ind. Med. *50* (1993), 317–324
2. Bryant, M. S., Osterman-Golkar, S.: Hemoglobin Adducts as Dosimeters of Exposure to DNA-Reactive Chemicals. CIIT *11* (1991), 1–12
3. Brugnone, F., Perbellini, L., Pasini, F., Bertolucci, G. B., DeRosa, E.: Ethylene oxide exposure: Biological monitoring by analysis of alveolar air and blood. Int. Arch. Occup. Environ. Health. *28* (1986), 105–112
4. Calleman, C. J., Ehrenberg, L., Jansson, B., Osterman-Golkar, S., Segerbäck, D., Svensson, K., Wachtmeister, C. A.: Monitoring and risk assessment by means of alkyl groups in hemoglobin in persons occupationally exposed to ethylene oxide. J. Environ. Pathol. Toxicol. *2* (1978), 427–442
5. Denk, B.: Abschätzung des kanzerogenen Risikos von Ethylen und Ethylenoxid für den Menschen durch Speziesextrapolation von der Ratte unter Berücksichtigung der Pharmakokinetik. Dissertation, GSF-Bericht 20/90, München 1990
6. Denk, B., Filser, J. G.: Abschätzung des durch Ethylen und Ethylenoxid bedingten kanzerogenen Risikos für den Menschen – Vergleich mit dem Risiko durch endogenes Ethylen. In: Schuckmann, R., Schopper-Jochum, S. (eds.): Berufskrankheiten, krebserzeugende Arbeitsstoffe, Biological Monitoring. 80. Jahrestagung der Deutschen Gesellschaft für Arbeitsmedizin e.V., 28.–31. Mai 1990, Gentner Verlag, Stuttgart 1991, pp. 397–401
7. Dunkelberg, H.: Carcinogenic activity of ethylene oxide and its reaction products 2-chloroethanol, 2-bromoethanol, ethylene glycol and diethylene glycol. I. Carcinogenicity of ethylene oxide in comparison with 1,2-propylene oxide after subcutaneous, administration in mice. (Ger.) Zbl. Bakt. Hyg. I. Abt. Orig. B. *174* (1981), 383–404
8. Dunkelberg, H.: Carcinogenicity of ethylene oxide and 1,2-propylene oxide upon intragastric administration to rats. Br. J. Cancer *46* (1982), 924–933
9. Ehrenberg, L., Hiesche, K. D., Osterman-Golkar, S., Wennberg, I.: Evaluation of genetic risks of alkylating agents: tissue doses in the mouse from air contaminated with ethylene oxide. Mutat. Res. *24* (1974), 83–103
10. Ehrenberg, L., Osterman-Golkar, S., Segerbäck, D., Svensson, K., Calleman, C. J.: Evaluation of genetic risks of alkylating agents. III. Alkylation of hemoglobin after metabolic conversion of ethene to ethene oxide in vivo. Mutat. Res. *45* (1977), 175–184
11. Farmer, P. B., Neumann, H.-G., Henschler, D.: Estimation of exposure of man to substances reacting with macromolecules. Arch. Toxicol. *60* (1987), 251–260
12. Filser, J. G., Bolt, H. M.: Inhalation pharmacokinetics based on gas uptake studies VI. Comparative evaluation of ethylene oxide and butadiene monoxide as exhaled reactive metabolites of ethylene and 1,3-butadiene in rats. Arch. Toxicol. *55* (1984), 219–233
13. Filser, J. G., Denk, B., Törnqvist, M., Kessler, W., Ehrenberg, L.: Pharmacokinetics of ethylene in man; body burden with ethylene oxide and hydroxyethylation of hemoglobin due to endogenous and environmental ethylene. Arch Tox. *66* (1992), 157-163

14. Föst, U., Marczynski, B., Kasemann, R., Peter, H.: Determination of 7-(2-hydroxyethyl)guanine with gas chromatography/mass spectrometry as a parameter for genotoxicity of ethylene oxide. Arch. Toxicol. Suppl. *13* (1989), 250–253
15. Föst, U., Hallier, E., Ottenwälder, H., Bolt, H. M., Peter, H.: Distribution of Ethylene Oxide in Human Blood and its Implications for Biomonitoring. Human & Experimental Toxicology *10* (1991), 25–31
16. Gardner, M. J., Coggon, D., Panett, B., Harris, E. C.: Workers exposed to ethylene oxide: a follow up study. Br. J. Ind. Med. *46* (1989), 860–865
17. Garman, R. H., Snellings, W. M., Maronpot, R. R.: Brain tumors in F-344 rats associated with chronic inhalation exposure to ethylene oxide. Neurotoxicology *6* (1985), 117–138
18. Garman, R. H., Snellings, W. M., Maronpot, R. R.: Frequency, size and location of brain tumours in F-344 rats chronically exposed to ethylene oxide. Food Chem. Toxicol. *24* (1986), 145–153
19. Hattis, D.: A pharmacokinetic/mechanism-based analysis of the carcinogenic risk of ethylene oxide. Center for Technology, Policy and Industrial Development at the Massachusetts Institute of Technology, Cambridge 1987
20. Hagmar L., Welinder, H., Linden, K., Attewell, R., Osterman-Golkar, S., Törnqvist, M.: An epidemiological study of cancer risk among workers exposed to ethylene oxide using hemoglobin adducts to validate environmental exposure assessments. Int. Arch. Occup. Environ. Health *63* (1991), 271–277
21. Hogstedt, C., Rohlen, O., Berndtsson, B. S., Axelson, O., Ehrenberg, L.: A cohort study of mortality and cancer incidence in ethylene oxide production workers. Br. J. Ind. Med. *36* (1979), 276–280
22. Hogstedt, C., Aringer, L., Gustavsson, A.: Ethylene oxide and cancer – Review of the literature and follow-up of two studies (Swed.) Arbete Hälsa *49* (1984), 1–32
23. Hogstedt, C., Aringer, L., Gustavsson, A.: Epidemiological support for ethylene oxide as a cancer causing agent. J. Am. Med. Assoc. *255* (1986), 1575–1578
24. Kolman, A., Segerbäck, D., Osterman-Golkar, S.: Estimation of the cancer risk of genotoxic chemicals by the rad-equivalence approach. In: Bartsch, H., Hemminki, K., O'Neill, I.K. (eds.) Methods for detecting in DNA damaging agents in humans: application in cancer epidemiology and prevention. IARC Scientific Publications, No. 89. IARC, Lyon 1988
25. Latarjet, R., Averbeck, D., Levy, S., Poirier, V.: Quantitative comparison of genotoxic effects of atomic energy and fossil-fuelled energy. Radequivalences for ethylene, ethylene oxide and formaldehyde – consequences for decisions at Government level. Proc. Int. Symp. on Health Impacts on Different Sources of Energy, International Atomic Energy Agency. No. IAEM-SM-254/49, Vienna 1981
26. Lynch, D. W., Lewis, T. R., Moorman. W. J., Burg, J. R., Groth, D. H., Khan, A., Ackerman, L. J., Cockrell, B. Y.: Carcinogenic and toxicological effects of inhaled ethylene oxide and propylene oxide. Toxicol. Appl. Pharmacol. *76* (1984), 69–84
27. Morgan, R.W., Claxton, K. W., Divine, B. J., Kaplan, S. D., Harris, V. B.: J. Occup. Med. *23* (1981), 767
28. National Toxicology Program: Toxicology and Carcinogenesis Studies of Ethylene Oxide (CAS No. 75-21-8) in B6C3Fl Mice (Inhalation Studies) (NTP TR 326; NIH Publ. No. 86-2582), Research Triangle Park, NC (1986)
29. Neumann, H. G.: Hemoglobin binding in control of exposure to and risk assessment of aromatic amines. In: Bartsch, H., Hemminki, K., O'Neill, I. K. (eds.): Methods for detecting DNA damaging agents in humans: applications in cancer epidemiology and prevention. IARC Scientific Publications, Nr. 89. IARC, Lyon 1988, pp. 157–165
30. Osterman-Golkar, S., Ehrenberg, L., Segerbäck, D., Hällstöm, I.: Evaluation of genetic risks of alkylating agents. II. Hemoglobin as a dose monitor. Mutat. Res. *34* (1976), 1–10
31. Osterman-Golkar, S.: Tissue doses in man: Implications in risk assessment. In: Hayes, A. W., Schnell, R. C., Miya, T. S. (eds.): Developments in the Science and Practice of Toxicology Elsevier, Amsterdam 1983, pp. 289–298
32. Passingham, B. J., Farmer, P. B., Bailey, E., Brooks, A. G. F., Yates, D. W.: 2-Hydroxyethylation of Hemoglobin in man. In: Bartsch, H., Hemminki, K., O'Neill, I. K. (eds): Methods for detecting DNA-damaging agents in humans: application in cancer epidemiology and prevention. IARC Scientific Publications, No. 89. IARC, Lyon 1988, pp. 279–285
33. Potter, D., Blair, D., Davies, R., Watson, W. P., Wright, A. S.: The relationship between alkylation of hemoglobin and DNA in Fisher 344 rats exposed to (^{14}C)ethylene oxide. Arch. Toxicol. Suppl. *13* (1989), 254–257
34. Segerbäck, D.: Alkylation of DNA and hemoglobin in the mouse after exposure to ethene and ethene oxide. Chem.-Biol. Interact. *45* (1983), 139

35. Snellings, W. M., Weil, C. S., Maronpot, R. R.: A two-year inhalation study of the carcinogenic potential of ethylene oxide in Fisher 344 rats. Toxicol. Appl. Pharmacol. *75* (1984), 105–117
36. Thiess, A. M., Frentzel-Beyme, R., Link, R., Stocker, W. G.: Mortality study on employees exposed to alkylene oxides (ethylene oxide/propylene oxide) and their derivatives. In: Prevention of Occupational Cancer – International Symposium. Occupational Safety and Health Series No. 46, International Labour Office, Geneva 1981, pp. 249–259
37. Törnqvist, M., Osterman-Golkar, S., Kautiainen, A., Jensen, S., Farmer, P. B., Ehrenberg, L.: Tissue doses of ethylene oxide in cigarette smokers determined from adduct levels in hemoglobin. Carcinogenesis *7* (1986), 39–42
38. Törnqvist, M., Gustafsson, B., Kautiainen, A., Harms-Ringdahl, M., Granath, F., Ehrenberg, L.: Unsaturated lipids and intestinal bacteria as sources of endogenous production of ethene and ethylene oxide. Carcinogenesis *10* (1989), 39–42
39. van Sittert, N. J., DeJong, G., Clare, M. G., Davies, R., Dean, B. J., Waren, L. J., Wright, A. S.: Cytogenetic, immunological, and hematological effects in workers in an ethylene oxide manufacturing plant. Br. J. Ind. Med. *42* (1985), 19–26
40. Wong, O., Trent, L. S.: An epidemiological study of workers potentially exposed to ethylene oxide. B. J. Ind. Med. *50* (1993), 308–316

Authors: K. Norpoth, H. M. Bolt
Approved by the Working Group: 5th May 1994

Hydrogen fluoride and inorganic fluorine compounds (Fluorides)

BAT	7.0 mg fluoride/g creatinine Sampling time: end of shift 4.0 mg fluoride/g creatinine Sampling time: prior to next shift
Date of evaluation	1983
Substances	Hydrogen fluoride Hydrofluoric acid Inorganic fluorides
MAK	
Fluorides	2.5 mg/m^3 (calculated as fluorine)
Fluorides and hydrogen fluoride where both are simultaneously present	2.5 mg/m^3
hydrogen fluoride	3 ml/m^3 (ppm) 2 mg/m^3

1 Metabolism and Kinetics

The extraordinarily reactive element fluorine exists in elementary form only under certain conditions. It has, despite high toxicity, no practical-toxicological meaning. Its character as an irritant gas is the most important of the effects of elementary fluorine intoxication (1). The conspicuous changes in the tracheal, bronchial and alveolar epithelia after inhalation of fluorine involve tissue necrosis (2), apparently a result of the fluoridation of proteins.

Under the physiological conditions in the respiratory tract (humidity, temperature) after inhalation of elementary fluorine approx. 10 % hydrogen fluoride is formed (3) so that the possible internal fluoride exposure is therefore greatly below the fluoride exposure resulting from direct hydrogen fluoride or fluoride intoxication.

The absorption, distribution, retention and excretion of hydrogen fluoride and its inorganic compounds in the human organism have been investigated by numerous research groups (4–7).

The uptake of hydrogen fluoride and its inorganic compounds takes place via the respiratory tract, the skin and the gastro-intestinal tract. Acute exposures to hydrogen fluoride or fluoride ions cause, after a dose-dependent latent period, local damage to the skin and mucous membranes. After chronic exposure they lead to changes in

Essential BAT Value Documentations. DFG, Deutsche Forschungsgemeinschaft

ISBN 3-527-31477-6

the skeletal system and in the teeth due to binding of the calcium. In calcium metabolism fluoride can cause both the formation of osteoporosis (decalcification of the bones) and also, via an increased heterotopic deposition of calcium salts, osteosclerosis (8).

In the physiological concentration range of approx. 1 mg/day, fluorides are necessary in the body as essential trace elements for the calcification of the bone and hardening of the enamel of the teeth. An adult takes in between 0.5 and 5 mg as fluoride anions daily with food.

In the adult organism with an intake of fluoride with food of less than 0.4 mg fluoride/day the plasma fluoride concentration is between 0.01 and 0.04 mg/l (9, 10). This plasma value increases after a single oral dose of 1.5–10 mg fluoride (3.3–22 mg NaF) within 30 minutes to a plasma fluoride value of 0.06–0.4 mg/l and then decreases with a half-life between 2.0 and 9.0 hours.

In blood plasma approx. 72 % of the total blood fluoride content is present (11) without protein binding in the form of free fluoride ions (12). Both with healthy and osteoporotic patients approx. 50–70 % of the internal fluoride exposure (fluoride body burden) is excreted with an approx. 12-hour biological half-life via the urine, approx. 10 % via the faeces and approx. 20 % via perspiration. The excretion rate is said to decrease with increasing internal fluoride exposure (13, 14). Part of the internal fluoride exposure is deposited long-term in the skeleton (12, 15, 16). With increasing fluoride exposure the bone deposit seems to increase marginally (14).

The norm value of the fluoride content in the bone (hip bone) of unexposed adults not exposed is approx. 1 mg fluoride/g bone ash. Even without additional industrial exposure the fluoride content of the bone increases physiologically with increasing age (17). The threshold limit value of pathological fluoride exposure in the bone is approx. 4.0 mg fluoride/g bone ash (18). Increased internal fluoride exposures can block essential calcium metabolism (possibly also carbohydrate metabolism) by chemical binding to calcium and magnesium ions and the consequent inhibition of important enzymes (19, 20–22).

2 Critical Toxicity

In industrial practice at present above all occasional accidents still lead to acute exposures to high doses of gaseous fluorides (HF) with irritation of the mucous membranes in the eyes, nose and respiratory tract.

The possible effects of external fluoride exposures should be differentiated as acute illness due to local skin burns, irritation of the respiratory tract, as well as gastrointestinal effects and chronic damage with characteristic effects on the bone system (fluorosis, osteosclerosis) (23).

Local exposure to low concentrations of hydrogen fluoride and hydrofluoric acid, but also to the hydrogen fluorides formed by the hydrolysis of labile fluorides, causes local reddening and burning of the skin. In higher concentrations these substances penetrate the skin and lead to ulceration and necrosis. The most severe systemic effects of intoxication are caused by the inhibition of essential enzymes. After oral intake burning occurs in the mouth, oesophagus and stomach. The inhalation of fluorides as gases or dusts leads to coughing, sometimes also to laryngeal and bronchial spasms, shortness of breath. The symptoms can subside after low concentrations (10–20 ml/m^3) and return after a latent period of 10–25 hours with coughing, shortness of breath, bronchitis, cyanosis and lung oedema. With higher concentrations the latent period is shorter or is lacking completely.

Chronic occupational exposure to more than 10–80 mg fluoride/day can cause fluorosis after several years (8). This characteristic disturbance of the mineral metabolism leads in the bone system with the hardening and solidification of the compacta to the stiffening of joints and the spine, to brittleness of the nails etc. (24, 25)

The acute intake of 1.5 g hydrofluoric acid leads to immediate death of an adult (26), while on the other hand for sodium fluoride 5–10 g is the minimum lethal dose.

Blood fluorine concentrations of on average 8.0 mg/l (2.6–16) led in 10 cases after inhalation or absorption to death (27).

The long-term fluoride deposition in the bones with the development of fluorosis are to be regarded as the chronic toxic effects of hydrogen fluoride and its inorganic compounds which are relevant for the evaluation of a BAT value. The critical target organ is thus the skeletal system.

3 Exposure and Effects

Within the framework of the exposure and effect concept, the concentration of the hydrofluoric acid and fluorides in the air of the workplace leads to the external exposure of the test persons. Their maximum permitted value is regulated by the appropriate MAK value. On this basis the acute toxic effects of hydrogen fluoride or hydrofluoric acid, which include extremely painful inflammation of the skin and the mucous membranes and which can quickly spread by further diffusion of the undissociated acid, are confined exclusively to accidents. The internal fluoride exposure should be limited to within the exposure range stipulated in the BAT concept due to the toxic effects of higher fluoride concentrations, as with chronic exposure fundamental changes in the bone structure in the sense of osteosclerosis, osteoporosis and mixtures of these forms of osteopathy can occur (28–30). As in particular the speed of the renal excretion of the fluorides is limited, chronic fluoride exposures lead to extensive fluoride deposition in the bones. The extent of fluorosis can be ascertained by a combination of histological investigations and microchemical fluoride determination in bone biopsies from the crest of the ilium (18).

Generally the physiological fluoride concentration in the bone increases with increasing age. The fluoride in drinking water can also lead to increased bone fluoride values. The identification of fluoride in the bones is the only indicator able to recognise chronic fluoride exposure after the end of exposure in every case and before the detection of damage is possible by X-ray examination (31). The determination of the fluoride content in human bones (32) is not a method for routine health surveillance because the necessary samples must be obtained by biopsy (17). Rather, the possible internal fluoride body burden must be determined by other biological indicators, whereby the fluoride analysis in the blood and/or urine samples has proved appropriate for the correlating evaluation of internal fluoride exposure (10, 14, 33). A direct linear relationship between the external fluoride exposure and the renal fluoride excretion was ascertained. Furthermore, it has been proven that in the dynamic metabolic equilibrium, mainly after at least 3 working days, the fluoride concentration of a single post-shift urine sample significantly correlated with the daily total fluoride excretion. With increasing external fluoride exposure, combined with increasing internal fluoride exposure, the amount of the urinary fluoride excretion does not increase proportionately any more. An increased fluoride deposition in the organism is the consequence. Thus, individual urinary fluoride values, even if they are measured in the post-shift urine, can only determine the acute fluoride exposure but cannot give any sufficient indication of the extent of a long-term internal fluoride exposure. This circumstance is independent of whether the monitoring of the internal fluoride exposure is carried out in 24-hour urine or in spontaneous urine samples after the end of an exposure phase (4).

A differentiation between acute and chronic fluoride exposure can only take place by multiple measurement of the urinary fluoride levels which provide an indication of the possible fluoride body burden.

In the extensive literature (34) of almost exclusively animal-experimental studies the correlations of internal fluoride exposure, with among other things effects on the bone metabolism, the blood coagulation system, and with very differing enzyme activities in the liver metabolism, have been investigated and demonstrated mainly for unphysiological, chronic internal exposure doses greatly over 10 ml/m^3 fluoride which are not found in practice.

Effect parameters that can be used in practice are not available at present. The continuous monitoring of the urinary fluoride excretion of persons exposed to fluoride guarantees an adequate prevention in the detection of lower values.

4 Selection of the Indicators

The fluoride concentrations in whole blood as well as in urine can be regarded as indicators of internal fluoride exposure (12, 33). The fluoride determination in the urine is preferred in practice as an indicator of internal fluoride exposure for exposed employees (14, 35). The additional or even exclusive determination of fluoride concentrations in the plasma is not very meaningful due to the short half-life. It is recommended in a few cases for estimating current fluoride exposures (36, 37), the differential diagnosis of metabolic disturbances (38–41), the monitoring of exposure with anaesthetics containing fluorine (42) and the direct monitoring of therapy of accidental fluorine intoxications (26, 27, 43, 44).

In the urine samples of unexposed test persons, fluoride concentrations between 0.2 and 3.2 mg/l with a clear dependency on the fluoride uptake with food could be detected (33). The normal fluoride-blood or fluoride-plasma concentration is 0.01 to 0.04 mg/l (9, 10). During chronic external fluoride exposure of 2.65 mg $fluoride/m^3$

(the MAK value is 2.5 mg/m^3) the urinary fluoride excretion increases on average to 4.5 mg/l (2.1 – 14.7 mg/l) (33).

The evaluation of internal fluoride effects is at present causing much controversy without any relevant occupational medical conclusion being apparent. The significant internal fluoride exposure is determined via the urinary fluoride excretion as there is a good correlation between the external fluoride exposure and the renal fluoride excretion as well as between the fluoride concentration of a post-shift urine sample and the daily excretion of internal fluoride exposure, especially in the dynamic metabolic equilibrium after at least 3 working days. No statistical correlation, however, combines the urinary fluoride excretion with the internal fluoride exposure caused by long-term, chronic fluoride exposure (14).

In the occupational medical health surveillance of test persons with significant indications of greatly increased internal fluoride exposure, after accidental fluoride intoxication or chronic urinary fluoride excretion of over 10 mg/g creatinine for example, the determination of the serum calcium level (45, 46) and the urinary calcium excretion (46, 47) should be included as a matter of principle for the preventive evaluation of internal fluoride effects.

5 Methodology

For the determination of the fluoride content in plasma and urine the DFG Commission for the Investigation of Health Hazards of Chemical Compounds in the Work Area in the Working Group "Analytische Chemie" ("Analytical Chemistry") in the loose-leaf collection "Analysen in biologischem Material" ("Analyses of Hazardous Substances in Biological Materials") has compiled a collection of tested analytical methods (48). The most suitable procedure is the ion selective electrode. For statistical quality control according to the TRgA 410 (regulation of hazardous chemical compounds in the work area) control materials (urine) are available (49).

The determination of the calcium in the plasma and urine can take place photometrically according to well-known clinical-chemical determination methods (e.g. Boehringer, Mannheim).

All internal exposures due to hydrofluoric acid, hydrogen fluoride or the various fluorides are described together as internal fluoride exposure and are determined and evaluated in the form of the fluoride anion (F^-).

6 Evaluation of the BAT Value

The BAT value for internal fluoride exposure must be oriented to the chronic fluoride effects such as fluorosis, osteosclerosis and osteoporosis.

Pharmacokinetic investigations have shown that the amount of fluoride deposited in the bones is relatively independent of the amount of the daily fluoride uptake (12, 15, 16). With exclusively hydrogen fluoride exposure the fluoride urinary excretion rate is said, however, to decrease with an increasing hydrogen fluoride dose. The fluoride not excreted is deposited mainly in the bones (14).

In numerous investigations on groups exposed to fluoride, tolerable urinary fluoride concentrations between 2.0 and 8.0 mg fluoride/l urine have been described (50–55).

Lauwerys (1975) (35) formulated a tolerable exposure range of 4.0–5.0 mg fluoride/l urine, however, without investigation of the correlation between external and internal fluoride exposure.

Then further investigations were based both on exact fluoride analysis in biological material (urine, plasma, bones) and radiological and histological bone examinations. In the "Schlegel study" (1974) (56) the fluorosis resulting from the effect of internal fluoride exposure on the skeleton was divided into 4 grades of severity and the fluoride levels found correlated directly with the duration of the fluoride exposure.

NIOSH published in 1975 and 1976 (5, 6) a comprehensive evaluation of all the available studies on hydrogen fluoride and fluoride exposure in the industrial field. The tolerable internal and external fluoride exposures were compared in each case. The result of this evaluation was the statement that persons occupationally exposed to fluoride below a fluoride exposure of 2.5 mg F^-/m^3 air show a fluoride excretion in the post-shift urine of less than 7.0 mg/l. In the next pre-shift urine less than 4.0 mg/l urine was excreted. With this excretion rate no fluorosis or illnesses due to fluorine are to be observed.

It has been taken into account that the maximum values of the urinary fluoride excretion do not usually occur until 2–3 hours after the end of the shift. The urine samples should be collected after at least 3 days exposure.

A very extensive investigation (57), described later, on the internal and external exposure in an aluminium factory led to comparable results. 56 workers with 10–43 years of exposure at an external fluoride exposure level of 2–3 mg fluoride/m^3 were examined for about 15 years. Within the 15-year period the average urinary excretion amounted to 7.71 mg fluoride/l urine in the post-shift urine and 2.78 mg fluoride/l urine in pre-shift urine without diagnosis of a change in the skeleton due to fluorine. From this investigation it was deduced that at least in the aluminium industry internal fluoride exposures up to a maximum 8.0 mg fluoride/l post-shift urine can also be tolerated long-term without fluoride-specific risks (57).

Under the specific exposure conditions of the aluminium industry apparently only approx. 45 % of the inhaled fluorides are absorbed while contact with pure hydrogen fluoride leads to complete absorption and thus to a much higher internal fluoride exposure.

Taking as a basis the correlations between external exposure and internal exposure repeatedly demonstrated in the extensive investigations and epidemiological studies of the NIOSH reports, including the evaluation of the dose-dependent fluoride body burden, and taking into consideration the results of occupational medical and epidemiological investigations, a BAT value is established for internal fluoride exposure as a pair of values on the condition that internal exposures up to

7.0 mg fluoride/g creatinine in post-shift urine

are only to be tolerated if after a pause in work of at least 16 hours, at the most, however, 24 hours, the internal fluoride exposure amounts at the most to

4.0 mg fluoride/g creatinine in the next pre-shift urine

measured in each case as the fluoride anion (F^-) concentration.

As a rule the additional pre-shift urine value should only then be determined if the post-shift urine value measured first is above 4.0 mg fluoride/g creatinine.

As this BAT value documentation is oriented mainly to the chronic effects of the relevant occupational medical internal fluoride exposure a differentiation in the exposures due to hydrogen fluoride and fluoride can be dispensed with.

The relating of the urinary excretion of fluoride to g creatinine is necessary as a very large number of workplaces at which fluoride exposure occurs are high-temperature workplaces. According to the experience of the DFG Commission for the Investigation of Health Hazards of Chemical Compounds in the Work Area, at high-temperature workplaces with fluoride exposure the creatinine concentration is on average 1.9 g creatinine/l urine compared to an average urinary excretion of 1.2 g creatinine/l urine. Neglecting the concentration of the urine at high-temperature workplaces would thus, with a large number of those exposed, lead to urine concentrations that seem too high if taken absolutely. For this reason standardisation with creatinine has been used for the BAT value of the fluorides.

A BAT value for elementary fluorine cannot at present be established either with occupational-medical or animal-experimental experience. A field study that was carried out, in which an average fluoride excretion in the urine of 1.1 mg/l could be observed with 57 workers in a chemical plant during an 8-year average external exposure of 0.3 – 1.4 ml elementary fluorine/m^3, at least gives an indication of the possible fluoride levels after elementary fluorine exposure (58).

7 Interpretation of the Data

The high half-life of internal fluoride exposure of approx. 12 to a maximum of 24 hours can cause a marked fluoride cumulation during the usual work shifts.

With workers with an external fluoride exposure up to the level of the present MAK value a sufficient correlation between the internal fluoride exposure and urinary fluoride excretion is only observed after three consecutive working days of a shift (14).

In the 4-shift system at present usual in industry with the weekly change between three work shifts and one free shift each employee receives, only after 3 continuous working weeks of 21 working days, with his free week the possibility of eliminating to a large extent the acquired cumulative fluoride body burden.

For the certain determination of representative and interindividually comparable fluoride exposures the sampling of urine should be carried out after at least 3, better after 4 uninterrupted working days, for all workers of a shift at the same time, at the shift change. Usually the collection of the post-shift urine is begun on a Thursday and after a work-free pause of at least 16, at the most, however, 24 hours on the directly following day the collection of the pre-shift urine is carried out. The urine sample collection should take place under contamination-free conditions, preferably after washing and in private clothes, if possible in a works medical department. The maximum exposure time of each test person can be determined from which shift he belongs to.

For reasons of practicability this monitoring of the internal fluoride exposure can only rarely take place in portioned 24-hour urine samples but has to be carried out in spontaneous urine samples (14). They should be related to the creatinine content. Urine samples with creatinine concentrations below 0.5 and over 2.5 g/l should only then be evaluated if their fluoride content corresponds to the long-term individual fluoride level of the test person.

The BAT pair of values for internal fluoride exposures limits their maximum values at the end of an exposure phase (shift period). The follow-up measures necessary after exceeding the BAT values should be arranged by the occupational physician responsible. In any case the internal fluoride exposure of the test person concerned should be monitored repeatedly at definite times until the BAT values are no longer exceeded (59).

Occupational medical health surveillance of persons exposed to fluorine, hydrogen fluoride and fluorides should otherwise be carried out in the Federal Republic of Germany according to the berufsgenossenschftlicher Grundsatz G34 (1981) (guideline issued by the Employers' Liability Insurance Association). Here the time intervals for the follow-up examinations are also given. With borderline values more frequent monitoring might be appropriate (60).

8 References

1. Keplinger, M. L.: Toxicol. Appl. Pharmacol. *14* (1969), 192
2. Ricca, P. M.: Arch. Environ. Health *12* (1966), 399
3. Ricca, P. M.: Am. Ind. Hyg. Ass. J. *31* (1970), 22
4. WHO: Fluorides and Human Health, World Health Organization, Geneva 1970
5. NIOSH: Criteria for a recommended standard. Occupational Exposure to inorganic Fluorides. HEW Publication Nr. 76–103 (1975)
6. NIOSH: Criteria for recommended standard Occupational Exposure to Hydrogen Fluorides. HEW Publication Nr. 76–143 (1976)
7. National Academy of Sciences, "Fluorides" Washington, DC 1971
8. Roholm, K.: quoted acc. Baader E. W. Handbuch der gesamten Arbeitsmedizin II/1 Berufskrankheiten, Verlag Urban u. Schwarzenberg, Berlin, München, Wien 1961
9. Baselt, R. C.: Biological Monitoring Methods for Industrial Chemicals, Davis, California 1980, pp. 140–143
10. Zober, A., Schiele, R.: 18. Jahrestagung der Deutschen Gesellschaft für Arbeitsmedizin – Arbeitsmedizinisches Kolloquium des Hauptverbandes der Gewerblichen Berufsgenossenschaften. H. Loskant (ed.) Gentner, Stuttgart 1978, pp. 69–75
11. Charlson, C. H., Armstrong, W. D., Singer, L.: Proc. Soc. Exp. Biol. Med. *104* (1960), 235–239
12. Ekstrand, J., Alvan, G., Boreus, L. O., Norlin, A.: Environ. J. Clin. Pharmacol. *12* (1977), 311–317
13. Eichler, O., Farah, A., Herken, H., Welch, A. D.: Handbuch der experimentellen Pharmakologie XX/1, Pharmacology of Fluorides. Springer Verlag, Heidelberg, Berlin, New York 1966
14. Zober, A., Geldmacher v. Mallinckrodt, M., Schaller, K. H.: Int. Arch. Occup. Environ. Health *40* (1977), 13–24
15. McClure, F. J., Mitchell, H. H., Hamitten, T. S., Kinser, C. A.: J. Ind. Hyg. Toxicol. *27* (1945), 159–170
16. Spencer, H., Osis, D., Waitrowski, E.: Clin. Chem. *21* (1975), 613–618

17. Schellmann, B., Zober, A.: Int. Arch. Occup. Environ. Health *35* (1975), 233–244
18. Franke, J., Auermann, E.: Int. Arch. Arbeitsmed. *29* (1972), 85–94
19. Zipkin, I., McClure, F. J., Lee, W. A.: Arch. oral Biol. *2* (1960), 190
20. Sporn, A., Dinu, I., Stonesau, L.: Rev. Roum. Biochim. *7* (1970), 299
21. Weber, Ch. W., Reid, B. L.: Toxicol. Appl. Pharmacol. *14* (1969), 420
22. Knaus, R. M., Dost, F. N., Wang, C. H.: Abstr. 11th. Ann. Meet. Soc. Toxicol., Williamsburg, Virginia Nr. 127 (1972)
23. Valentin, H., Lehnert, G., Petry, H., Weber, G., Wittgem, H., Woitowitz, H. J.: Arbeitsmed. Bd. 2: Berufskrankheiten, G. Thieme Verlag, Stuttgart 1979
24. Hodge, H. C., Smith, F. A.: J. Occup. Med. *19* (1977), 12–39
25. Waldbott, G. L.: Vet. Hum. Toxicol. *21* (1979), 4–8
26. Curry, A. S.: Brit. Med. J. *1* (1962), 687–689
27. Speaker, J. H.: J. For. Sci. *21* (1976), 121–126
28. Weidmann, S. M., Weatherell, J. A., Jackson, D.: Proc. Nutr. Soc. *22* (1963), 105–110
29. Minder, W.: In: T. Gordonoff (ed.) Toxikologie des Fluors, Verlag Schwabe & Co., Basel/Stuttgart 1964, pp. 80–90
30. Krishnamachari, K., Krishnaswany, K.: Lancet II (1973), 877–879
31. Zober, A.: 14. Jahrestagung der Deutschen Gesellschaft für Arbeitsmedizin. G. Lehnert, D. Szadkowski, H. J. Weber (eds.) Gentner, Stuttgart 1975
32. Zober, A., Schellmann, B.: Z. Klin. Chem. Klin. Biochem. *13* (1975), 197–201
33. Derryberry, O. M., Bartholomew, M. D., Fleming, R.: Arch. Environ. Health *6* (1963), 503–511
34. De Bruin, A.: Biochemical Toxicology of Environmental Agents, Elsevier/North-Holland Biomedical Press 1976, pp. 1172–1193
35. Lauwerys, R.: Scand. J. Werk, Environ. Health *1* (1975), 139–173
36. Hosking, D. J., Chamberlain, M. J.: Clin. Science *42* (1972), 152–161
37. Mazze, R. J., Calverley, R. K., Smith, M. T.: Anesthesiology *46* (1977), 265–271
38. Stookey, G. K., Crane, D. B., Muhler, I. C.: Proc. Soc. Exp. Biol. Med. *115* (1964), 295
39. Taves, D. R.: Fred. Proc. *29* (1970), 1185
40. Jowsey, J., Riggs, B. L., Kelly, P. J., Hoffmann, D. J.: Am. J. Med. *53* (1972), 43
41. Friedmann, S. A., Raizner, A. E., Rosen, H.: Ann. Int. Med. *76* (1972), 41
42. Palahniuk, R. J., Cumming, M.: Canad. Anaesth. Soc. J. *22* (1975), 291–297
43. Gettler, A. O., Ellerbrook, L.: Am. J. Med. Sci. *197* (1939), 625–638
44. Greendyke, R. M., Hodge, H. C.: J. For. Sci. *9* (1964), 383–390
45. Chaika, P. A.: Vop. Pitan. *27* (1968), 29
46. Srikantia, S. G., Siddiqui, A. H.: Clin. Sci. *28* (1965), 477
47. Macuch, P., Kortus, J., Balazova, G.: Brit. J. Ind. Med. *25* (1968), 131
48. Zober, A., Schaller, K. H.: Fluorid in Serum. In: D. Henschler (ed.): Analytische Methoden zur Prüfung gesundheitsschädlicher Arbeitsstoffe. Bd. 2: Analysen in biologischem Material. Deutsche Forschungsgemeinschaft, 6. Lieferung, VCH Verlagsgesellschaft, Weinheim 1982
49 Angerer, J., Schaller, K. H., Heinrich, R.: ASP *16* (1981), 125–127
50. Gerarde, H. W.: Fed. Proc. *19* (1960), 22–25
51. Gage, J. C. in: C. P. Steward, A. Stollmann: Toxicology. Academic Press, New York, London 1961
52. Elkins, H. B.: Pure Appl. Chem. *3* (1961), 269–273
53. Eagers, R. Y.: Toxic Properties of Inorganic Fluorine Compounds, Elsevier, Amsterdam, London, New York 1969
54. Hodge, H. C., Smith, F. A.: J. Air. Poll. Contr. Assoc. *20* (1970), 226–232
55. Neefus, J. D., Cholak, J., Saltzman, B. E.: Am. Ind. Hyg. Assoc. J. *31* (1970), 96–99
56. Schlegel, H. H.: Sozialmed. Präventivmed. *19* (1974), 269–274
57. Dinman, B. D., Bovard, W. J., Bonney, T. B., Cohen, J. M.: J. Occup. Med. *18* (1976), 7–25
58. Lyon, J. S.: J. Occup. Med. *4* (1962), 199
59. Massmann, W.: Zentralbl. f. Arbeitsmed. *31* (1981), 484–488
60. BG-Grundsatz: G34, 1981, Hauptverband der gewerblichen Berufsgenossenschaften e. V., A. W. Gentner Verlag, Stuttgart

Author: J. Lewalter
Approved by the Working Group: 10. 11. 1983

Lead and its compounds (except lead arsenate, lead chromate and alkyllead compounds)

BAT for women older than 45 years and for men (for women younger than 45 years see Addendum)	400 µg lead/l blood
Date of evaluation	2000
CAS No. (metallic lead)	7439-92-1
Formula (metallic lead)	Pb
Atomic weight (metallic lead)	207.2
Melting point (metallic lead)	327.4°C
Boiling point (metallic lead)	1740°C
Vapour pressure at 970°C (metallic lead)	1.33 mbar
MAK [last established: 2000]	Carcinogen category 3B

The following occupational-medical, toxicological documentation applies for exposure to metallic lead, lead oxides and lead salts. Not taken into account is exposure to covalent lead compounds (e.g. alkyllead compounds), or lead salts with an anion (e.g. lead arsenate, lead chromate), which are carcinogenic or of suspected carcinogenicity.

1 Pharmacokinetics

There are numerous studies available of the absorption, distribution, retention and excretion of lead in the human organism. Particular reference is made to Chamberlain 1985, Skerfving 1993, US Environmental Protection Agency 1986, and WHO 1995.

Essential BAT Value Documentations. DFG, Deutsche Forschungsgemeinschaft

ISBN 3-527-31477-6

1.1 Absorption

Lead and its inorganic compounds are absorbed by the human organism via the lungs and gastrointestinal tract. At the workplace inhalation is the most important route of absorption. In 1995 the WHO reviewed the current data for the absorption of lead (WHO 1995).

1.2 Elimination

The absorbed lead is eliminated mainly (75–80 %) with the urine and in smaller amounts via gastrointestinal excretion (WHO 1995). The rate of elimination is relatively slow. It is very difficult to give a biological half-life because of the constantly decreasing availability of the depot in the bones. The "Task Group on Metal Accumulation" gives a half-life for lead in human bones of about 10 years (TGMA 1973).

1.3 Metabolism

The absorbed lead immediately enters the blood stream. About 95 % of the blood lead is bound to the erythrocyte membrane and is distributed in this form in the organism. In the body the lead is present as a displaceable and an irreversibly bound fraction (Baloh 1974).

- The rapid exchange pool represents the biologically effective body burden. It correlates with the blood lead concentration, i.e. the lead concentration in the blood is in equilibrium with the lead concentration in soft tissue.
- Lead readily passes the placental barrier. Foetal blood therefore has more or less the same lead concentration as the maternal blood (Haas *et al.* 1972, Roels *et al.* 1978).
- Lead also passes the blood–brain barrier, but is not thought to accumulate in the brain.
- 90 % of the lead bound in the body is contained in the bones and teeth.

2 Critical Toxicity

The literature on the toxicology of lead and its compounds in experiments with animals and in man was reviewed in the occupational-medical, toxicological documentation of the MAK value (Henschler 1977, Greim 2002). There is also extensive data in Environmental Health Criteria 165, "Inorganic lead" from the International Programme on Chemical Safety (IPCS) of the WHO (1995).

In the occupational-medical, toxicological documentation of the MAK value (Greim 2002) the current data for the toxic effects of lead on reproduction, fertility, genotoxicity and carcinogenicity are presented in detail. The MAK documentation also describes the effects on the kidneys, the blood pressure, the haematopoietic system and the thyroid gland in man.

For the setting of the BAT value, the critical effect of lead is the effect on the central nervous system. The most sensitive parameter for the toxic effects of lead and its compounds, with the exception of the alkyl compounds, is the decrease in performance in behavioural tests. The data from current studies relevant for setting the threshold limit value are described below in Section 3.2. For other effects of lead and its compounds on health, the reader is referred to the occupational-medical, toxicological documentation of the MAK value (Henschler 1977, Greim 2002).

3 Exposure and Effects

3.1 Relationship between external and internal exposure

As far as it is known, there is no clearcut relationship between the external and internal exposure to lead. There are many reasons for this. The main reason is that, unlike for the determination of lead in the air (current exposure), the lead concentration in blood represents the long-term uptake of lead and the total body burden. In addition to the inhalation of lead, the substance can be ingested from contaminated hands and with drinks and food. A BAT value cannot, therefore, be evaluated on this basis.

3.2 Relationships between internal exposure and effects

As already explained in Section 2, the BAT value must be evaluated on the basis of the relationship between the blood lead concentration and the neurotoxic effects of lead compounds. The most sensitive parameter for the toxic effects of lead in men and women is the decrease in performance in behavioural tests.

3.2.1 Neurophysiological effects

The most important results published since 1980 from neurophysiological studies of persons exposed to lead at work are described below.

19 studies published between 1970 and 1984 were evaluated in a review (Ehle 1986). Most of the studies report a slight reduction in nerve conduction velocity (about 7 %) at blood lead concentrations below 600 µg/l. Correlation with clinical symptoms was not found in any study. The author emphasises that in most of the studies no relationship was detected between the nerve conduction velocity and blood lead concentrations below 700 µg/l. The reduced nerve conduction velocities in general are of no clinical relevance and are not considered to be a "sub-clinical" manifestation (Ehle 1986).

In a review published in 1990, Davis and Svendsgaard evaluated 32 studies in which various nerve conduction velocities were determined in persons exposed to lead at the workplace. In general, reduced nerve conduction velocities were found. In a meta-analysis the authors combined the results of the studies and calculated the magnitude of the effects. They concluded that the nerve conduction velocity in persons exposed to lead is reduced and the effect is most pronounced in the median nerve (Davis and Svendsgaard 1990). In their analysis the authors draw attention to two longitudinal studies whose results, however, are inconsistent (Seppäläinen *et al.* 1983, Spivey *et al.* 1980). While Seppäläinen *et al.* (1983) described significant reductions in nerve conduction velocity in 89 employees of a factory producing batteries with blood lead concentrations of about 300 to 500 µg/l and an observation period of 4 years, Spivey *et al.* (1980) could not find any significant differences between control persons and 69 lead smelters (blood lead concentration 600 to 800 µg/l) over a period of 12 to 18 months.

An evaluation of lead and its inorganic compounds by a WHO committee (1995) included a description of the peripheral neurotoxic effects (WHO 1995). The conclusion of the committee that the nerve conduction velocity changes at blood lead concentrations as low as 300 µg/l is based purely on the study of Seppäläinen *et al.* (1983). The fact that this finding could not be confirmed in other studies is mentioned by the WHO committee, but is not critically analysed from a methodological point of view.

There are only few more recent studies which investigate the relationships between occupational exposure to lead and peripheral nerve function.

Chia *et al.* (1996a, 1996b) investigated 72 employees from a factory producing batteries; the mean blood lead concentration of the workers was found to be 369 µg/l (range 73 to 685 µg/l). The authors found significant differences between the nerve conduction velocities of the median nerve and ulnar nerve in the employees and those in control persons, without values lower than normal being found on a group basis (Chia *et al.* 1996a). Clinical findings are not reported. On the basis of the results of the 3-year longitudinal study the authors concluded that a cumulative blood lead concentration of less than 400 µg/l does not cause any neurophysiological changes (Chia *et al.* 1996b).

Kovala *et al.* (1997) determined the nerve conduction velocities of the median nerve and sural nerve in 60 workers from a factory producing batteries. The exposure was evaluated by determining the blood lead concentration (mean concentration 331 µg/l, highest concentration 1014 µg/l) over the whole exposure period and the bone lead concentration (tibia) (mean 26 mg/kg). Weak negative correlations, which were not statistically significant, were found between the exposure parameters and the nerve conduction velocity. A threshold value was not given.

There are also studies in which various electrophysiological parameters (evoked potentials, such as e.g. VEP, BAEP, P 300, electrocardiogram) and body sway (posturography) were determined in persons exposed to lead (Chia *et al.* 1994, Chia *et al.* 1996c, Fujimura *et al.* 1998, Kovala *et al.* 1997, Murata and Araki 1991, Murata *et al.* 1993, Teruya *et al.* 1991, Yokoyama *et al.* 1997). It was shown that lead can influence not only the peripheral nerve fibres, but also the vegetative nervous system, functions of the spinal cord and the central nervous system. It is not possible to make a definitive statement on the clinical relevance of these effects or on whether they are to be considered adverse. Threshold concentrations can also not be defined.

According to a Japanese working group, copper and zinc seem to have antagonistic effects on the sub-clinical effects of lead on peripheral nervous functions (Araki *et al.*

1987, Murata *et al.* 1987). With regard to neurophysiological changes, a recent study found that lead mobilized using EDTA is a more sensitive parameter of lead exposure than is the blood lead concentration (Yokoyama *et al.* 1998).

The polyneuropathy induced by lead progresses with increasing exposure. The course of the disorder depends mainly on the severity of the initial lesion (Triebig 1984). In earlier stages complete regression can be expected within a few months (Krigman *et al.* 1980, WHO 1995).

In summary, it is possible to detect effects on functions of the peripheral and autonomous nervous system at blood lead concentrations in the range of 300 to 500 µg/l on a group basis, but effects which can be described as adverse occurred consistently only at blood lead concentrations above 600 to 700 µg/l.

3.2.2 Toxic effects on behaviour

3.2.2.1 Database

There are numerous epidemiological studies of the behavioural effects of exposure to lead. The data from the 1980s and 1990s indicate that effects on behaviour can be detected for occupational exposure in the range above 300 µg/l blood.

The following summary takes into account 30 publications; different publications concerning the same study were taken as one, so that in total 24 studies were included. 22 publications provide information on the current effects of lead exposure on the basis of cross-sectional studies, 5 publications describe long-term effects on the basis of longitudinal studies.

3.2.2.2 Documentation of the studies

The studies included in the evaluation are summarized in Tables 1a–d, 2a–2c and 3 at the end of this chapter.

3.2.2.3 Methodological evaluation of the studies

In an evaluation of 28 publications covering 21 studies of exposure to lead, Balbus-Kornfeld *et al.* (1995) conclude that no definitive statement can be made about the possible adverse effects of cumulative exposure to lead on the central nervous system in man because the extent of cumulative exposure has not been adequately studied. The effects found in the studies may be merely transitory or reversible and are therefore of limited meaning for the evaluation of health effects. This view is not shared by the present authors, as in the argumentation for the setting of a threshold limit value also current effects are seen as potential early signs of long-term effects.

We agree with the above authors, however, that on the basis of the evaluation criteria for studies of behavioural toxicology (DFG 1997) various studies have methodological shortcomings. The comparability of the groups with regard to age, sex and education is taken into consideration by most of the researchers, but there are critical exceptions. In the studies of Haenninen *et al.* (1978) and Jeyaratnam *et al.* (1986) the control groups are older, in Williamson and Teo (1986) and Yokoyama *et al.* (1998) the control groups are younger. Only some of the studies include these group features in the further analysis (Baker *et al.* 1983, 1984, 1985, Braun and Daigneault 1991, Campara *et al.* 1984, Chia *et al.* 1997, Haenninen *et al.* 1978, Hogstedt *et al.* 1983, Lindgren *et al.* 1996, Maizlish *et al.* 1995, Mantere *et al.* 1984, Parkinson *et al.* 1986, Repko *et al.* 1978, Spivey *et al.* 1979, Stollery *et al.* 1989, Valciukas *et al.* 1978, Zimmermann-Tansella *et al.* 1983), so that confounding effects cannot be excluded in the other studies.

In the studies of Braun and Daigneault (1991), Campara *et al.* (1984) Zimmermann-Tansella *et al.* (1983), Baker *et al.* (1983, 1984, 1985) and Grandjean *et al.* (1978) the difference in the results between the exposed persons and the control group in the vocabulary test suggests a different premorbid intelligence. In Baker *et al.* (1983, 1984, 1985) and Braun and Daigneault (1991) the small difference in the results of this test suggests it is of less importance. The different premorbid intelligence is clearer in the groups investigated by Repko *et al.* (1978).

Another methodological problem is the comparability of the activities within the exposed groups or between the exposed persons and controls. This aspect is not taken into consideration in many of the studies, which might be due to the fact that the activities of workers are assumed to be comparable. This aspect is included in the evaluation of Stollery *et al.* (1989), Maizlish *et al.* (1995), Haenninen *et al.* (1978), Baker *et al.* (1983, 1984, 1985), Valciukas *et al.* (1978), Williamson and Teo (1986), Lindgren *et al.* (1996), Österberg (1997) and Haenninen *et al.* (1998). There may be differences between the groups investigated by Campara *et al.* (1984), Zimmermann-Tansella *et al.* (1983), Repko *et al.* (1978), Braun and Daigneault (1991) and Valciukas *et al.* (1980). The meaning of the variable “activity” for the determination of performance is demonstrated in the study of Lindgren *et al.* (1996). It was discovered that the duration of employment acts as a suppressor variable, as the duration of employment was connected with further training and thus also promotion to higher positions.

The consumption of alcohol and drugs, and previous illnesses, also as exclusion criteria, were taken into consideration by most of the authors (exceptions: Repko *et al.* (1978), Banks and Stollery (1988), Dotzauer (1990), Valciukas *et al.* (1980), Haenninen *et al.* (1978), Valciukas *et al.* (1978), Jeyaratnam *et al.* (1986)). Stollery *et al.* (1989), Braun and Daigneault (1991), Haenninen *et al.* (1998), Arnvig *et al.* (1980) and Williamson and Teo (1986) took only alcohol consumption into consideration.

As a result of the methodological limitations with regard to premorbid intelligence, doubts about the meaningfulness of the studies of Braun and Daigneault (1991), Campara *et al.* (1984), Zimmermann-Tansella *et al.* (1983), Baker *et al.* (1983, 1984, 1985) and Grandjean *et al.* (1978) are justified. As the importance of premorbid intelligence with regard to its invariance to toxic effects is, however, not completely clear (Balbus-Kornfeld *et al.* 1995, Haenninen *et al.* 1998), these studies should be included in the evaluation “with discretion”. The study of Repko *et al.* (1978) should not be included because of differences in premorbid intelligence.

Also in the studies of Dotzauer (1990), Spivey *et al.* (1979), Valciukas *et al.* (1978, 1980), Haenninen *et al.* (1978), Jeyaratnam *et al.* (1986) and Williamson and Teo (1986) there are methodological shortcomings with regard to the comparability of the groups. There are differences in alcohol consumption, previous illnesses and the age-matching of the persons in the groups. Therefore also these studies should be included in the evaluation only "with discretion". The shortcomings in the evaluation of Banks and Stollery (1988) with regard to alcohol consumption make this study unsuitable for the evaluation of effects of lead.

3.2.2.4 Summary of behavioural effects after occupational exposure to lead

In the evaluation of the meaningfulness of the findings listed in Tables 1a–d and 2a–c, it must be borne in mind that several areas of performance were taken into consideration by most authors, but well-being and subjective complaints were investigated much less often and there are no data on current changes in well-being. The data for symptoms and well-being come from a smaller database and cannot achieve the same significance for the evaluation as the data on performance.

3.2.2.4.1 Effects on performance

Perceptual discrimination was determined specifically in 5 studies, but is covered by numerous other test procedures e.g. in the attention tests. A meta-analysis of the available results for visual interference revealed no significant effects for the groups investigated. The numerous deficits in performance in attention tests do not, however, exclude the possibility that lead-induced impairments in performance can be detected also in tests for perceptual discrimination.

Learning and memory was investigated in 20 studies. Not affected by exposure to lead is long-term memory, i.e. the recollection of things learnt earlier in life. Effects can be seen, however, in the areas of short-term memory and retention of verbal and senseless material. Meta-analysis[1] revealed a marked effect ($d = -0.39$) on the short-term retention of verbal information for an average current blood lead concentration of 400 µg/l. Deficits in performance occur frequently in the active recollection of figural material and remembering numbers. An effect on the remembering of numbers could not be shown after meta-analysis using the overall scores for the memory span (reproducing digits forwards and backwards). The determination of a total score for memory span is open to criticism, because it involves association of different cognitive processes (Lezak 1995).

Concentration and attention were also investigated in 20 studies. With only a few exceptions, vigilance was found to be impaired by exposure to lead. Also complex searching and association performance, as demanded in the digit-symbol test and trail-making test, are affected. The meta-analysis for the digit-symbol test yielded for a group

[1] Meta-analysis can be used to summarise studies with the same methods and approaches. The strength of the effect (effect size) for the relationships investigated is determined ($d = 0.20$ /50 /80 as a slight/moderate/strong effect). The negative values here mean that the results in the control group were more favourable than in the exposed group. The analysis was carried out according to the procedure of Fricke and Treinies (1985). For the calculations and results see Meyer-Baron and Seeber (2000)

of studies (average current blood lead concentration 450 µg/l) an effect size of $d = -0.25$, for a second group of studies (average current blood lead concentration 460 µg/l) an effect size of $d = -1.04$.

Other cognitive processes such as verbal expression, encoding and concluding are dealt with in 17 studies. Concluding and visuo-constructive abilities, which are called for e.g. in the Mosaic test, verbal expression and figural intelligence are repeatedly found to be impaired. Meta-analysis revealed an effect size of $d = -0.30$ for visuo-constructive performance at an average current blood lead concentration of 420 µg/l. For verbal expression, as a result of the heterogeneous results, analysis is only possible for a subgroup of studies (average current blood lead concentration 480 µg/l) and yielded a value of $d = -0.58$. For methodological reasons it is not possible to demonstrate an overall effect in the area of logical thinking.

Motor processes were investigated in 19 studies and found with various test procedures to be impaired. In addition to sensorimotor velocity, also dexterity and co-ordination are affected. For an average current blood lead concentration of 450 µg/l meta-analysis revealed an effect size of $d = -0.20$ for the finger dexterity of the dominant hand.

3.2.2.4.2 Symptoms and changes in personality

Data on well-being and/or complaints are given in 12 studies. The changes recorded include mood and emotions, and neurological, neurovegetative and gastrointestinal symptoms. One of the main areas studied is the complex annoyance, tension, irritability, animosity and conflicts. In addition, adverse effects on drive and subjective loss of memory and concentration are frequently mentioned. The main motor complaints are unsteadiness and weakness in the extremities. Two authors who investigated this aspect noted an increase in accidents at work.

3.2.3 Discussion of the effects

To summarise, the studies repeatedly revealed impairments in performance as a result of exposure to lead at current blood lead concentrations of < 700 µg/l, e.g.

- in the area of learning and memory for short-term retention of verbal information at an average blood lead concentration of 400 µg/l and an effect size of $d = -0.39$,
- in the area of attention and association performance for the digit-symbol test at average blood lead concentrations of 460 µg/l and 480 µg/l, and effect sizes of $d = -1.04$ and $d = -0.25$,
- in the area of more complex cognitive functions for the Mosaic test and verbal expression at an average blood lead concentration of 420 µg/l and $d = -0.30$, and 450 µg/l and $d = -0.58$,
- in the area of sensorimotor functions for finger dexterity at an average of 450 µg/l and $d = -0.20$.

In addition, mood changes, lack of drive and an increase in the number of cases of impairment of motor functions were found.

A more general evaluation of the effects can take either of two directions: it can be based on age-related changes or on statistical reference values. With regard to *age-related changes*, in the study of Campara *et al.* (1984) impaired performance was found in association tests (digit-symbol test) at a current blood lead concentration of 460–600 µg/l corresponding to an age-related change of about 25 years.

With regard to *statistical reference values*, an effect size of $d = -0.20$ means that an increase in the blood lead concentration in the exposed groups relative to the normal value in the control group causes a decrease in the test parameter corresponding to one fifth of the standard deviation of the test performance. For the results of the digit-symbol test in the described meta-analysis, this means that in the studies included in the meta-analysis at a current average blood lead concentration of 460 µg/l a decrease in performance of $d = -1.04$ was found; this corresponds to around one standard deviation in the test score. Theoretically a person's test performance would fall e.g. statistically from the 92nd percentile in the normal distribution to the 24th percentile. Relative to the normal results in the digit-symbol test for the age group, this is indicative of a decrease in performance corresponding to ageing by about 50 years. For the digit-symbol test at current average blood lead concentrations of 480 µg/l (an effect size of $d = -0.25$) the other group of authors found a change corresponding to a quarter of the standard deviation for the normal population. This effect size indicates that a person would fall e.g. from the 92nd percentile to the 82nd. In terms of age, this decrease in performance corresponds to ageing by at least 10 years. If we compare the above with the data of Campara *et al.* (1984), the lead-induced decrease in performance in the digit-symbol test can be regarded as verified and its extent confirmed for a current blood lead concentration in the range of 400–500 µg/l. The other effects can be interpreted in the same way.

As these are not individual findings but effects determined in meta-analyses, the necessity of resetting the threshold limit value is evident. Irrespective of this, the reversibility of the effects is first to be discussed below.

3.2.4 The reversibility of exposure-related changes

The results of studies of the reversibility of the effects are contradictory. Two studies found the effects to be reversible. In the study of Yokoyama *et al.* (1988) the decrease in performance was found to be reversible after the exposure to lead was reduced (blood lead concentration at the time of the first investigation 400–640 µg/l, after 2 years 260–590 µg/l). This result applied to 19 exposed persons. In the study of Baker *et al.* (1985) the reduced exposure (blood lead concentration at the time of the first investigation 500–800 µg/l, after 1 year 370–670 µg/l) led to a marked improvement in the variable mood/emotion without a corresponding change in the performance variables. The authors attributed this to the fact that in the first investigation the symptoms were exaggerated. Because the changes occurred only in the group with the highest level of exposure, the improvements in mood scores could be seen as the result of a reduction in exposure. These effects were seen in 10–12 persons.

It speaks against the reversibility of the effects that in 7 studies dose–response relationships reveal closer correlation in some cases to the accumulated levels (IBL), average exposures (TWA) and to indicators of long-term exposure, such as zinc protoporphyrin (ZPP) than to the current level of lead exposure (Valciukas *et al.* 1980, Haenninen *et al.* 1978, Valciukas *et al.* 1978, Baker *et al.* 1985, Österberg 1997, Chia *et al.* 1997, Spivey *et al.* 1979). This is also clear from the results of Lindgren *et al.* (1996), which showed that despite the lack of a relationship with the current blood lead concentrations, a dose–response relationship could be determined between performance parameters and the total exposure over the employment period. Also the study of Haenninen *et al.* (1998) revealed that in the group with higher level exposure the correlation between performance and the cumulative exposure to lead is better than that with the current exposure level, or that a relationship could only be detected to the cumulative exposure to lead. However, this study identifies a closer correlation of the performance in the group with low-level exposure with the current blood lead concentration. Such differentiation is possibly reflected in the results of Maizlish *et al.* (1995), in which the correlations with the current blood lead concentration are mostly higher.

To summarise, there is evidence from the available studies of clear and long-term behavioural deficits also at current blood lead concentrations < 70 μg/l.

3.2.5 Discussion

It must first of all be noted that none of the studies consider sex-specific differences in the effects. The studies investigated almost exclusively male persons and where (a few) women took part in the study no differentiation is made. Thus, the question of possible sex-specific differences in the effects is not treated in the following discussion.

The mean current blood lead concentration at which effects were detected in performance or personality variables was found to be 310 to about 500 μg/l in the studies cited. When blood lead concentrations determined over a longer period are taken into consideration, values of 290–530 μg/l are associated with statistically verified effects on performance and personality. The study of Lindgren *et al.* (1996) reports on the lowest levels of exposure with statistically verified effects, but only on a group basis. With mean current exposures of about 280 μg/l, but long-term 400 μg/l, a dose–response relationship was found between the effects on performance and an index of cumulative long-term exposure. Changes in performance affected attention, association and sensorimotor functions. Evidence of effects on performance below the level of 400 μg/l were also found on a group basis in Chia *et al.* (1997) (exposed versus control groups: 370 versus 60 μg/l) and in Mantere *et al.* (1984) (310 versus 110 μg/l). All three of the above studies are designated in Tables 1a–c as those which use more than one current blood lead concentration.

If the results of the meta-analysis of Meyer-Baron and Seeber (2002) are taken as the basis for discussing a threshold limit value, the concentration associated with slight and moderate effect sizes for the given performance parameters is in the range of 400–480 μg/l (see Section 3.2.3). The meta-analysis shows that in analogy to age-related changes even these small effect sizes are responsible for a change in test performance corresponding to a 10-year age difference. These changes should be regarded as relevant for health.

Effects on performance that can generally be reproduced begin at an average concentration of 400 μg/l. An evaluation of 30 publications revealed three studies which indicate effects also in the range from about 300 µg/l. In view of this, a BAT value of 400 µg lead/l blood is at present justified. When other publications become available, this value must be reviewed to determine whether and to what extent there is evidence of reproducible effects, in particular in the range between 300 and 400 µg/l.

4 Selection of the Indicators

For several years there has been a consensus of opinion in occupational medicine that the recognition of increased absorption of lead at the workplace must be based mainly on laboratory analysis of specimens from exposed persons. There is a wide spectrum of both exposure and effect parameters available for this purpose. These can be classified as follows:

Parameters of internal exposure
Determination of the lead concentration in biological materials:
- blood lead concentration
- amount of lead excreted with the urine
- amount of lead in bones
- amount of lead excreted with the urine after provocation with complexing agents.

Parameters of effect
Disturbance of porphyrin synthesis is the main biological parameter used to detect the effects of lead. These disturbances are best recognized in man in effects on haematological parameters.
- in blood: δ-aminolaevulinic acid dehydratase (ALA-D), erythrocyte porphyrins (EPs) and zinc protoporphyrins (ZPPs)
- in urine: δ-aminolaevulinic acid (ALA-U).

At present, the lead concentration in blood is the most reliable and practicable parameter for monitoring persons exposed to lead. It is the most specific parameter for evaluating the internal exposure to lead. Effect parameters can no longer be recommended, either for methodological or practical reasons, or for reasons of inadequate sensitivity in view of the fact that the levels of exposure to lead at the workplace are lower than in the past.

5 Methods

Quantitative determination of the lead concentration in whole blood can be carried out using atomic absorption spectrometry, voltammetry and ICP-MS. Reliable and tested methods for these three analytical techniques are included in the series "Analyses of

Hazardous Substances in Biological Materials" (Angerer and Schaller 1985, 1988, 1999) published by the DFG Commission for the Investigation of Health Hazards of Chemical Compounds in the Work Area. Voltammetric analysis is very sensitive, but also very time-consuming and is therefore not used routinely (Ostapczuk 1992). Because special apparatus is needed, ICP-MS is also not used routinely (Delves and Campbell 1988, Gercken and Barnes 1991).

Today graphite furnace atomic absorption spectrometry (GF-AAS) with Zeeman compensation is used almost exclusively. Usually, after dilution and the addition of a matrix modifier, the blood is analysed directly. For a description of current GF-AAS methods for determining lead in blood the reader is referred to the literature (Christensen and Kristiansen 1993, D'Haese *et al.* 1991, Miller *et al.* 1987, Jacobson *et al.* 1991, Jin *et al.* 1990, Shuttler and Delves 1986, Angerer and Schaller 1985, Parson and Slavin 1993).

The description of a tested method for the determination of blood lead can be found in Volume 1 "Biological Monitoring of Chemical Exposure in the Workplace" (WHO 1996).

The determination of lead in blood must be carried out under conditions of statistical quality control. There are various commercially available control samples for internal quality control (WHO 1996). External quality control programmes which include the determination of blood lead in the occupational-medical and environmental-medical range are offered twice a year in Germany (Schaller *et al.* 1995, Lehnert *et al.* 1998, 1999).

6 Background Exposure

The internal exposure to lead in the general population has decreased considerably in recent years. At present the following reference values (95th percentiles) are given for the population of Germany by the Umweltbundesamt (Federal Environmental Agency):
- Women aged 25–69 years: 90 µg/l
- Men aged 25–69 years: 120 µg/l.

The median values are in the range from 30–40 µg/l (Ewers *et al.* 1999).

7 Evaluation of the BAT Value

The most sensitive parameter for the toxic effects of lead in men and women is the decrease in performance in behavioural tests. Effects on performance that can generally be reproduced begin at an average blood lead concentration of 400 µg/l. Other end points of lead toxicity, in particular effects on the peripheral nervous system and the kidneys, only become relevant in exposure ranges which are much higher.

It can therefore be assumed that a threshold limit value based on the avoidance of central nervous effects also offers protection against adverse effects on the peripheral nervous system and the kidney system, including potential nephrocarcinogenicity. Similar conclusions can therefore also be drawn for other toxic effects of lead, such as haem synthesis and effects on blood pressure.

There is considerable uncertainty about lead-induced adverse effects on reproduction in man. There is evidence that for men only blood lead concentrations above 400 µg/l may be associated with impairment of fertility.

Another consideration for the setting of threshold limit values at the workplace is the existence of background levels resulting from general environmental sources, and which are present also without occupational exposure (see "Kommission Human-Biomonitoring des Umweltbundesamtes" (Ewers *et al.* 1999)).

Under these circumstances the BAT value for women older than 45 years and for men has been changed to

400 µg lead per l blood

For women younger than 45 years the previous BAT value of 300 µg lead per litre blood has been reduced to 100 µg lead per litre blood (see Addendum).

The values must be reassessed if sufficient evidence should become available that behavioural effects may occur even at exposure levels in the range between 100 and 400 µg/l blood. The Commission recommends the BAT value for women older than 45 years and for men be set at 400 µg/l blood for the following reasons:

- There is evidence of beginning effects at a current blood lead range between 300 and 400 µg/l in 3 of the around 30 publications evaluated. It cannot be excluded that the effects may have been caused by earlier much higher levels of lead exposure. This will have to be borne in mind in the evaluation of further publications.
- The BAT value is conceived as a threshold limit value for the individual (ceiling value). On the basis of the existing data a value of 400 µg/l therefore seems justified.

8 Interpretation of Data

Occupational-medical health surveillance of persons exposed to lead and its inorganic compounds is carried out in Germany in accordance with guideline G2 issued by the Berufsgenossenschaft (Employers' Liability Insurance Association). Here the intervals between follow-up examinations and for additional biological monitoring are also given. With borderline findings more frequent monitoring may be necessary.

Because lead has a long half-life in the human organism, the blood samples may be taken at any time.

Abbreviations used in Tables 1a-d, 2a-c and 3:

PbB_{max}	=	maximum level of lead in blood
PbB	=	level of lead in blood
cumPb	=	cumulative level of lead in blood
AM	=	arithmetic mean
CBLI	=	cumulative blood lead index
SD	=	standard deviation
TWA-PbB	=	time-weighted average level of lead in blood
IBL	=	cumulative blood lead over the whole period of employment
ALA-D	=	δ-aminolaevulinic acid dehydratase
ALA-U	=	δ-aminolaevulinic acid in urine
ZPP	=	zinc protoporphyrin
MPb	=	lead in urine mobilized by calcium disodium ethylenediaminetetraacetate (CaEDTA)
EPI	=	Eysenck Personality Inventory

Blood lead values are given in µg/100 ml
The parameters for lead exposure have been rounded, mostly to two significant figures
N.B. "Tests/variables": these are generally procedures, also symptom and mood scales are given.

Table 1a. Epidemiological studies of occupational exposure to lead included in the evaluation of a threshold limit value (cumulative exposure to lead)

Exposed group/ control group	Exposure variables	Tests/ variables	Significant differences between the groups	Significant correlations, dose/effect	Checks for confounders	Evaluation of the study
Haenninen *et al.* 1998						
exposed: 54 workers/ battery factories (43 men/11 women)		12/22	high versus low (PbB_{max}): • digit-symbol test • embedded figures • spatial memory • tiredness (**tests in reverse order**)	*in the total group*: with cumulative PbB (whole working life): • digit-symbol test • embedded figures • spatial memory • similarities with maximum PbB (whole working life): • digit-symbol test • embedded figures • spatial memory • similarities • Mosaic test with average PbB over the whole working life (is an indicator of current exposure here): • Santa Ana co-ordination (dominant hand) • digit-symbol *at low exposure levels*: with maximum PbB (whole working life): • embedded figures • symptoms (tiredness) • mood variables (tension, depression, helplessness) with cumulative PbB (whole working life): • mood variables (helplessness)	comparability of the groups with regard to: • working conditions • ethnic provenance • mother tongue • social status • job no diseases of the central nervous system no exposure to other neurotoxic substances no excessive alcohol consumption investigator unaware of level of exposure consideration of the influence of: • age • sex • education	satisfactory consideration of confounders

Table 1a. continued

Exposed group/ control group	Exposure variables	Tests/ variables	Significant differences between the groups	Significant correlations, dose/effect	Checks for confounders	Evaluation of the study
				with average PbB over the whole working life (is an indicator of current exposure here): • Mosaic test • similarities • mood variables (helplessness) with cumulative PbB in the last 3 years: • digit-symbol test • Mosaic test • spatial memory • memory span for digits *at high exposure levels*: with cumulative PbB (whole working life:) • embedded figures with maximum PbB (whole working life): • digit-symbol (memory)		
Chia *et al.* 1997						
exposed: 50 workers/ battery factory controls: 97 workers/ garage	• current PbB: exposed: 37/13–65 (geometric mean/range) controls: 6/2–12 (geometric mean/range) • cumPb (cumulative PbB, 1979–1997)	8/12	exposed versus controls: Santa Ana co-ordination (not dominant hand) grooved pegboard (2 variables) memory span for digits (forwards)	> 35 years of age: with current PbB: • trail making A (better with increasing lead level) with cumulative PbB: • digit-symbol • trail making A	controls had no exposure to neuro-toxic substances no continuous medication exclusion criteria: • previous illness • regular alcohol consumption	on the whole satisfactory consideration of confounders

Table 1a. continued

Exposed group/ control group	Exposure variables	Tests/ variables	Significant differences between the groups	Significant correlations, dose/effect	Checks for confounders	Evaluation of the study
	exposed: 264/176/10–1146 (median/AM/ range)		pursuit aiming (correct answers) trail making (A and B)		both groups unaware of purpose of the study investigator unaware of level of exposure same examination time for all persons (8–10 am) consideration of the influence of: • age • education • ethnic provenance • nicotine consumption • alcohol consumption	
Österberg 1997						
exposed: 38 workers/ lead smelting controls: 19 workers/ machine factory	• current PbB: low: 34/17–55 (median/range) high: 38/19–50 (median/range) controls: 4/1–7 (median/range) • CBLI (cumulative blood lead index)/µmol/l × month: low: 143/27–477 (median/range) high: 233/74–948	9/47	low/high versus control group; **controls worse!** • drawing figures (time for not dominant hand) • marking mid-points (time for not dominant hand)	with current PbB: • continuous graphic performance (errors) • acute symptoms (2 variables e.g. irritation) with CBLI: • Bourdon-Wiersma (omissions/errors) • remembering faces (errors) • activity (higher in controls) with maximum PbB: • Bourdon-Wiersma (errors) • long-term symptoms (e.g. concentration)	three parallel groups with regard to: • age • education • job comparability of the groups with regard to • alcohol consumption • nicotine consumption no relevant previous illnesses computer tests	consideration of all relevant confounders; it is questionable, however, whether groups are comparable enough with regard to premorbid intelligence (results not given)

Table 1a. continued

Exposed group/ control group	Exposure variables	Tests/ variables	Significant differences between the groups	Significant correlations, dose/effect	Checks for confounders	Evaluation of the study
	• max. PbB: low: 57/34–78 (median/range) high: 63/46–90 (median/range) • bone lead					
Lindgren *et al.* 1996						
exposed: 467 male workers/lead smelting	• current PbB: 28/8 (AM/SD) range ? • TWA PbB: 40/4–66 (AM/range) • IBL (cumulative blood lead over the whole period of employment): 765/0.6–1626 µg × y × dl^{-1} (AM/range) low: 269/195–66 (AM/SD) moderate: 821/122–66 (AM/SD) high: 1228/145 (AM/SD)	9/14	low versus high: • digit-symbol test • logical memory (short-term) • trail making (2 variables) • Purdue pegboard (dominant hand) low versus moderate: not clear from the data	not investigated	no significant differences with regard to: • speech • slight neurological disturbances consideration of significant differences with regard to: • age • education • depression • alcohol consumption exclusion criteria: • severe neurological diseases • recent psychiatric illness consideration of the suppressor variable duration of employment investigator unaware of level of exposure investigations at the beginning of the shift	appropriate inclusion of all relevant confounders in the analysis

Table 1b. Epidemiological studies of occupational exposure to lead which fulfil the criteria for inclusion in the evaluation of a threshold limit value (repeated determination)

Exposed group/ control group	Exposure variables	Tests/ variables	Significant differences between the groups	Significant correlations, dose/effect	Checks for confounders	Evaluation of the study
Stollery *et al.* 1989						
exposed: 86 workers/battery factory/printing industry	• current PbB: low: < 20 moderate: 21–40 high: 41–80 range 5–72 • ALA-U: group 1: 2.5 group 2: 4.0 group 3: 5.7 range 0.5–22 mg/l • ZPP	5/28	high versus moderate + low: • forming and remembering categories (identifying objects which belong in one class and those which do not, difficult choices) • choice reaction (number of attempts; decision time; speed of movement)	with current PbB: • forming and remembering categories (identifying objects which belong in one class and those which do not, difficult choices) • choice reaction (number of attempts; decision time; speed of movement)	consideration of the influence of: • exposure duration • age • age left school • sleep • alcohol consumption • job • stress/arousal comparability of the groups with regard to: • ethnic provenance • regional provenance computer tests	consideration of previous illnesses unclear consideration of the age on leaving school is possibly an inadequate way of checking the level of premorbid intelligence
Stollery *et al.* 1989						
exposed: 70 workers	• average PbB at 3 investigation times within 8 months: low: 14/–20 (AM/range) moderate: 31/21–40 (AM/range) high: 52/41–80 (AM/range) • ALA-U • ZPP	5/28	high versus low: • logical thinking (reaction time reduced in group with high exposure, errors not reduced in high group) • forming and remembering categories (errors in learning)	with current PbB: • logical thinking (errors) • forming and remembering categories (errors in learning) • choice reaction (decision time; speed of movement, items skipped at high speeds) with ZPP: • forming and remembering categories with ALA-U: • forming and remembering categories	see above	see above

Table 1b. continued

Exposed group/ control group	Exposure variables	Tests/ variables	Significant differences between the groups	Significant correlations, dose/effect	Checks for confounders	Evaluation of the study
Yokoyama *et al.* 1998						
exposed: 19 workers/ foundry controls: 12 workers/ foundry (same company) after 2 years 17/10	• current PbB: exposed: 30–64 (range) controls: 8–20 (range) high: 40–64 low: 30–39 controls: 8–20 • current PbB after 2 years: high: 26–59 ** low: 24–39 controls: 8–14 • lead in urine (MPb)	5/5	Investigation 1: high versus low: • completing pictures high versus controls: • completing pictures Investigation 2: none found	in the exposed persons at the time of investigation 1: with current PbB: • completing pictures with MPb: • completing pictures with ALA-D: • completing pictures in the exposed persons at the time of investigation 2: not reported	comparability of the groups with regard to: • age • education • alcohol consumption no exposure to other neurotoxic substances no relevant previous illnesses no alcohol or drugs consumed on the day of the test	controls younger exposed group drinks more as the effect on performance disappears after the level of lead exposure is lowered both these points seem to be of little importance
Mantere *et al.* 1984						
exposed: 24 employees /battery factory after 1 year: 24 (6 women) after 2 years: 16 (6 women) after 4 years: 11 (5 women) controls: 33 workers (4 women)/cable production/power plant after 1 year: 33 after 2 years: 31	• current PbB: exposed: 16/7–30 (AM/SD) after 1 year: 31/13–49 (AM/SD) after 2 years: 31/14–46 (AM/SD) after 4 years: 29/17–45 (AM/SD) controls: 11/1–21 (AM/SD)	8/12	at beginning of exposure, exposed versus controls: • none after 1 year exposed versus controls: • Mosaic test (deterioration) • Santa Ana coordination (deterioration) after 2 years exposed versus controls: • Mosaic test (deterioration)	not investigated	exclusion criteria: • (other) neurotoxic exposure • previous illnesses comparability with regard to: • education • alcohol consumption • medicine consumption • nicotine consumption	consideration of confounders on the whole satisfactory (unclear about sex and job) exposed persons with higher level of performance in the initial test deteriorate less and/or have greater improvements in performance

Table 1b. continued

Exposed group/ control group	Exposure variables	Tests/ variables	Significant differences between the groups	Significant correlations, dose/effect	Checks for confounders	Evaluation of the study
after 4 years: 10 (4 women)	after 1 year: 11/6–18 (AM/SD) after 2 years: 11/5–21 (AM/SD) after 3 years: 7/4–12 (AM/SD) • TWA–PbB (1–4 years): exposed: constant 29 (AM) controls: 11 (AM) after 4 years: 8 (AM) low: ≤ 27 high: > 27 • ZPP		• Santa Ana coordination (deterioration) • memory span for digits (deterioration) after 4 years exposed versus controls: • determination of significance not carried out as number of persons too small at the beginning of exposure high versus controls/low versus controls: • none after 1 year high versus controls/low versus controls: • none after 2 years high versus controls: Mosaic test after 2 years low versus controls: Mosaic test Santa Ana coordination (**only in the low group**)		consideration of the influence of: • age • performance in initial test examiner unaware of level of exposure	

Table 1c. Epidemiological studies of occupational exposure to lead which fulfil the criteria for inclusion in the evaluation of a threshold limit value (TWA)

Exposed group/ control group	Exposure variables	Tests/ variables	Significant differences between the groups	Significant correlations, dose/effect	Checks for confounders	Evaluation of the study
Maizlish *et al.* 1995						
exposed: 43 workers/ lead smelting controls: 47 workers/ glass factory	• current PbB: exposed: 43/12/9–68 (AM/SD/range) controls: 15/6 (AM/SD) < 10 4 % 10–25 44 % 25–39 20 % 40–61 26 % 61–81 6 % • maximum PbB (1986–1993): exposed: 60/20 (AM/SD) controls: 15/6 (AM/SD) • TWA-PbB: exposed: 48/12 (AM/SD) controls: 15/6 (AM/SD)	7/14	exposed versus controls: • symptoms reported in the year before the study (concentration, annoyance or agitation without reason, exceptional tiredness, painful joints)	with current PbB > PbB_{max} & TWA with current PbB: • POMS (tension/anxiety, animosity, tiredness, depression) with maximum PbB: • POMS (animosity, depression) TWA PbB: • POMS (animosity, depression)	comparability of the groups with regard to: • job • geographical provenance consideration of the influence of: • age • education • alcohol consumption • earlier exposure to solvents • state of health examiner not 'blind'	• consideration of confounders satisfactory • as a result of the dismissal of many persons exposed long-term shortly before the study was carried out, it is questionable whether the group was representative (healthy worker effect?)
Parkinson *et al.* 1986						
exposed: 288 workers/ 3 battery factories controls: 181 workers/ chassis production	• current PbB: exposed: 40/13 (AM/SD) range ? controls: 7/3 (AM/SD) range ?	17/18	none	with current PbB: • psychosocial variable (conflicts) with ZPP: • psychosocial variable (annoyance at the workplace)	comparability of the groups with regard to: • ethnic provenance • psychiatric history • drug/alcohol abuse	• despite group comparison, the exposure levels for the controls were not given exactly (≤35) • adequate inclusion of all relevant confounders in the analysis

Table 1c. continued

Exposed group/ control group	Exposure variables	Tests/ variables	Significant differences between the groups	Significant correlations, dose/effect	Checks for confounders	Evaluation of the study
	• TWA-PbB: 49/12 (AM/SD) • maximum PbB: 79/29 (AM/SD) • PbB > 60: 0.23/0.22 (AM/SD) • ZPP			with TWA–PbB: • psychosocial variables (conflicts, 2 variables) • trait–annoyance • number of accidents at work • Mosaic test **(better with increasing exposure)** with maximum PbB: • psychosocial variables (conflicts, annoyance at the workplace) with PbB > 60: • psychosocial variables (conflicts, 2 variables) • number of accidents at work	consideration of the influence of: • age • education • income controls had no known exposure to neurotoxic substances exclusion criteria: • relevant neurological or other illnesses	
Ryan *et al.* 1987						
		18/21	exposed versus controls: • psychomotor velocity/manual dexterity factor • grooved pegboard (2 variables) • embedded figures (time, **in reverse order**)	not investigated		

Table 1c. continued

Exposed group/ control group	Exposure variables	Tests/ variables	Significant differences between the groups	Significant correlations, dose/effect	Checks for confounders	Evaluation of the study
Hogstedt *et al.* 1983						
exposed: 49 workers who took part in occupational-medical health check-ups/lead smelting/battery factory controls: 27 industrial workers who took part in occupational-medical health check-ups/wire industry/ turnery/munitions factory	• current PbB: exposed: 42 (AM) controls: 15 (AM) • TWA-PbB: exposed: 48 (AM) highest individual value 65 of 14 persons one had a value > 69 range 27–69 high: > 53 low: 27–52 controls: < 21 • ZPP	15/7	low versus controls: • memory factor • learning factor high versus controls: • memory factor • simple reaction time high + low versus controls: • memory factor • learning factor **(here there were also decreases in performance from high to low)** • simple reaction time • irritability	significance unclear	comparability of the groups with regard to: • alcohol consumption • previous illnesses • exposure to solvents consideration of the influence of: • age only persons with the same level of schooling were allowed to take part similar examination times for all examiner aware whether the persons were exposed or belonged to the controls	• the lack of differences in verbal tests indicate comparable premorbid intelligence • consideration of confounders largely satisfactory • differences in the number of shift workers between the exposed and control groups may have led to underestimation of the effects, as shift workers generally had poorer performance

Table 1d. Epidemiological studies of occupational exposure to lead in the evaluation of a threshold limit value (single determination of current blood lead)

Exposed group/controls	Exposure variables	Tests/ variables	Significant differences between the groups	Significant correlations, dose/effect	Checks for confounders	Evaluation of the study
Pasternak *et al.* 1989						
exposed: 24 workers/ production of electrical components controls: 29 workers/same company	77 % exposure ≤ 3 years last 18 months without notable exposure • exposure years × median PbB: exposed: 128/156/19–680 (AM/SD/range) • PbB_{max}: exposed: 67/14/48–105 (AM/SD/range) • exposure years × median ZPP: exposed: 439/556/22–2008 (AM/SD/range) • ZPP_{max}: 265/136/39557 (AM/SD/range)	27/35	exposed versus controls: • tapping (2×) • memory span for digits (forwards) • visual memory • deletion test • dynamometer (only for the women) • anxiety • tiredness • confusion	• not investigated	exclusion criteria: • intake of psycho-active substances • previous illnesses comparability of the groups with regard to: • age • sex • ethnic provenance • family status • level of education/ premorbid intelligence • alcohol consumption • computer experience computer tests investigator unaware of level of exposure	• results of the vocabulary test indicate comparable premorbid intelligence • consideration of confounders largely satisfactory • no data for the exposure of the controls
Arnvig *et al.* 1980						
exposed: 9 workers/ battery factory	current PbB: 69/58–82 (mean/range)	17/22	• could not be investigated, as no controls available	• not investigated	average premorbid intelligence no relevant previous illnesses no excessive alcohol consumption both tests carried out at the same times for all in some cases consideration of the influence of: • age	• inclusion of the relevant confounders • inappropriately small number of samples • as a result of the exceptionally poor performance of those investigated and reported observations (impression of pre-senile dementia) it is questionable whether the group was representative

Table 2a. Epidemiological studies of occupational exposure to lead which are to be used with discretion in the evaluation of a threshold limit value (repeated determination)

Exposed group/ control group	Exposure variables	Tests/ variables	Significant differences between the groups	Significant correlations, dose/effect	Checks for confounders	Evaluation of the study
Dotzauer 1990						
exposed: 47 employees/ battery factory controls: 14 employees after 18 months: exposed: 11	• current PbB: controls: < 30 low: 40–60 high: > 60 range ? • ALA–U (µmol/100ml): controls: < 39 low: 76 high: > 76.4	4/11	high versus low + controls: • recognition of faces high + low versus controls: • choice reaction (errors/tempo self-determined) significant improvements after 18 months: • aiming • d2 • recognition of figures • choice reaction (hits/tempo self-determined)	with current PbB: • choice reaction (hits and errors/tempo self-determined, errors/ tempo predetermined) with ALA–U: • aiming (errors) • choice reaction (errors/tempo self-determined, errors/ tempopredetermined)	comparability of the groups with regard to: • age • education investigator unaware of level of exposure	• alcohol consumption and job not considered as confounders • previous illnesses not taken into consideration • it is not possible to check whether the consideration of other confounders was appropriate • no data for the exposure at the second investigation
Baker *et al.* 1983/1984/1985						
exposed: 99 workers/ foundry controls: 61 workers/ assembly line in the second year of investigation: 43/34 in the third year of investigation: 38/19	in the first year of investigation: current PbB: 0–20 16 % 21–40 61 % 41–60 18 % 61–80 5 % range 3–80 • TWA PbB (12 months)	15/23	in the first year of investigation: significance not investigated	in the first year of investigation: with current PbB: • vocabulary test • finding similarities • mental control • POMS (annoyance, depression, tiredness, confusion) with TWA–PbB: • continuous performance	comparability of the groups with regard to: • ethnic provenance • job • wage consideration of the influence of: • education • age • sex	• no comments on the significance of group differences in the first year of investigation

Table 2a. continued

Exposed group/ control group	Exposure variables	Tests/ variables	Significant differences between the groups	Significant correlations, dose/effect	Checks for confounders	Evaluation of the study
	in the second year of investigation: • current PbB: range 7–59 in the third year of investigation: • current PbB: range 8–50 • maximum PbB (15 months) • TWA–PbB (15 months) • quadratic mean • TWA min > 40 • ZPP			• POMS (annoyance, depression, tiredness, confusion) in the second year of investigation: with TWA/quadratic mean/TWA min >40 > current PbB/max PbB with current PbB: • pair-associated learning with TWA–PbB: • pair-associated learning • finding similarities • vocabulary test • Santa Ana (both hands) • POMS (annoyance, depression, vitality, confusion) with quadratic mean: • pair-associated learning • Santa Ana (both hands) • POMS (annoyance, depression, vitality, confusion) with maximum PbB: • pair–associated learning • POMS (annoyance) with TWA min >40: • pair-associated learning • Santa Ana (both hands) • POMS (annoyance, depression, confusion)	for mood variables consideration of the influence of: • job exclusion criteria: • increased alcohol consumption • drug abuse • exposure to solvents • previous illnesses double blind study	• the correlations with the vocabulary test makes it seem questionable that confounders were adequately considered for premorbid intelligence. It is recognizable from the results, however, that the difference is not large

Table 2b. Epidemiological studies of occupational exposure to lead which are to be used with discretion in the evaluation of a threshold limit value (TWA)

Exposed group/ control group	Exposure variables	Tests/ variables	Significant differences between the groups	Significant correlations, dose/effect	Checks for confounders	Evaluation of the study
Braun & Daigneault 1991						
exposed: 41 workers/ lead smelting (30 no longer exposed for up to 84 months) controls: 37 workers/ printing, copying service	• maximum PbB: exposed: 87/22/49–158 (mean/SD/range) TWA–PbB: exposed: 53/8/30–66 (mean/SD/range)	12/23	exposed versus controls: • simple reaction time (scatter of the reaction time/length of the reaction time) • grip strength (exposed group better)	with TWA–PbB: • tapping (not dominant hand) • tapping (right foot) • grip strength (dominant/ not dominant hand) • grooved pegboard (dominant/not dominant hand) • motor performance factor with maximum PbB: • tapping (not dominant hand) • grooved pegboard (dominant/not dominant hand)	exclusion criteria: • poor performance in a vocabulary test • ethnic provenance • neurological/ psychiatric and other relevant previous illnesses • exposure to other heavy metals comparability of the groups with regard to: • age • years of schooling • alcohol consumption • other chemical exposures • calculation test • body weight • height	• the mixing of persons no longer exposed for 7 years with those currently exposed does not seem sensible in view of the uncertainty about the reversibility of lead-induced effects • the analysis of other toxic exposures indicates that the results may be confounded by other exposures (excluded only for controls)
Haenninen *et al*. 1978						
exposed: 49 workers/ battery factory/ machine factory (10 women) controls: 24 workers/ battery factory/ electronics factory	• current PbB: exposed: 32/11 (AM/SD) controls: 12/4 (AM/SD) range ? • maximum PbB: exposed: 50/12(AM/SD)	13/29	exposed versus controls: • tiredness • sleep disturbances • absence • depression • lability • neurovegetative symptoms • gastrointestinal complaints	with TWA > maximum PbB > current PbB with current PbB: • repetition of spoken numbers • Santa Ana co-ordination (right hand) with TWA–PbB: • Mosaic test • visual reproduction	comparability of the groups with regard to: • sex • education • job exposed persons tended to be younger neuroticism taken into account	• inadequate consideration of confounders (age distribution) • alcohol consumption and previous illnesses not considered as confounders

Table 2b. continued

Exposed group/ control group	Exposure variables	Tests/ variables	Significant differences between the groups	Significant correlations, dose/effect	Checks for confounders	Evaluation of the study
	• TWA–PbB: exposed: 38/9 (AM/SD)		• neurological symptoms I • neurological symptoms II • neuroticism high versus low (only for symptoms and EPI): • absence • gastrointestinal symptoms • neurological symptoms II	• Santa Ana co-ordination (right, left, both hands) with maximum PbB: • Santa Ana co-ordination (right, left, both hands)		

Table 2c. Epidemiological studies of occupational exposure to lead which are to be used with discretion in the evaluation of a threshold limit value (single determinations of current blood lead level)

Exposed group/ control group	Exposure variables	Tests/ variables	Significant differences between the groups	Significant correlations, dose/effect	Checks for confounders	Evaluation of the study
Jeyaratnam *et al.* 1986						
exposed: 49 workers/ lead processing controls: 36 workers	• current PbB (AM/SD): exposed: 49/15 controls: 15/3 range ?	9/18	exposed versus controls: • digit-symbol test • Bourdon-Wiersma (speed) • trail-making (A) • Santa Ana co-ordination (right, left hand) • flicker fusion frequency • simple reaction time • subjective symptoms (anxiety, depression, lack of concentration, forgetfulness, headaches, dizziness)	not investigated	level of education comparable significant differences with regard to: • age	• inadequate consideration of confounders (controls older) makes the results seem more meaningful • alcohol consumption, job and previous illnesses not considered as confounders • exposure only estimated for controls
Williamson & Teo 1986						
exposed: 59 male workers/battery factory, lead smelting controls: 49 men, 10 women	• current PbB: exposed: 49/13/ 25–82 (median/ SD/range) controls: ? • current PbB also as the mean value in 3 years	9/20	exposed vs. controls: • flicker fusion frequency • simple reaction time • visual pursuit (slower at both speeds) • hand steadiness (2 variables) • sensory memory (3 variables) • Sternberg short-term memory (2 speed variables)	with current PbB: • sensory memory (1 variable)	no significant differences with regard to: • age • type of job • duration of employment • level of education • cigarette consumption • alcohol consumption no toxic exposure of the controls	• questionable whether consideration of the confounder age was adequate (despite a lack of significance, median of the controls 4.5 years lower) • previous illnesses not considered as confounders • data for the exposure of the controls not given

Table 2c. continued

Exposed group/ control group	Exposure variables	Tests/ variables	Significant differences between the groups	Significant correlations, dose/effect	Checks for confounders	Evaluation of the study
			• pair-associated learning/short-term reproduction (number of reproductions, number of attempts, success)			• groups not comparable with regard to sex
Campara *et al.* 1984/Zimmermann-Tansella *et al.* 1983						
exposed: 40 workers/ battery factory controls: 20 male nurses	• current PbB: controls: 20/6/11–27 (AM/SD/range) low: 32/3/26–35 (AM/SD/range) high: 52/5/46–60 (AM/SD/range) • maximum PbB: low: < 40 high: < 60	16/34	high versus low: • finding similarities • vocabulary test • digit-symbol test • completing pictures • deletion test (2 error variables) • Rey Osterrieth • SSQ22 (in particular motor disturbances) • general performance • logical thinking high versus controls: • copying symbols • finding similarities • vocabulary test • digit-symbol test • completing pictures • deletion test (2 error variables) • Rey Osterrieth • SSQ22 (in particular motor disturbances, paraesthesia and weakness in the extremities) low versus controls: • motor disturbances	with current PbB: • finding similarities • vocabulary test • digit-symbol test • completing pictures • sorting cards (decision time) • general performance • logical thinking • SSQ20 (physical symptoms) • group of gastrointestinal symptoms • group of neurological symptoms	comparability of the groups with regard to: • family status • distance to workplace • chronic illnesses • duration of employment • age • schooling • neuroticism/extraversion no participants with • increased alcohol consumption • drug abuse in the last 6 months • relevant previous neurological or psychiatric illnesses investigator unaware of level of exposure same examination time	• job not considered as a confounder • the relationship between the vocabulary test results and blood lead concentration indicates that the different kinds of jobs are also linked with a different premorbid intelligence and the results could be confounded by this

Table 2c. continued

Exposed group/ control group	Exposure variables	Tests/ variables	Significant differences between the groups	Significant correlations, dose/effect	Checks for confounders	Evaluation of the study
Valciukas *et al.* 1980						
exposed: 141 workers/ cable processing New York/cable production New York/lead smelting California controls: 265 persons from Michigan who took part in health check-ups	• current PbB (AM/SD): exposed: cable processing 28/6 cable production 39/11 lead smelting 51/12 range: < 30– > 80 • ZPP	3/4	not carried out	with ZPP > current PbB: with current PbB: • Mosaic test (in the group of lead smelters) • summarized performance index (in the group of lead smelters) with ZPP: • embedded figures (in the group of cable producers) • summarized performance index (in the group of cable producers) • Mosaic test (in the group of lead smelters) • digit-symbol test (in the group of lead smelters) • embedded figures (in the group of lead smelters) • summarized performance index (in the group of lead smelters)	consideration of the influence of: • age • education investigator unaware of level of exposure	• lack of current PbB for controls less important as no group comparison was carried out • alcohol consumption, job and previous illnesses not considered as confounders
Spivey *et al.* 1979						
exposed: 69 workers/ lead smelting, processing controls: 35 workers/ aluminium smelting, processing	• current PbB: exposed: 61/13 (AM/SD) controls: 22/2 (AM/SD) • ALA-D	1/3	exposed versus controls: • neurological symptoms (difficulties in calculating, dejection, dizziness,	with current PbB: • total number of symptoms with ALA-D: • total number of symptoms	exclusion criteria: duration of employment < 1 year comparability of the groups with regard to: • job	• very careful selection of the groups with regard to exposure conditions/ job

Table 2c. continued

Exposed group/ control group	Exposure variables	Tests/ variables	Significant differences between the groups	Significant correlations, dose/effect	Checks for confounders	Evaluation of the study
			concentration difficulties, wobbly handwriting, weakness in the hands) • other symptoms (painful joints, metallic taste, nocturia, racing heartbeat, watery eyes (not allergic))		• previous illnesses • alcohol consumption • nicotine consumption importance of differences unclear for: • age • schooling significant differences with regard to: • exposure to arsenic and cadmium (is presented as being in the normal range) consideration of the influence of: • ethnic provenance • arsenic • schooling	• positive is that other toxic exposures were checked; it is unclear whether differences are influenced by the level of premorbid intelligence • that the symptoms decrease with increasing duration of employment could also indicate that habituation/compensation effects occur
Grandjean *et al.* 1978						
exposed: 42 workers/ battery factory/lead processing/radiator repair/cable production controls: 22 workers/ oil mill	• current PbB: exposed: 46/13–88 (median/range) controls: 17/11–27 (median/range) • ZPP • lead in hair	14/30	exposed versus controls (2-sided test!): • visual production/ reproduction **(exposed better)** • continuous graphic performance (time) • tapping (not dominant hand) • number learning **(exposed better)**	(only within the exposed group) with current PbB: • visual production (learning) • number learning • Wechsler intelligence test (general understanding, arithmetic, finding similarities, memory span for digits, digit-symbol, picture completion, Mosaic test, verbal IQ, performance IQ, total IQ)	comparability of the groups with regard to: • education • sex the influence of age taken into account in the Wechsler intelligence test no participants with relevant previous neurological or psychiatric illnesses	• significant difference in premorbid intelligence (vocabulary test) in the exposed and control groups • inadequate consideration of the confounder alcohol consumption is of less importance as the exposed group drink less

Table 2c. continued

Exposed group/ control group	Exposure variables	Tests/ variables	Significant differences between the groups	Significant correlations, dose/effect	Checks for confounders	Evaluation of the study
			• Wechsler intelligence test (general knowledge, general understanding, arithmetic, finding similarities, vocabulary, digit-symbol, Mosaic test, ordering pictures, verbal IQ, performance IQ, total IQ)	with ZPP: • visual production (learning) • continuous graphic performance (errors, time) • Wechsler intelligence test (general understanding, finding similarities, memory span for digits, digit-symbol, Mosaic test, verbal IQ, performance IQ, total IQ)	different number of slight head injuries alcohol consumption lower in the exposed group examiner aware whether the persons were exposed or belonged to the controls	
Valciukas *et al.* 1978						
exposed: 90 workers/ lead smelting (1 woman) controls: 25 workers/ steel works 99 workers/paper factory 93 farmers	• current PbB: exposed: < 40 17 % 40–59 61 % 60–79 20 % > 80 1 % controls: < 40 94 % 40–59 6 % range: < 30–> 80 • ZPP	4/5	exposed versus controls: • Mosaic test • digit-symbol test • embedded figures	with ZPP > PbB: with ZPP: • Mosaic test • digit-symbol test • embedded figures with current PbB: • Mosaic test • embedded figures with exposure duration: • digit-symbol test • embedded figures • Santa Ana co-ordination (both hands)	comparability of the groups with regard to: • sex • ethnic provenance • job • life-style consideration of the influence of: • education • age investigator unaware of level of exposure exclusion criteria controls: good state of health no exposure to neurotoxic substances	• alcohol consumption and previous illnesses not considered as confounders

Table 3. Epidemiological studies of occupational exposure to lead which are not of use for the evaluation of a threshold limit value

Exposed group/ control group	Exposure variables	Tests/ variables	Significant differences between the groups	Significant correlations, dose/effect	Checks for confounders	Evaluation of the study
Banks & Stollery 1988						
exposed: 40 workers/ printing industry controls: ? workers/ printing industry (same company)	• current PbB: exposed: 31 (mean?) controls: 15 (mean?)	1/3	exposed versus controls in the current comparison: • logical thinking (errors) exposed versus controls in the course of the year: • logical thinking (errors decrease in the exposed, similar to the controls) • logical thinking (reaction time dependant on difficulty of the task, no improvement in the exposed)	with current PbB (only in the exposed group, with the blood lead level which changed over the course of the year): • logical thinking (errors in complex tasks)	comparability of the groups with regard to: • age on leaving school • sleep • stress comparability questionable as not analysed for: • age • alcohol consumption • arousal • waking time	• previous illnesses and job not considered as confounders • age on leaving school is not a reliable indicator of the level of premorbid intelligence • although waking time and alcohol consumption differ greatly in the exposed and control groups and correlate significantly/highly significantly with the errors, it is not recognizable that they were included in the analysis as confounders; it cannot be excluded that the effects have to be attributed to this • the levels of exposure given provide only an inexact impression

Table 3. continued

Exposed group/ control group	Exposure variables	Tests/ variables	Significant differences between the groups	Significant correlations, dose/effect	Checks for confounders	Evaluation of the study
Repko *et al.* 1978						
exposed: 85 workers/ battery factory (81 men, 4 women) controls: 55 workers/ production of illuminants, repair workshops, unemployed persons (46 men/9 women)	• current PbB: exposed: 46 controls: 18 range ? • ALA-D: exposed: 27 units/l red blood cells controls: 23 units/l red blood cells • ALA-U: exposed: 0.7 controls: 0.3 • lead in urine • free erythrocyte protoporphyrin	6/53	exposed versus controls: • eye-hand co-ordination (1 variable) • simple reaction time (1 variable) • pure tone auditory thresholds (7 variables/ 6 frequencies) • tone decay (7 variables) • enjoyment-disgust, **high in controls!** • annoyance, **higher in controls!** • accidents at work	with ALA-U: • pure tone auditory thresholds (1 variable) • tone decay (1 variable) with ALA-D: • tone decay (2 variables)	exclusion criteria: • lead exposure • exposure to toxic substances comparability of the groups with regard to: • age • sex • ethnic provenance • lack of inclination to answer in the sense of a social desirability in some cases consideration of the influence of: • sex group differences with regard to education	• as a result of the use of an unsuitable test, the extent of the difference in the level of education in the groups was underestimated • different confounders (job, alcohol consumption, previous illnesses) were not considered • positive is that inclination was checked, in the sense of a social desirability to answer, a tendency that could not be detected

9 References

Angerer J, Schaller KH (Eds) (1985) Lead in blood. in: Analyses of hazardous substances in biological materials, Vol. 1, VCH, Weinheim

Angerer J, Schaller KH (Eds) (1988) Lead in blood and urine. in: Analyses of hazardous substances in biological materials, Vol. 2, VCH, Weinheim

Angerer J, Schaller KH (Eds) (1999) Lead, ICP-MS collective method. in: Analyses of hazardous substances in biological materials, Vol. 6, Wiley-VCH, Weinheim

Araki S, Murata K, Aono H (1987) Central and peripheral nervous system dysfunction in workers exposed to lead, zinc and copper. Int Arch Occup Environ Health 59: 177–187

Arnvig E, Grandjean P, Beckmann J (1980) Neurotoxic effects of heavy lead exposure determined with psychological tests. Toxicol Lett 5: 399–404

Baker EL, Feldman R, White R, Harley J (1983) The role of occupational lead exposure in the genesis of psychiatric and behavioral disturbances. Acta Psychiatr Scand 67: 38–48

Baker EL, Feldman RG, White RA, Harley JP, Niles CA, Dinse GE, Berkey CS (1984) Occupational lead neurotoxicity: a behavioural and electrophysiological evaluation-study design and year one results. Br J Ind Med 41: 352–361

Baker EL, White RA, Pothier LJ, Berkey CS, Dinse GE, Travers PH (1985) Occupational lead neurotoxicity: Improvement in behavioral effects after reduction of exposure. Br J Ind Med 42: 507–516

Balbus-Kornfeld JM, Stewart W, Bolla KI, Schwartz BS (1995) Cumulative exposure to inorganic lead and neurobehavioural test performance in adults: an epidemiological review. Occup Environ Med 52: 2–12

Baloh RW (1974) Laboratory diagnosis of increased lead absorption. Arch Environ Health 28: 198–208

Banks HA, Stollery BT (1988) The longitudinal evaluation of verbal-reasoning in lead workers. Sci Total Environ 71: 469–476

Braun CMJ, Daigneault S (1991) Sparing of cognitive executive functions and impairment of motor functions after industrial exposure to lead: A field study with control group. Neuropsychol 5: 179–193

Campara P, D'Andrea F, Micciolo R, Savonitto C, Tansella M, Zimmerman-Tansella C (1984) Psychological performance of workers with blood-lead concentration below the current threshold limit value. Int Arch Occup Environ Health 53: 233–246

Chamberlain AC (1985) Prediction of response of blood lead to airborne and dietary lead from volunteer experiments with lead isotopes. Proceedings of the Royal Society B 224: 149–182

Chia SE, Chua LH, Ng TP, Foo SC, Jeyaratnam J (1994) Postural stability of workers exposed to lead. Occup Environ Med 51: 768–771

Chia SE, Chia HP, Ong CN, Jeyaratnam J (1996a) Cumulative blood lead levels and nerve conduction parameters. Occup Med 46: 59–64

Chia SE, Chia K-S, Chia HP, Ong CN, Jeyaratnam J (1996b) Three-year follow-up of serial nerve conduction among lead-exposed workers. Scand J Work Environ Health 22: 374–380

Chia SE, Chia HP, Ong CN, Jeyaratnam J (1996c) Cumulative concentrations of blood lead and postural stability. Occup Environ Med 53: 264–268

Chia SE, Chia HP, Ong CN, Jeyaratnam J (1997) Cumulative blood lead levels and neurobehavioral test performance. Neurotoxicology 18: 793–804

Christensen JM, Kristiansen J (1993) Lead. in: Handbook on metals in clinical chemistry. Marcel Dekker Inc., New York

D'Haese PCD, Lamberts LV, Liang L, Van de Vyver FL, De Broe ME (1991) Elimination of matrix and spectral interferences in the measurement of lead and cadmium in urine and blood by ET-AAS with deuterium background correction. Clin Chem 1991; 37: 1583–1588

Davis JM, Svendsgaard DJ (1990) Nerve conduction velocity and lead: A critical review and meta-analysis, in: BL Johnson (Ed.) Advances in neurobehavioral toxicology: Applications in environmental and occupational health. Lewis Publishers, Chelsea, Mi 373–376

Delves HAT, Campbell MJ (1988) Measurements of total lead concentrations and of lead isotope ratios in whole blood by use of inductively coupled plasma source mass spectrometry. J Anal Atom Spectr 3: 343–348

DFG (Deutsche Forschungsgemeinschaft) Seeber A, Bolt HM, Gelbke HP, Miksche L, Pawlik K, Rüdiger HW, Triebig G, Ziegler-Skylakakis K (1997) Verhaltenstoxikologie und MAK-Grenzwertfestlegungen. Wissenschaftliche Arbeitspapiere. Wiley-VCH Verlag, Weinheim

Dotzauer H (1990) Bleiexposition und psychische Leistungen – Ein Diskussionsbeitrag zu Dosis-Wirkungsbeziehungen nach kurzer Expositionsdauer. Z ges Hyg 36: 271–273

Ehle AL (1986) Lead neuropathy and electrophysiological studies in low level lead exposure – a critical review. Neurotoxicology 7: 203–216

Ewers U, Krause C, Schulz C, Wilhelm M (1999) Reference values and human biological monitoring values for environmental toxins. Int Arch Occup Environ Health 72: 255–260

Fricke R, Treinis G (1985) Einführung in die Metaanalyse. Huber, Bern

Fujimura Y, Araki S, Murata L, Sakai T (1998) Assessment of peripheral, central and autonomic nervous system functions in two lead smelters with high blood lead concentrations: A follow-up study. J Occup Health 40: 9–15

Gercken B, Barnes RM (1991) Determination of lead and other trace element species in blood by size exclusion chromatography and inductively coupled plasma/mass spectrometry. Anal Chem 63: 283–287

Grandjean P, Arnvig E, Beckmann J (1978) Psychological dysfunctions in lead-exposed workers – relation to biological parameters of exposure. Scand J Work Environ Health 4: 295–303

Greim H (Ed.) (2002) Lead and its inorganic compounds, apart from lead arsenate and lead chromate. in: Occupational toxicants, Vol. 17, Wiley-VCH, Weinheim

Haas Th, Wieck AG, Schaller KH, Mache K, Valentin H (1972) Die usuelle Bleibelastung bei Neugeborenen und ihren Müttern. Zbl Bakt Hyg I Abt Orig B 155: 341–349

Haenninen H, Aitio A, Kovala T, Luukhouen R, Matihainen E, Maumela T, Erkkitä J, Riihimäki V (1998) Occupational exposure to lead and neuropsychological dysfunction. Occup Environ Med 55: 202–209

Haenninen H, Hernberg S, Mantere P, Vesanto R, Jalkanen M (1978) Psychological performance of subjects with low exposure to lead. JOM: 683–689

Henschler D (Ed.) (1977) Blei und seine Verbindungen (berechnet als Pb) außer Bleiarsenat, Bleichromat und Alkylbleiverbindungen. Gesundheitsschädliche Arbeitsstoffe, Toxikologisch-arbeitsmedizinische Begründungen von MAK-Werten, 5. Lieferung, Verlag Chemie, Weinheim

Hogstedt C, Hane M, Bodin A, Agrell L (1983) Neuropsychological test results and symptoms among workers with well-defined long-term exposure to lead. Br J Ind Med 40: 99–105

Jacobson BE, Lockitch G, Quigley G (1991) Improved sample preparation for accurate determination of low concentrations of lead in whole blood by graphite furnace analysis. Clin Chem 37: 515–9

Jeyaratnam J, Boey K, Ong C, Chia C, Phoon W (1986) Neuropsychological studies on lead workers in Singapore. Br J Ind Med 43: 626–629

Jin Z, Shougui J, Shikum C, Desen J, Chahvalarle D (1990) Direct determination of lead in human blood and selenium cadmium, copper, zinc in serum by electrothermal atomic absorption spectrometry using Zeeman effect background correction. Fresenius J Anal Chem 337: 877–881

Kovala T, Matikainen E, Mannelin T, Erkkilä J, Riihimäki V, Hänninen H, Aitio A (1997) Effects of low level exposure to lead on neurophysiological functions among lead battery workers. Occup Environ Med 54: 487–493

Krigman M, Bouldin TW, Mushak P (1980) Lead. in: Spencer PS, Schaumburg HH (Eds) Experimental and clinical neurotoxicology. Williams & Wilins, Baltimore, 490–507

Lehnert G, Angerer J, Schaller KH (1998) Statusbericht über die externe Qualitätssicherung arbeits- und umweltmedizinisch-toxikologischer Analysen in biologischen Materialien. Arbeitsmed Sozialmed Umweltmed 33: 21–26

Lehnert G, Schaller KH, Angerer J (1999) Report on the status of the external quality-control programs for occupational-medical toxicological analyses in biologicals in Germany. Int Arch Occup Environ Health 72: 60–64

Lezak MD (1995) (Ed.) Neuropsychological assessment. New York: Oxford University Press, 3rd edition

Lindgren K, Masten V, Ford D, Bleecker M (1996) Relation of cumulative exposure to inorganic lead and neuropsychological test performance. Occup Environ Med 53: 472–477

Maizlish N, Parra G, Feo O (1995) Neurobehavioral evaluation of Venezuelan workers exposed to inorganic lead. Occup Environ Med 52: 408–414

Mantere P, Haenninen H, Hernberg S, Luukkonen R (1984) A prospective follow-up study on psychological effects in workers exposed to low levels of lead. Scand J Work Environ Health 10: 43–50

Meyer-Baron M, Seeber A (2000) A meta-analysis for neurobehavioural results due to occupational lead exposure with blood lead concentrations < 70 μg/100 ml. Arch Toxicol 73: 510–518

Miller DT, Paschal DC, Gunter EW, Strand PE, D'Angelo J (1987) Determination of lead in blood using electrothermal atomization absorption spectrometry with L'Vov platform and matrix modifier. Analyst 112: 1701–4

Murata K, Araki S, Aono H (1987) Effects of lead, zinc and copper absorption on peripheral nerve conduction in metal workers. Int Arch Occup Environ Health 59: 11–20

Murata K, Araki S (1991) Autonomic nervous system dysfunction in workers exposed to lead, zinc, and copper in relation to peripheral nerve conduction: a study of R–R interval variability. Am J Ind Med 20: 663–671

Murata K, Araki S, Yokoyama K, Uchida E, Fujimura Y (1993) Assessment of central, peripheral, and autonomic nervous system functions in lead workers: neuroelectrophysiological studies. Environ Res 61: 323–336

Ostapczuk P (1992) Direct determination of cadmium and lead in whole blood by potentiometric stripping analysis. Clin Chem 38: 1995–2001

Österberg K (1997) A neurobehavioural study of long-term occupational inorganic lead exposure. Sci Tot Environ 201: 39–51

Parkinson D, Ryan C, Bromet E, Connell M (1986) A psychiatric epidemiologic study of occupational lead exposure. Am J Epidemiol 123: 261–269

Parson PJ, Slavin W (1993) A rapid Zeeman graphite furnace atomic absorption spectrometric method for the determination of lead in blood. Spectrochim Acta 48B: 925–39

Pasternak G, Becker CE, Lash A, Bowler R, Estrim W, Law D (1989) Cross-sectional neurotoxicology study of lead-exposed cohort. Clin Toxicol 27: 37–51

Repko JD, Corum CR, Garcia PD, Jones LS (1978) The effects of inorganic lead on behavioural and neurologic function (US Dept of Health, Education, and Welfare, National Institute for Occupational Safety and Health). Cincinnatti: DHEW (NIOSH)

Roels H, Hubermont G, Buchet JP, Lauwerys R (1978) Placental transfer of lead, mercury, cadmium, and monoxide in women. III. Factors influencing the accumulation of heavy metals in the placenta and the relationship between metal concentration in the placenta and in maternal and cord blood. Environ Res 16: 236–247

Ryan CM, Morrow L, Parkinson D, Bromet E (1987) Low level lead exposure and neuropsychological functioning in blue collar males. Int J Neurosci 36: 29–39

Schaller KH, Angerer J, Lehnert G (1995) Current status of the external quality assurance programmes of the German Society for Occupational and Environmental Medicine. Toxicol Lett 77: 213–217

Seppäläinen AM, Hernberg S, Vesanto R, Kock B (1983) Early neurotoxic effects of occupational lead exposure: a prospective study. Neurotoxicol 4: 181–192

Shuttler IL, Delves HAT (1986) Determination of lead in blood by atomic absorption spectrometry with electrothermal atomization. Analyst 111: 651–60

Skerfving S (1993) Inorganic lead. in: Beije B, Lundberg P (Eds) Criteria documents from the Nordic expert group 1992. Arbeite och Hälsa 1: 125–238

Spivey G, Brown CP, Baloh RW (1979) Subclinical effects of chronic increased lead absorption – a prospective study. J Occup Med 21: 423–429

Spivey GH, Baloh RW, Brown P, Browdy BL, Campion DS, Valentine JL, Morgan DE, Culver BD (1980) Subclinical effects of chronic increased lead absorption – a prospective study. J Occup Med 22: 60–612

Stollery B, Banks H, Broadbent D, Lee W (1989) Cognitive functioning in lead workers. Br J Ind Med 46: 698–707

Teruya K, Sakurai H, Omae K, Higashi T, Muto T, Kaneko Y (1991) Effect of lead on cardiac parasympathetic function. Int Arch Occup Environ Health 62: 549–553

Task Group on Metal Accumulation TGMA (1973). Environ Physiol Biochem 3: 65–107

Triebig G (1984) Schwere Blei-Polyneuropathie. Fortschr Med 102: 485–488

US Environmental Protection Agency. (1986) Air quality criteria for lead. EPA–600/8–83/028aF, Vols I–IV, Environmental Protection Agency, Environmental Criteria and Assessment Office, Research Triangle Park, N.C

Valciukas JA, Lilis R, Eisinger J, Blumberg WE, Fischbein A, Selikoff IJ (1978) Behavioural indicators of lead neurotoxicity: results of a clinical field survey. Int Arch Occup Environ Health 41: 217–236

Valciukas JA, Lilis R, Singer R, Fischbein A, Anderson HA, Glickman L (1980) Lead exposure and behavioral changes: Comparisons of four occupational groups with different levels of lead absorption. Am J Ind Med 1: 421

WHO (World Health Organization) (1995) Inorganic lead. IPCS (International Programme on Chemical Safety). Environmental Health Criteria 165, WHO, Geneva

WHO (1996) Biological monitoring of chemical exposure in the workplace, Guidelines, Volume 1. WHO – HPR – OCH 1996.1, WHO, Geneva

Williamson A, Teo R (1986) Neurobehavioral effects of occupational exposure to lead. Br J Ind Med 43: 374–380

Yokoyama K, Araki S, Murata K, Morita Y, Katsuno N, Tanigawa T, Mori N, Yokata J, Ito A, Sakata E (1997) Subclinical vestibulo-cerebellar, anterior cerebellar lobe and spinocerebellar effects in lead workers in relation to concurrent and past exposure. Neurotoxicol 18: 371–380

Yokoyama K, Araki S, Aono H, Murata K (1998) Calcium disodium ethylenediaminetetraacetate-chelated lead as a predictor for subclinical lead neurotoxicity: follow-up study on gun-metal foundry workers. Int Arch Occup Environ Health 71: 459–464

Zimmerman-Tansella C, Campara P, D'Andrea F, Savonitto C, Tansella M (1983) Psychological and physical complaints of subjects with low exposure to lead. Human Toxicology 2: 615–23

Authors: H.M. Bolt, K.H. Schaller

Approved by the Working Group: 19.01.2000

Lead and its compounds, Addendum (except lead arsenate, lead chromate and alkyllead compounds)

BAT for women younger than 45 years	100 µg lead/l blood
Date of evaluation	2003

10 Re-evaluation of the BAT Value for Lead for Women below 45 Years of Age

More recent studies of the toxic effects of lead on reproduction in women and a reduction in the exposure to lead of the general population have made necessary the re-evaluation of the previous BAT value of 300 µg lead per litre blood for women younger than 45 years.

10.1 Exposure and effects

The current data for the developmental toxicity of lead can be found in the supplement to the MAK documentation for lead and its inorganic compounds, apart from lead arsenate and lead chromate (Greim 2002). Discussed there are the results of prospective studies of children (longitudinal studies) which determined the relationship between blood levels in prenatal or perinatal maternal blood or in umbilical cord blood and data for postnatal cognitive development. Seven birth cohorts were evaluated, which are presented in the MAK documentation (see Table 1 at the end of this addendum). Cross-sectional studies, which are primarily of environmental relevance, were not taken into consideration.

The seven studies evaluated are summarized in the MAK documentation (Greim 2002) as follows:

The meta-analyses of the prospective studies which have been carried out, which analysed only postnatal blood lead levels, can contribute only little to answering our question of the significance of prenatal and perinatal exposure to lead on later cognitive development (Pocock *et al.* 1994, WHO 1995).

"In spite of intensive efforts to standardize the methods used (body burden, measurement of effects, relevant confounders), the prospective studies are so different that a truly concurrent picture of the effects of lead cannot really be expected (WHO 1995). The various cohorts differ markedly in the correlates reflecting opportunities for cognitive development. The average maternal IQ in the Boston study cohort was, for

Essential BAT Value Documentations. DFG, Deutsche Forschungsgemeinschaft

ISBN 3-527-31477-6

example, 121, that in the Cleveland study cohort only 75; this reflects enormous socio-economic and familial differences. The nature of the exposure to lead also differs markedly in the various studies. It includes exposure via paint containing lead in dilapidated slum areas (Cincinnati), exposure mainly via traffic in cities like Sydney and Boston, exposure in the drinking water in one city (Glasgow), and emissions from lead smelters (Port Pirie, Kosovo).

For these reasons it is hardly surprising that the results are discrepant. The results of the seven prospective studies are inconsistent if, as is necessary in the present context, the effect only of the prenatal and perinatal exposure to lead is considered as the predictor for cognitive development. Three of the studies revealed no such relationship (Glasgow, Port Pirie, Sydney). In three other studies (Boston, Cleveland, Cincinnati) a significant negative association was determined at the age of six months. In the Kosovo study this association was detected in samples from children aged 48 months but not from younger children. In four of the studies (not in Sydney, Glasgow or Cleveland) mainly relationships between cognitive development and postnatal lead exposure were found and these are in accordance in this respect with the results of most cross-sectional studies (not discussed here).

Thus it is still not clear whether specifically prenatal or perinatal exposure to lead is relevant for a persistent impairment of later cognitive development; the clearest evidence was obtained in the Boston study in which 100 µg/l blood was the effect threshold (Bellinger *et al.* 1991). The impairment persists, however, for at most 24 months. Prenatal and postnatal blood lead levels are necessarily correlated, so that a negative correlation between prenatal or perinatal blood lead levels and postnatal development could also be detected postnatally. Then it would be justified to doubt that maternal exposure to lead can affect the later cognitive development of her child and to conclude that the developmental toxicological data indicate that changes in the BAT value for women of child-bearing age are not necessary. However, the quantitative situation is unclear and more epidemiological studies are necessary" (Greim 2002).

The available literature shows that a scientifically grounded value, based on a threshold concentration for foetal effects, still cannot be evaluated. Effects can be seen even at low levels of exposure; a threshold concentration for such effects can probably not be determined. This view is further supported by the most recent studies (Canfield *et al.* 2003, Rogan and Ware 2003, Selevan *et al.* 2003, Walkowiak *et al.* 1998).

10.2 Background exposure

Exposure situation in Germany

The internal exposure to lead in the general population has decreased considerably in recent years. The following reference values were given for the German population for the years 1990/92 (95th percentiles) by the "Kommission Human-Biomonitoring des Umweltbundesamtes" (Federal Environmental Agency, UBA) (Krause *et al.* 1996):

- Women aged 25 to 69 years: 90 µg/l
- Men aged 25 to 69 years: 120 µg/l

In the meantime, the level of lead in blood has decreased further in Germany. The environmental survey from 1998 yielded the following reference values (95th percentiles):

- Women aged 18 to 69 years: 62 µg/l
- Men aged 18 to 69 years: 79 µg/l

The median value was in the range of 27 to 36 µg/l (Becker *et al.* 2002).

The Federal Environmental Agency commission therefore set the following reference values on the basis of the 3rd environmental survey (Becker *et al.* 2002, UBA 2002):

- Women (18–69 years): 70 µg/l *
- Men (18–69 years): 90 µg/l *

International situation

In the "Tracy project", in 1996 the blood lead levels in the general population world-wide were evaluated. Ten studies were selected which were suitable for evaluation as regards the analysis and definition of the population group. They concluded that no general reference values for the blood lead level can be given, as the lead concentrations in blood depend greatly on the sampling time. As a result of the elimination of lead from motor fuels, there has been a constant decrease in blood lead levels (Herber 1999). In Sweden, for example, they fell from 60 µg lead per litre blood in 1978 to 25 µg/l in a period of 15 years. The study showed that numerous factors, such as age, sex, ethnic origin, food, drinking and smoking habits, hobbies, the season and year of sampling, residential area and geographical origin influence the lead levels in the general population (Gerhardsson *et al.* 1996). In the NHANES (National Health and Nutrition Examination Survey) report of the CDC (2003), for the female American general population a 95th percentile of 40 µg/l blood was evaluated. This value is based on the analysis of 4057 blood samples, taken in the period 1999–2000 in the United States.

11 Re-evaluation of the BAT Value

For a re-evaluation of the BAT value for women younger than 45 years the following points are relevant:

- As for the BAT value for women older than 45 years and for men, only the lead concentration in blood can be used as a biomarker. The exposure range in discussion disqualifies the use of effect parameters, such as the excretion of δ-aminolaevulinic acid in urine (ALA-U) and the concentration of the erythrocyte porphyrins, for occupational-medical health monitoring. Determination of the activity of ALA-D (δ-aminolaevulinic acid dehydratase) in blood as a monitoring parameter is not practicable.
- A scientifically grounded BAT value for the blood lead level in women of child-bearing age cannot at present be evaluated, as a clear threshold concentration cannot be defined. In the Boston longitudinal study, however, an effect threshold of 100 µg/l is assumed (Bellinger *et al.* 1991). The need for a stricter limitation of exposure for women of child-bearing age (below 45 years) compared to for women not of child-bearing age (45 years and above) and men is evident for the reasons given above and

---

* When using the updated reference values, an analytical uncertainty of ± 20 % must be taken into account.

from a preventive point of view. As already stipulated in the occupational-medical, toxicological documentation for the previous BAT value of 300 µg/l blood, in view of the general considerations women of child-bearing age should not be exposed to a much greater degree than the average population (Henschler and Lehnert 1989). On the basis of the environmental survey from 1998, currently for the German general population a blood lead concentration for women (18–69 years of age) of 62 µg/l is given as the 95th population percentile. A blood lead concentration of 70 µg/l is the resulting reference value.

In analogy to the BAT value for women younger than 45 years evaluated in 1987, on the basis of the current background exposure of the general population and taking into consideration the findings in a longitudinal study which gives an effect threshold of 100 µg/l, a BAT value has been set of

100 µg lead per l blood

12 References

Baghurst PA, McMichael AJ, Wigg NR, Vimpani GV, Robertson EF, Roberts RJ, Tong SL (1992) Environmental exposure to lead and children's intelligence at the age of seven years. The Port Pirie cohort study. New Engl J Med 327: 1279–1284

Becker K, Kaus S, Krause C, Lepom P, Schulz C, Seiwert M, Seifert B (2002) German environmental survey 1998 (GerES III): environmental pollutants in blood of the German population. Int J Hyg Environ Health 205: 297–308

Bellinger DC, Needleman HL, Leviton A, Waternaux C, Rabinowitz MB, Nichols ML (1984) Early sensory-motor development and prenatal exposure to lead. Neurobehav Toxicol Teratol 6: 387–402

Bellinger D, Leviton A, Needleman H, Waternaux C, Rabinowitz M (1986) Low-level lead exposure and infant development in the first year. Neurobehav Toxicol Teratol 8: 151–161

Bellinger D, Leviton A, Waternaux C, Needleman H, Rabinowitz M (1987) Longitudinal analyses of perinatal and postnatal lead exposure and early cognitive development. N Engl J Med 316: 1037–1043

Bellinger D, Sloman J, Leviton A, Rabinowitz M, Needleman HL, Waternaux C (1991) Low-level lead exposure and children's cognitive function in the preschool years. Pediatrics 87: 219–227

Canfield RL, Henderson Jr. CR, Cory-Slechta DA, Cox C, Jusko TA, Lanphear BP (2003) Intellectual impairment in children with blood lead concentrations below 10 µg per deciliter. N Engl J Med 348: 1517–1526

CDC (Centers for Disease Control and Prevention) (2003) Second national report on human exposure to environmental chemicals. NCEH Pub. No. 02-0716, National Center for Environmental Health, Division of Laboratory Sciences, Atlanta, Georgia

Cooney GH, Bell A, Mcbride W, Carter C (1989) Neurobehavioural consequences of prenatal low level exposure to lead. Neurotoxicol Teratol 11: 95–104

Dietrich KN, Krafft KM, Bornschein RL, Hammond PB, Berger O, Succop PA, Bier M (1987) Low level fetal lead exposure effect on neurobehavioral development in early infancy. Pediatrics 80: 721–730

Dietrich KN, Succop PA, Bornschein RL, Krafft KM, Berger O, Hammond PB, Buncher CR (1990) Lead exposure and neurobehavioral development in later infancy. Environ Health Perspect 89: 13–19

Dietrich KN, Succop PA, Berger OG, Hammond PB, Bornschein RL (1991) Lead exposure and the cognitive development of urban preschool children: the Cincinnati lead study cohort at age 4 years. Neurotoxicol Teratol 13: 203–211

Dietrich KN, Succop PA, Berger OG, Keith RW (1992) Lead exposure and the central auditory processing abilities and cognitive development of urban children: the Cincinnati lead study cohort at age 5 years. Neurotoxicol Teratol 14: 51–56

Dietrich KN, Berger OG, Succop PA, Hammond PB, Bornschein RL (1993) The developmental consequences of low to moderate prenatal and postnatal lead exposure: intellectual attainment in the Cincinnati lead study cohort following school entry. Neurotoxicol Teratol 15: 37–44

Ernhart CB, Wolf AW, Kennard MJ, Erhard P, Filipovich HF, Sokol RJ (1986) Intrauterine exposure to low levels of lead: the status of the neonate. Arch Environ Health 41: 287–291

Ernhart CB, Morrow-Tlucak M, Marler MR, Wolf AW (1987) Low level lead exposure in the prenatal and early preschool periods: early preschool development. Neurotoxicol Teratol 9: 259–270

Ernhart CB, Morrow-Tlucak M, Wolf AW (1988) Low level lead exposure and intelligence in the preschool years. Sci Total Environ 71: 453–459

Ernhart CB, Morrow-Tlucak M, Wolf AW, Super D, Drotar D (1989) Low level lead exposure in the prenatal and early preschool periods: intelligence prior to school entry. Neurotoxicol Teratol 11: 161–170

Gerhardsson L, Kazantzis G, Schutz A (1996) Evaluation of selected publications on reference values for lead in blood. Scand J Work Environ Health 22: 325–331

Greim H (Ed.) (2002) Lead and its inorganic compounds, apart from lead arsenate and lead chromate. in: Occupational toxicants, Vol. 17, Wiley-VCH, Weinheim

Henschler D, Lehnert G (Eds) (1989) Arbeitsmedizinisch-toxikologische Begründungen von BAT-Werten, 4. Lieferung, VCH, Weinheim

Herber RFM (1999) Review of trace element concentrations in biological specimens according to the TRACY protocol. Int Arch Occup Environ Health 72: 279–283

Krause C, Babisch W, Becker K, Bernigau W, Helm D, Hoffmann K, Nöllke P, Schulz C, Schwabe R, Seiwert M, Thefeld W (1996) Umwelt-Survey 1990/92, Band Ia: Studienbeschreibung und Human-Biomonitoring: Deskription der Spurenelementgehalte in Blut und Urin der Bevölkerung der Bundesrepublik Deutschland. WaBoLu-Hefte 1/1996, Werbung und Vertrieb, Berlin

McMichael AJ, Baghurst PA, Wigg NR, Vimpani GV, Robertson EF, Roberts RJ (1988) Port Pirie cohort study: environmental exposure to lead and children's abilities at the age of four years. N Engl J Med 319: 468–475

Moore MR, Bushnell IWR, Goldberg Sir A (1989) A prospective study of the results of changes in environmental lead exposure in children in Glasgow. in: Smith MA, Grant LD, Sors AI (Eds) Lead exposure and child development. An international assessment. Published for the Commission of the European Community and the US Environmental Protection Agency, Kluwer Academic Publishers, Dordrecht, 371–378

Pocock SJ, Smith M, Baghurst P (1994) Environmental lead and children's intelligence: a systematic review of the epidemiological evidence. BMJ 309: 1189–1197

Rogan WJ, Ware JH (2003) Exposure to lead in children – how low is low enough? N Engl J Med 348: 1515–1516

Selevan SG, Rice DC, Hogan KA, Euling SY, Pfahles-Hutchens A, Bethel J (2003) Blood lead concentration and delayed puberty in girls. N Engl J Med 348: 1527–1536

UBA (Umweltbundesamt) (2002) Bekanntmachungen des Umweltbundesamtes – Addendum zur "Stoffmonographie Blei – Referenz- und Human-Biomonitoring-Werte" der Kommission "Human-Biomonitoring" Stellungnahme der Kommission "Human-Biomonitoring" des Umweltbundesamtes. Bundesgesundheitsbl Gesundheitsforsch Gesundheitsschutz 45: 752–753

Vimpani GV, Baghurst PA, Wigg NR, Robertson EF, McMichael AJ, Roberts RR (1989) The Port Pirie cohort study – cumulative lead exposure and neurodevelopmental status at age two years: Do HOME scores and maternal IQ reduce apparent effects of lead on Bayley mental scores? in: Smith MA, Grant LD, Sors AI (Eds) Lead exposure and child development. An international assessment. Published for the Commission of the European Community and the US Environmental Protection Agency, Kluwer Academic Publishers, Dordrecht, 332–344

Walkowiak J, Altmann L, Krämer U, Sveinsson K, Turfeld M, Weishoff-Houben M, Winneke G (1998) Cognitive and sensorimotor functions in 6-year-old children in relation to lead and mercury levels: adjustment for intelligence and contrast sensitivity in computerized testing. Neurotox Teratol 20: 511–521

Wasserman G, Graziano JH, Factor-Litvak P, Popovac D, Morina N, Musabegovic A, Vrenezi N, Capuni-Paracka S, Lekic V, Preteni-Redjepi E, Hadzialjevic S, Slavkovich V, Kline J, Shrout P, Stein Z (1992) Independent effects of lead exposure and iron deficiency anemia on developmental outcome at age 2 years. J Pediatr 121: 695–703

Wasserman GA, Graziano JH, Factor-Litvak P, Popovac D, Morina N, Musabegovic A, Vrenezi N, Capuni-Paracka S, Lekic V, Preteni-Redjepi E, Hadzialjevic S, Slavkovich V, Kline J, Shrout P, Stein Z (1994) Consequences of lead exposure and iron supplementation on childhood development at age 4 years. Neurotoxicol Teratol 16: 233–240

WHO (World Health Organization) (1995) Inorganic lead. Environmental Health Criteria 165, Geneva

Wigg NR, Vimpani GV, McMichael AJ, Baghurst PA, Robertson EF, Roberts RJ (1988) Port Pirie cohort study: childhood blood lead and neuropsychological development at age two years. J Epidemiol Community Health 42: 213–219

Authors: K.H. Schaller, H.M. Bolt
Approved by the Working Group: 23.07.2003

Table 1. Prospective studies of toxic effects on reproduction in women (Greim 2002)

Authors, year of publication	Country	Test persons Age (years)	N	Lead exposure	Variables	Results
Bellinger *et al.* 1984, 1986, 1987, 1991	Boston, MA	birth to 10	249	level of lead in umbilical cord blood (low: 1–8 µg/dl, high: 14.6 µg/dl) 6, 12, 24 months (low: < 10 µg/dl, high: > 10 µg/dl)	Bayley scales (MDI, PDI), McCarthy scales GCI, WISC-R	1) significant inverse relationship between the level of lead in umbilical cord blood and the Bayley MDI at all times up to 24 months; 2) non-significant relationships between the blood lead level and the Bayley MDI at the age of 6 months; 3) significant negative relationship between the 24 month blood lead level and the 57 month McCarthy scale; the prenatal effects of lead remain significant at 57 months for low SES children, for those with a simultaneous higher blood lead level and for boys; 4) inverse relationship between the WISC-R and the blood lead level at 24 months
Dietrich *et al.* 1987, 1990, 1991, 1992, 1993	Cincinnati, OH	birth to 6.5	305	level of lead in umbilical cord blood (x = 8 µg/dl), blood lead level (24–60 months)	Bayley scales, K-ABC, WISC-R	significant negative relationship between the umbilical cord lead level and 6 month Bayley MDI, not significant at the age of 24 months, K-ABC not significant at 4 years, significant at 5 years; inverse relationship at the age of 6.5 years between the WISC-R and the postnatal blood lead level
Ernhart *et al.* 1986, 1987, 1988, 1989	Cleveland, OH	birth, follow-up studies at 6 months, 1, 2, 3 and 4 years and 10 months	162	level of lead in umbilical cord blood (x = 5.8 µg/dl), blood lead level (6 months to 4 years)	Brazelton Neonatal Behavior Assessment Scale, Graham/ Rosenblith test for newborn babies, Bayley scales, WPSSI	prenatal lead level negatively significant for 2 neonatal parameters (others not significant); with 6 month Bayley scale, not significant with 1, 2, 3 year Bayley scale and the WPPSI after adjustment for confounders
Moore *et al.* 1989	Glasgow, UK	birth, maternal PbB, follow-up study (24 months)	151	high: > 300 µg/l medium: 150–200 µg/l low: < 100 µg/l	Bayley scales	no significant group differences at the age of 12 and 4 months

Table 1. continued

Authors, year of publication	Country	Test persons Age (years)	N	Lead exposure	Variables	Results
Wigg *et al.* 1988 McMichael *et al.* 1988, Baghurst *et al.* 1992, Vimpani *et al.* 1989	Port Pirie, Australia	birth to 7	537	level of lead in umbilical cord blood (x = 8.8 µg/dl), blood lead level over 7 years, level of lead in teeth at the age of 7 years	Bayley scales, McCarthy GCI, WISC-R	significant inverse relationship between the 6 month blood lead level and 2 year Bayley MDI, relationship between the level of lead in umbilical cord blood and the Bayley MDI not significant; significant inverse relationship between the blood lead at the age of 2 and 3 years and McCarthy GCI at the age of 4 years; the index for the cumulative blood lead concentration shows the greatest inverse relationship to the GCI score at the age of 4 years; the WISC-R has a significant inverse relationship to the level of lead in blood and teeth at the age of 7 years
Wasserman *et al.* 1992, 1994	Kosovo (formerly Yugoslavia), towns with smelting works and towns with low lead exposure	birth to 4	392	lead level (x = 35.5 µg/dl smelting towns) (x = 8.4 µg/dl towns with low lead exposure)	Bayley MDI, McCarthy GCI	lead effects (confounded) with anaemia, lead effects lower than the anaemia effects at the age of 2 years; significant lead–GCI relationship at the age of 4 years; lead-related behavioural disturbances
Cooney *et al.* 1989	Sydney, Australia	birth to 5	318	level of lead in umbilical cord blood (x = 8.1 µg/dl)	Bayley MDI	non-significant relationship between blood lead level and MDI after covariable adjustment

Abbreviations: BNBAS: Brazelton Neonatal Behaviour Assessment Scale; BSID: Bayley Scales of Infant Development; GCI: General Cognitive Index; K-ABC: Kaufman-Assessment Battery of Children; MDI: Mental Development Index; MSCA: McCarthy Scales of Children's Abilities; PDI: Psychomotor Development Index; SES: Socio Economic Status; WISC-R: Wechsler Intelligence Scale for Children-Revised; WPPSI: Wechsler Preschool and Primary Scale of Intelligence; PbB: blood lead level

Lead and its compounds (except lead arsenate, lead chromate and alkylated compounds)

BLW for women older than 45 years for men	400 µg lead/l blood Sampling time: no restrictions
Date of evaluation	2005
BLW for women younger than 45 years	100 µg lead/l blood Sampling time: no restrictions
Date of evaluation	2005

13 Evaluation of BLW Values

Lead has been classified in Category 3 B for carcinogenic substances in the workplace due to occurrence of genotoxic effects. In addition to genotoxic effects there is also a suspicion of occurrences of tumours, which is discussed in some of the studies. The previous MAK value of 100 µg/m^3 has been withdrawn, and thus the BAT value has to be withdrawn, too.

In the case of lead however, one must consider that the previous BAT values of 400 µg/l blood for women older than 45 years and for men, and the BAT value of 100 µg/l blood for women younger than 45 years are based on toxic effects. This includes neurotoxic (and also behavioural) effects, which are of considerable relevance for the occupational hygiene concerns. The present BAT values have therefore been carried over as BLW values. Especially the prevention of neurotoxic effects is of great importance for lead-exposed persons and can be achieved by observing the BLW values. This also applies to the minimizing of reproductive toxic effects. Therefore, the BLW values have been set at

400 µg lead/l blood (for women older than 45 years and for men)
100 µg lead/l blood (for women younger than 45 years)

The importance of occupational-medical health surveillance including biological monitoring has to be stressed.

Author: H.M. Bolt
Approved by the Working Group: 23.05.2005

Essential BAT Value Documentations. DFG, Deutsche Forschungsgemeinschaft

ISBN 3-527-31477-6

Methanol

BAT	30 mg methanol/l urine Sampling time: end of the working week, 2nd half of the shift
Date of evaluation	1983
Synonyms	Methyl alcohol Carbinol
Formula	CH_3OH
Molecular weight	32.04
Melting point	−94 °C
Boiling point	64.7 °C
Vapour pressure at 20 °C	128 hPa
MAK	200 ml/m^3 (ppm) 260 mg/m^3

1 Metabolism and Kinetics

There are comprehensive reviews by Treon (1936) (1), Browning (1965) (2), Tephly et al. (1974) (3), Rowe and McCollister (1982) (4) and in the research report from the Deutsche Gesellschaft für Mineralölwissenschaft und Kohlechemie e. V., DGMK-Forschungsbericht 260-07 (1982) (5).

1.1 Metabolism

The biological transformation of methanol takes place in three steps:

I Oxidation of methanol to formaldehyde
II Oxidation of formaldehyde to formic acid
III Oxidation of formic acid to carbon dioxide and water

In addition formic acid and formaldehyde are built into amino acids and other endogenous substances (IIa and IIIa). The metabolism of methanol in humans (according to Forth et al., 1980 (6)) can be represented as follows:

Essential BAT Value Documentations. DFG, Deutsche Forschungsgemeinschaft

ISBN 3-527-31477-6

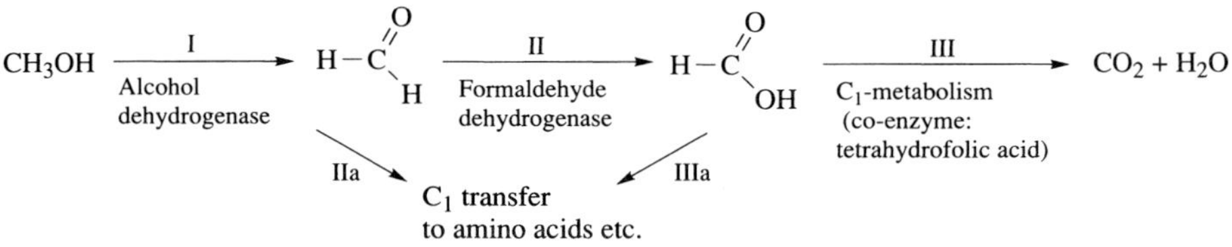

Notes to I: The oxidation of methanol (3, 7 – 10) is catalysed by the alcohol dehydrogenase (ADH) of the liver (7).

Von Wartburg et al. (1965) (11) as well as Blair and Vallee (1966) (9) discovered, however, that the human liver ADH oxidised methanol at a speed which amounted to only 12 or 11% of that for ethanol. Through ethanol the methanol oxidation is inhibited competitively so that a simultaneous exposure to ethanol leads to an increased methanol excretion via the lungs and urine (12, 13).

Notes to II: With regard to the oxidation of formaldehyde, the investigations by Goodman and Tephly (1971) (14) showed the existence of a specific NAD and GSH dependent formaldehyde dehydrogenase (FDH) in the liver of humans. Malorny et al. (1965) (15) discovered, after the findings of Matthies (1957/58) (16, 17) had already indicated the existence of a FDH in the erythrocytes of humans, that also in the erythrocytes of human blood formaldehyde can be transformed to formic acid.

For the elimination from the blood after intravenous formaldehyde application Rietbrock (1965/69) (18, 19) quotes as the half-life in various animal species 1 min, McMartin et al. (1979) (20) for monkeys 1.5 min.

Notes to III: The oxidation of formic acid to carbon dioxide and water takes place within the bounds of the C1 metabolism with the participation of the co-enzyme tetrahydrofolic acid (21, 22).

With primates the folic acid content is low (22, 23) which results during methanol intoxication in the observed cumulation of formic acid. It varies interindividually, which might be one of the reasons for the differing sensitivity to methanol (24).

1.2 Kinetics

Methanol can enter the human organism in three ways: in liquid state by absorption via the gastro-intestinal tract (oral uptake) and the skin (percutaneous uptake) as well as in vapour form via the lungs (pulmonary uptake).

At the workplace, inhalation of the vapour plays an important role but there is often also skin contact with liquid methanol. Accidentally in rare cases there may even be oral intake.

Otherwise, most of the known cases of methanol intoxication are due to oral uptake (confusion with ethanol, ignorance of the dangers or suicide attempt).

The total amount of methanol retained after pulmonary uptake depends on the duration of exposure and respiratory minute volume.

Ferry et al. (1980) (25) calculated for an 8-hour exposure to 200 ml/m^3 a retained methanol dose of 2.6 g ($\cong$3.25 ml) – on the assumption of a total respiratory volume of 10 m^3 (i.e. RMV $\cong$20 l/min) and a 100% retention without exhalation.

With five volunteers who were exposed for 8 hours to methanol concentrations between 103 and 284 mg/m^3 ($\approx$80–220 ml/m^3) Šedivec et al. (1981) (26) found a pulmonary retention of 57.7% (extreme values 53.4 and 61.3%).

Scheuplein and Blank (1973) (27) investigated the permeability of the human epidermis and dermis on excised skin from a corpse (abdominal skin). A conversion of the flow rates found for pure methanol (dermis: 0.306 mg/cm^2/min, epidermis: 0.138 mg/cm^2/min) revealed data corresponding with the results of Dutkiewicz et al. (1980) (28). The latter authors observed in vivo with human skin (forearm) exposed for 60 min an average methanol absorption rate of 0.192 mg/cm^2/min and calculated from this that after a 2-minute submersion of a hand a dose of 170 mg would have entered the organism. This would correspond to about the dose that is absorbed during an 8-hour inhalation of 50 mg/m^3 methanol (c.f. 26). The authors conclude that the percutaneous absorption (note: after skin contact with liquid methanol) could be the main route of absorption for methanol.

Here they agree with Tada et al. (1975) (29) and Ferry et al. (1979) (30) who showed that – judging by the urinary methanol concentrations – at least with longer skin contact (4 h) relevant methanol amounts can be absorbed via small areas of skin.

Methanol distributes itself independent of the method of application very quickly to all tissues, whereby the methanol concentration of the various structures is closely related to their water content.

After oral methanol application, for blood methanol concentrations between 5 and 10 mg/dl, 1.3–1.6 times higher urinary methanol concentrations were measured (12, 25).

After inhalational methanol uptake Heinrich and Angerer (31) quote for concentrations in the blood between 1 and 10 mg/dl 2.2 and 1.1 times higher concentrations in the urine respectively.

The oxidation product formic acid accumulates in the organism (20, 22, 32, 33). The diffusion of the formic acid from the blood into the liquor depends on the pH value (23). An experimental acidification of the blood (corresponds to the metabolic acidosis during methanol intoxication) resulted in an increase in the formic acid concentration in the liquor and a decrease in the blood as the undissociated formic acid can permeate the blood-liquor barrier considerably more easily than the dissociated form.

The excretion of the unchanged substance via the lungs and urine as well as the metabolic break-down are part of the elimination procedure.

The pulmonary excretion of unchanged methanol amounted during the investigations by Dutkiewicz (1978) (34) and Dutkiewicz et al. (1980) (28) with oral application to 22% and with epicutaneous application to 16% of the dose taken in (in both cases over a time span of 5 h). In both cases the elimination had monophasic character with a half-life of 1.5 h. The percentage of the unchanged methanol excreted with the urine is considerably lower. Kendel and Ramanathan (1953) (35) found within 12 h an excretion in the urine of 1.3% of the applied dose. With a simultaneous ethanol dose the methanol excretion could be increased to about 2.8%.

Leaf and Zatman (1952) (12) registered after oral application an excretion of unchanged methanol in the urine of their test persons (also after about 12 h) of on average 0.7% of the applied amount. This could be increased by up to 4% by repeated ethanol doses.

Dutkiewicz et al. (1980) (28) quote even lower values: only 0.31 and 0.13% of the orally and epicutaneously applied doses respectively could be found unmetabolised in the urine.

Šedivec et al. (1981) (26) calculate from the course of the methanol excretion by their test persons (inhalation) a biological half-life of 1.5–2.0 h. This is in accordance with the half-life of 2.0–2.25 h for the methanol elimination from the blood ascertained by Ferry et al. (1979) (30) after oral methanol application.

Various authors describe first order kinetics for the elimination of methanol after low methanol doses and plasma levels (12, 30, 36). According to Ferry et al. (1979) (30) this elimination characteristic also applies to methanol levels such as are probably reached with occupational exposure. With the uptake of higher, acutely toxic doses the methanol elimination, however, takes place according to kinetics of zero order, i.e. with a constant speed independent of the concentration in the blood, whereby the capacity of the enzymatically controlled metabolic processes is exceeded (30, 36).

Formaldehyde is, after methanol application, due to its extremely short half-life, neither detectable in the urine nor in the expired air. The formic acid formed from methanol is only eliminated to a small extent, about 1.0% of the applied methanol dose, unchanged via the urine. The greatest part of the formic acid appears after oxidation as CO_2 in the expired air.

Malorny (1969) (37) quotes for humans after an oral formic acid dose a half-life of 45–46 min. Rietbrock (1969) (19) gives 55 min after i.v. injection of formate, emphasises however that the half-life is dependent upon the dose.

The limiting factor for the metabolic elimination of the formic acid is the folic acid content of the organism which is low in humans (see also section 1.1). Thus, with higher level methanol exposure the formic acid accumulates in the organism with subsequent effects.

2 Critical Toxicity

The effect of methanol on humans is among other things extensively described by Browning (1965) (2), Posner (1975) (38), in the NIOSH report (1976) (39), in Rowe and McCollister (1982) (4) and the DGMK report (1982) (5).

It has already been accepted for a long time that the impairment of the organ of vision typically observed with methanol intoxication as well as other CNS structures – in contrast to the narcotic effect – is to be attributed not to the methanol itself but to one of its metabolites.

However, the opinion as to which one is the toxic metabolite has changed recently. While Cooper and Kini (1962) (60) held formaldehyde to be responsible for the toxic effect of methanol, currently available data suggests that with great probability the formic acid is to be seen as the primary toxic agent (20, 41, 42).

The symptoms of acute methanol intoxication are independent of the mode of uptake (4).

It is characterised by 3 stages:

I narcotic effect (due to methanol itself)
II latent period (about 10–48 h)
III manifestation of the (probably due to the toxic metabolite formic acid) intoxication symptoms.

Stage III begins with unspecific disturbances in the general state of health (headache, dizziness, nausea etc.). With the increase of the formic acid concentration in the blood and the resulting metabolic acidosis there can be disturbances of consciousness up to severe coma and possibly death.

The characteristic initial symptom with regard to the eyes is blurred vision. With the increase in the visual impairment at first a scotoma or a central scotoma develops with corresponding losses of the field of vision. Finally transitory or irreversible blindness (wide, fixed pupils) can occur. The ophthalmoscopic findings during these phases range from hyperaemia of the optic disk to oedema of the optic disk to (often only temporary) pallor of the disk as signs of optic atrophy (43).

As symptoms resulting from acute methanol intoxication, further CNS impairments, in particular extrapyramidal symptoms similar to Parkinson's disease have been described (44–46).

The morphological counterpart of this is a bilateral putamen necrosis which has been found in autopsy repeatedly (47, 48) and in recent years, however, has also been able to be diagnosed in vivo with the help of computed tomography (46, 49).

The opinion that the repeated exposure to low-level doses or concentrations can also lead to symptoms of intoxication is not shared by all authors. Some publications, however do express that also with chronic low-level methanol exposure health effects can occur (2, 50–53). Impairment of the visual system as well as other CNS structures (acoustic degeneration; putamen necrosis with extrapyramidal symptoms similar to Parkinson's disease) are under discussion.

3 Exposure and Effects

As the typical toxic effect of methanol is not to be attributed directly to the substance itself but to a toxic metabolite, the "internal exposure" must be defined in biological material as the concentration of the corresponding metabolite (probably formic acid).

Various authors are of the opinion that the internal exposure is represented by the methanol concentration in biological material.

With chronic methanol exposure the effect appears predominantly as an impairment in the visual ability. Moreover, there can be impairment of other CNS structures.

3.1 Relationship between External and Internal Exposure

3.1.1 Formic Acid

Data on the relation of certain methanol concentrations in the ambient air to certain formic acid concentrations in the blood are rare in the literature. Baumann and Angerer (1979) (54) found with 20 workers who were subject to average methanol concentrations between 85 and 134 ml/m^3 a highly significant increase in the formic acid concentration in the blood from 0.32 $\pm$ 0.24 mg/dl to 0.79 $\pm$ 0.32 mg/dl blood after the shift. In a control group of 36 unexposed persons an interindividual variation range in the formic acid concentration in the blood of 0 to 20 mg/l was determined (55). In the study quoted first an increase in the formic acid concentration in the urine of 13.1 $\pm$ 3.9 mg/l before the shift to 20.2 $\pm$ 7.0 mg/l urine after the shift was determined in workers exposed to methanol. The concentrations of formic acid in the urine of 15 control persons at corresponding times amounted to 11.9 $\pm$ 5.6 mg/l and 11.7 $\pm$ 5.6 mg/l urine. Mraz et al. (1978) (56) were not able to register any increased formic acid concentrations in the urine in investigations with volunteers who were exposed for 8 h to methanol concentrations of approx. 75 or 150 ml/m^3.

In an investigation by Heinrich and Angerer (1982) (31) on 20 persons occupationally exposed to methanol (methanol concentration in the workplace air 37–231 ml/m^3) only 15% of the urinary formic acid concentrations measured with these persons were over the normal level. No correlation with the external exposure could be determined.

3.1.2 Methanol

Spasovski and Benčev (1969) (57) quote for a 6-hour inhalational exposure to 50 and 75 ml/m^3, blood methanol concentrations of 0.21 and 0.33 mg/dl, respectively. On this basis Ferry et al. (1980) (25) calculated for an 8-hour exposure to 200 ml/m^3 a value of almost 1 mg/dl blood: approx. 0.95 mg/dl for a half-life of 3.5 h (12) or approx. 0.9 mg/dl for 2.25 h (30).

Investigations by Heinrich and Angerer (1982) (31) on 20 persons exposed to a median methanol concentration over 8 hours of approx. 100 ml/m^3 (total range 37–231 ml/m^3) resulted in average blood methanol concentrations at the end of a working week of 0.89 $\pm$ 1.47 mg/dl (median value 0.36 mg/dl, total range $<$0.06–6.01 mg/dl) i.e. on average approx. 0.9 $\pm$ 1.5 mg/dl.

The methanol exposure did not lead in every case to a measurable increase in the blood methanol level. The median value was only 6 times as high as the detection limit (0.06 mg/dl). The methanol concentration in the blood of 26 unexposed control persons did not exceed this detection level. Majchrowicz and Mendelsohn (1971) (13) ascertained blood methanol concentrations below 0.1 mg/dl in 19 normal persons. After extensive drinking of methanol-free alcoholic beverages the methanol level was between 1.1 and 2.7 mg/dl, occasionally even over 4 mg/dl and more, which Majchrowicz and Mendelsohn attributed to a cumulation of endogenously formed methanol as a result of competitive inhibition of the methanol oxidation due to chronic ethanol consumption.

Spasovski and Benčev (1969) (57) observed in inhalation experiments with volunteers exposed for six hours that the methanol concentration in the urine varied almost linearly with the concentration in the air.

Various authors quote for certain methanol concentrations in the expired air corresponding methanol concentrations in the urine. Table 1 gives a summary.

Tab. 1: Relationship between external exposure and methanol concentration in the urine.

External methanol exposure ml/m^3	Duration of exposure	Internal methanol exposure concentration in urine (mg/l)	Comments	References
VP 1: – 540		7.8	These are values	Leaf and
– 560		10.5	corrected by the	Zatman (1952)
–1040		20.6	authors (acc. to	(12)
–1100	2.5 h	25.6	control value =	
VP 2: – 500		10.3	normal value on	
– 560		13.2	entering the ex-	
– 950		25.4	posure chamber)	
200 ("MAC")	8 h/day 5 days/week	approx. 4–8	Measurements "at the end of a day or a week"	Elkins (1954) (62)
125 (on average)		3	The measurements were carried out in	Treon (1963) (1)
		6	3 factories	
440 (on average)	not indicated	3.5		
		6.5		
2800 (on average)		9		
		16		
		44		
≅36		1.6 (1.3–1.84)		Spasovski and Benčev (1969) (57)
	6 h			
≅78		2.6 (2.0–3.6)		
			2 test persons	Tada et al. (1974) (64)
200 (110–360)	2 × 2 h/day interval: 2 h 3–4 days	10–14	These are average maximum values (peak values approx. 16 mg/l). normal values before the exposure: 0.5–4.5 mg/l	

Tab. 1: Continued.

External methanol exposure ml/m³	Duration of exposure	Internal methanol exposure concentration in urine (mg/l)	Comments	References
200 ("ACGIH TLV")	(8 h/day 5 days/week?)	< 5	Rough estimates due to the human experiments by Leaf and Zatman (1952) and Elkins (Treon, 1963; see above)	Lauwerys (1975) (68)
≅160 ≅230	8 h	6.5 9.5	4 test persons (each one went through both experiments) Normal value with 31 control persons: 0.32–2.61 (mean 0.73) mg/l.	Šedivec et al. (1981) (26)
200	8 h	≅6.5	Theoretical value on the basis of the results by Šedivec et al. (1981)	Heinrich and Angerer (1982) (31) Šedivec et al. (1981) (26)
			20 test persons	Heinrich and Angerer (1982) (31)
≅100	8 h (at the end of a week shift)	21.8 ± 20.0 (median value 19.2) (10.2 ± 7.3)	Analysis of the urine voided in the last 4 h (Analysis of the urine voided in the first 4 h) Normal values with 26 control persons: < 0.6–2.9 (mean 1.1 ± 0.9) mg/l.	
≅200	8 h (at the end of a week shift)	40	Estimate	

A comparison of the individual sets of data is made more difficult in that the duration of exposure differs greatly in some cases and also the conditions of exposure (additional dermal contact with methanol, respiratory minute volumes etc.) as well as the time interval of the urine sampling and the methods of determination were not uniform.

If one tries with the help of the data summarised in table 1 to deduce the methanol concentration which occurs in the urine after an exposure at levels of the order of magnitude of the MAK value (200 ml/m^3; 8 h/day; 5 days/week) a wide range of values results. Older publications up to 1981, obviously due to the method, allow urinary methanol concentrations between approx. 5 and 15 mg/l to be deduced after an exposure at the level of the MAK value.

With an optimised method Heinrich and Angerer (1982) (31) found an average methanol concentration of 21.8 ± 20.0 mg/l (median value 19,2 mg/l; total range < 0.6–57.3 mg/l) in the urine collected in the afternoon of the last 8-hour day of a week shift for a median methanol concentration in the workplace air of approx. 100 ml/m^3. The individual urinary methanol concentration was in the afternoon on average approx. 2.5 times higher than in the morning. With 12 unexposed control persons the urinary methanol concentrations were below the detection limit of 0.6 mg/l. With control persons who showed detectable methanol concentrations ethanol could also be detected gas chromatographically.

80% of the urinary methanol concentrations of the exposed persons were above the maximum concentration of the control group.

Heinrich and Angerer (1982) (31) determined by extrapolation that an exposure at the level of the MAK value (8 h, 200 ml/m^3) corresponds to a urinary methanol concentration of approx. 40 mg/l.

Baumann and Angerer (1979) (54) were able to determine an increase in the ethanol concentration during the shift in the alveolar air of workers exposed to methanol (85–134 ml/m^3), whereby there was no correlation with the air-methanol concentration.

3.2 Relationship between Internal Exposure and Effect

As there are only few indications of the relationship between internal and external exposure and effect after inhalational or percutaneous uptake as they occur at the workplace in the literature published so far, in the following treatise reference is made to the information obtained from (acute) oral cases of intoxication.

3.2.1 Formic Acid

In the literature there are merely a few details on the formic acid concentrations in the blood after acute oral methanol intoxication with a lethal outcome. The values quoted range between 5.7 and 104.7 mg/dl blood (48, 58, 59). Comparison and evaluation of these data is, however, difficult as it cannot be assumed that all the measurements were taken at the point in time of the highest formic acid concentration in the blood.

Details of the formic acid concentration in the blood associated with an impairment of the visual ability could not be gained from the literature available.

In cases of fatal oral methanol intoxication formic acid concentrations in the urine between 216 and 758 mg/dl are supposed to have been present (1, 60); such high values can hardly be of interest for the setting of a threshold limit value.

In the study by Heinrich and Angerer (1982) (31) the highest formic acid concentration in the urine measured at the end of the shift amounted to 121 mg/l. Further details are not to be gained from the literature.

3.2.2 Methanol

Knowledge of the methanol concentration in the blood and effects resulting from this has been gained exclusively from investigations of acute cases of oral intoxication. The methanol concentrations in the blood which are quoted in connection with the occurrence of toxic effects show a great variation in range. The reasons for this could include a different time span between the methanol uptake and blood methanol determination (58).

A selection of the lowest blood methanol concentrations mentioned in the literature which were measured in connection with toxic effects is given in table 2.

Furthermore, there are indications of probably non-toxic concentrations: Ferry et al. (1980) (25) registered during their experiments with volunteers at various opportunities blood methanol concentrations of 4 mg/dl without there being any symptoms. The highest value measured by Heinrich and Angerer (1982) (31) after inhalation of an average of 100 ml/m^3 (maximum 230 ml/m^3) was 6 mg/dl blood.

Data on the relationship between methanol concentrations in the urine and effects which are of interest with regard to the setting of a threshold limit value cannot be taken from the literature available. Merely some urinary methanol levels measured during some kinetic investigations give an indication of concentrations with which – over a relatively short period of time – obviously no toxic effects were observed.

Thus, in Tada et al. (1975) (29) 123.5 and 184.4 mg/l are the highest urinary methanol concentrations to be found. With test persons concentrations of over 90 and up to 47 mg/l have been determined without symptoms (12, 25).

Further information on the relationship between internal methanol exposure and effects can be gained indirectly via the MAK values.

As according to table 1, information as to the relationship between external exposure at the level of the MAK value and the corresponding methanol concentration in the urine is available or at least can be deduced, it would seem sensible to make conclusions on the probably harmless urinary methanol concentrations from this.

The urinary methanol concentrations which are quoted or can be deduced for an exposure at the level of the MAK value are not uniform but range between about 5 and 40 mg/l.

Tab. 2: Relationship between methanol concentration in blood and effects.

Methanol concentration in the blood (mg/dl)		Effect	References
5.0 12.0 39.7		severe metabolic acidosis	Keeney and Mellinkoff (1951) (69)
15.6 45.0 60.0 60.0 96.0 150.0	measured at the time of death	death (in one case blindness was observed beforehand)	
20		metabolic acidosis (this was a child)	Kahn and Blum (1979) (70)
19.4	measured about 50 h after uptake of methanol	transitory blindness; survived; with death 1.5 years later symmetrical putamen necrosis was diagnosed	Erlanson et al. (1965) (48)
27.5 27.7 86.0	measured about 50 h after uptake of methanol	death	
73		death	Naraqui et al. (1979) (71)
about 99		total blindness; symmetrical putamen necrosis	Aquilonius et al. (1980) (49)
110		blurred vision	Kane et al. (1968) (72)
120 130		death (blindness beforehand)	Bennett et al. (1953) (73)
3	measurement approx. 100 h after uptake of methanol	acidosis damage to the eyes	Gonda et al. (1978) (58)
25	approx. 40 h after uptake of methanol	acidosis damage to the eyes	
53 56	approx. 24 h after uptake of methanol	acidosis; only slight general symptoms (*no* impairment of vision)	
74 102	approx. 24 h approx. 40 h after uptake of methanol	acidosis; only temporary impairment of vision (blurred vision, photophobia)	

For methanol there are no suitable effect parameters available which indicate early enough the danger of a pathological change in the organism due to toxic influences.

On the other hand various internal exposure parameters have been examined for their usefulness (the formaldehyde concentration in biological material can, as discussed in sections 1 and 3, be dismissed as an indicator of internal exposure).

4.1 Formic Acid

(c.f. section 3.1.1)

A correlation between the air methanol concentration and the formic acid concentration in the blood could not be demonstrated (54). Furthermore, in the blood of control persons not occupationally exposed there was a large interindividual variation range of physiological formic acid concentrations (55) so that there was a large area of overlap between normal values and those after exposure.

The detection of formic acid in urine is not sensitive enough to be a monitoring parameter. A differentiation between methanol-induced and physiological levels is difficult. Moreover, other substances such as e.g. acetone (61) or methyl chloride as well as the consumption of certain foodstuffs can increase the formic acid concentration in the urine.

4.2 Methanol

(c.f. section 3.1.2)

In investigations by Heinrich and Angerer (1982) (31) the physiological normal values never exceed the detection limit of 0.06 mg/dl blood so that the authors – in agreement with Ferry et al. (1980) (25) – assume normal values of around 0.06 mg/dl and below (even after the consumption of beverages containing methanol). With the exposed persons, however, concentrations up to 6 mg/dl blood were measured from which a high diagnostic specificity can be read. On the other hand the sensitivity proved to be insufficient as not every individual blood methanol concentration increased measurably after exposure. The median value came to only 6 times the detection limit. Heinrich and Angerer therefore conclude that an 8-hour exposure to approx. 100 ml/m^3 cannot be determined with certainty in the individual case.

At an early date Elkins (1954) (62) ascertained in occasional measurements that persons who worked in the range of the greatest methanol vapour concentrations almost always showed the highest methanol concentrations in the urine.

Dutkiewicz and Blochowicz (1967) (63) found a linear relationship between the methanol dose retained in the organism and the average methanol concentration in the total shift urine, Spasovski and Benčev (1969) (57) an almost linear relationship between the methanol concentrations in the urine and the ambient air.

The use of the methanol concentration in the urine is also recommended by Tada et al. (1974) (64), Ferry et al. (1980) (25), Šedivec et al. (1981) (26) and by Heinrich and Angerer (1982) (31). The specificity of the methanol excretion is, in comparison to the other parameters, to be regarded as high. This also applies to the biological sensitivity. The sampling is simple.

No correlation was found between the methanol concentration in the alveolar air and in the ambient air. Moreover, as in practice there are often difficulties with regard to the exact sampling of alveolar air as well as the transport and storage of the samples (66) the methanol determination in the alveolar air has not proved suitable to date as a routine monitoring method.

5 Methodology

For the determination of the methanol concentration in the urine a tested gas chromatographic head space method is available which has proved to be practicable, analytically specific and sensitive, and produces reliable results.

A detailed description can be found in particular in Heinrich and Angerer (1982) (31). The detection limit is 0.6 mg/l.

6 Evaluation of the BAT Value

The most suitable biological parameter, according to currently available data for a biological monitoring of persons exposed to methanol is the methanol concentration in the urine (see section 4).

As, however, there are not sufficient data on the direct relationship between the methanol concentration in the urine and effect (see section 3.2.2) from which a BAT value could be determined, an indirect derivation via the MAK value (200 ml/m^3) must be carried out.

Most of the data published by 1981 were not gained by using optimised methods of analysis.

A field study resulted in a methanol excretion in the urine of around 20 mg/l (31) for an average air methanol concentration of approx. 100 ml/m^3. Assuming a linear correlation with exposure to concentrations near the MAK value a methanol excretion of 40 mg/l urine can be expected.

Under laboratory conditions at the end of an 8-hour exposure to 205 mg/m^3 ($\cong$160 ppm) and 300 mg/m^3 ($\cong$230 ppm) methanol, respectively, with 4 volunteers average methanol concentrations of 6.5 and 9.5 mg/l urine were found (26).

For the interpretation of these results it must be borne in mind that these investigations were carried out with persons at rest, while the field study on employees of a chemical company took place during physical work (31). The difference between the results of the two studies, in addition to the possibility of exposure due to skin contact and non-uniform time intervals of the sampling, should on the whole be due to the differences in the ventilation rates. The test persons investigated by Šedivec et al. (26) showed a ventilation rate of 10.5 l/min. If one takes a ventilation rate of 20 l/min for medium work as a basis, then for an exposure to 200 ml/m³ a value of around 20 mg methanol/l urine results.

Under consideration of both studies the BAT value has been set at

30 mg methanol/l urine

The urine samples are collected in the 2nd half of a shift at the end of the working week.

7 Interpretation of the Data

As stated in the above documentation the most suitable parameter for protection of the individual with occupational methanol exposure is the methanol concentration in urine.

In order to take into account the methanol cumulation during exposure the methanol concentration in the urine of the 2nd half of a shift at the end of a working week should be determined.

Occupational medical health surveillance of persons exposed to methanol should be carried out in the Federal Republic of Germany otherwise according to the berufsgenossenschaftlicher Grundsatz G10 (67) (guideline issued by the Employers' Liability Insurance Association). The time spans for follow-up investigations are also stated here. With border-line findings more frequent check-ups can be appropriate.

8 References

1. Treon, J. F.: Methyl alcohol. In: Patty's Industrial Hygiene and Toxicology, Vol. II. Interscience Publishers 1963
2. Browning, E.: Toxicity and metabolism of industrial solvents. Elsevier Publishing Company, Amsterdam – London – New York 1965, pp. 311 – 323
3. Tephly, T. R. et al.: Essays Toxicol. *5* (1974), 149 – 177
4. Rowe, V. K., McCollister, S. B.: Methanol. In: Patty's Industrial Hygiene and Toxicology, Vol. 2 C. Wiley-Interscience Publication 1982, pp. 4527 – 4708
5. DGMK: Deutsche Gesellschaft für Mineralölwissenschaft und Kohlechemie e. V., Forschungsbericht 260 – 07 (1982)
6. Forth, W. et al.: Allgemeine und spezielle Pharmakologie und Toxikologie. Bibliograph. Inst., Mannheim – Wien – Zürich 1980, p. 623
7. Goodman, J. I., Tephly, T. R.: Mol. Pharmacol. *4* (1968), 492 – 501
8. Von Wartburg, F. P. et al.: Biochemistry *3* (1964), 1775 – 1782
9. Blair, A. H., Vallee, B. L.: Biochemistry *5* (6) (1966), 2026 – 2034
10. Mani, J. C. et al.: Arch. Biochem. Biophys. *140* (1970), 52 – 59
11. Von Wartburg, J. P. et al.: Can. J. Biochem. *43* (1965), 889
12. Leaf, G., Zatman, L. J.: Brit. J. Ind. Med. *9* (1952), 19 – 31
13. Majchrowicz, E., J. M. Mendelsohn: J. Pharmacol. Exp. Ther. *179* (1971), 293 – 300
14. Goodman, J. I., Tephly, T. R.: Biochim. Biophys. Acta *252* (1971), 489 – 505
15. Malorny, G. et al.: Arch. Exp. Path. Pharmacol. *250* (1965), 419 – 436

16. Matthies, H.: Biochem. Z. *329* (1957), 421
17. Matthies, H.: Biochem. Z. *330* (1958), 169
18. Rietbrock, N.: Pharmacol. *259* (1965), 189–190
19. Rietbrock, N.: Arch. Exp. Path. Pharmacol. *263* (1969), 88–105
20. McMartin, K. E. et al.: Biochem. Pharmacol. *28* (1979), 645–649
21. Palese, M., Tephly, T. R.: J. Toxicol. Environ. Health *1* (1975), 13–24
22. McMartin, K. E. et al.: Alcohol Aldehyde Metab. Syst. *2* (1977), 429–440
23. Herken, W. et al.: Arch. Toxicol. *24* (1969), 214–228
24. Rietbrock, N. et al.: Biochem. Pharmacol. *20* (1972), 2613–2622
25. Ferry, D. G. et al.: Int. Arch. Occup. Environ. Health *47* (1980), 155–163
26. Šedivec, V. et al.: Int. Arch. Occup. Environ. Health *48* (1981), 257–271
27. Scheuplein, R. J., Blank, I. H.: J. Invest. Dermatal. *60* (1973), 286–296
28. Dutkiewicz, B. et al.: Int. Arch. Occup. Environ. Health *47* (1980), 81–88
29. Tada, O. et al.: J. Science of Labour *51* (1975), 143–253
30. Ferry, D. G. et al.: Toxicity of methanol/petrol mixtures. Alcohol fuels technology, 3rd Int. Symp., Asilomar, California; May 28–31, 1979, Vol. III
31. Heinrich, R., Angerer, J.: Int. Arch. Occup. Environ. Health *50* (1982), 341–349
32. Clay, K. L. et al.: Toxicol. Appl. Pharmacol. *34* (1975), 49–61
33. McMartin, K. E. et al.: Biochem. Med. *13* (1975), 319–333
34. Dutkiewicz, B.: Excerpta Med. Int. Congr. Ser. *440* (1978), 106–109
35. Kendal, L. P., Ramanathan, A. N.: Biochem. J. *54* (1953), 424–426
36. McQueen, E. G.: Toxicology of methanol/petrol blends, Alcohol fuels, Sydney, 9–11 August 1978, pp. 6–1 to 6–4
37. Malorny, G.: Z. Ernährungswiss. *9* (1969), 340–348
38. Posner, H. S.: J. Toxicol. Environ. Health *1* (1975), 153–171
39. NIOSH-Report: Occupational exposure to methyl alcohol. National Int. for Occupational Safety and Health. HEW Publication No. 76-148, 1976
40. Cooper, J. R., Kini, M. M.: Biochem. Pharmacol. *11* (1962), 405–416
41. Hayreh, M. M. S. et al.: Ocular toxicity of methanol: an experimental study. In: Neurotoxicity of the visual system. W. H. Merigen, B. Weiss (eds.). Raven Press, New York 1980, pp. 35–53
42. Martin-Amat, G. et al.: Toxicol. Appl. Pharmacol. *45* (1978), 201–208
43. Benton, C. D., Calhoun, F. P.: Trans. Am. Acad. Ophthalmol. Oto-Laryng. *56* (1952), 875–885
44. Riegel, H., Wolf, G.: Fortschr. Neurol. Psychiat. *34* (1966), 346–351
45. Guggenheim, M. A. et al.: Arch. Neurol. *24* (1971), 550–554
46. McLean, D. R. et al.: Can. J. Neurol. Sci. *5* (1978), 351
47. Orthner, H.: Die Methylalkoholvergiftung. Monographie (Heft 74), Springer Verlag, Berlin–Göttingen–Heidelberg 1950
48. Erlansan, P. et al.: Acta Med. Scand. *177* (4) (1965), 393–408
49. Aquilonius, S. H. et al.: J. Comput. Ass. Tomogr. *4* (4) (1980), 425–428
50. Führer, H.: Medizinische Toxikologie. 3. Auflage, Thieme Verlag, Stuttgart 1951, pp. 113–122
51. Burk, M.: Min. Mbl. Augenheilk. *130* (1957), 845–850
52. Garcia, J. H., Van Zandt, J. P.: Am. J. Pathol. *55* (1969), 5 a/6 a
53. Manufacturing Chemists' Association: Chemical safety data sheet SD-22: Methanol. Washington, D.C. 1970
54. Baumann, K., Angerer, J.: Int. Arch. Occup. Environ. Health *42* (1979), 241–249
55. Angerer, J.: Microchimica Acta (Wien) *2* (1977), 413–418
56. Mraz, M. et al.: Procov. Lék. *30* (9) (1978), 333–337
57. Spasovski, M., Benčev, I.: Hygiena i zdraveopazvane *12* (1969), 333–339
58. Gonda, A. et al.: Am. J. Med. *64* (1978), 749–758
59. Röe, O.: Pharmacol. Rev. *7* (1955), 399–412
60. Lund, A.: Acta Pharmacol. Toxicol. *4* (1948), 205–212
61. Baumann, K., Angerer, J.: Untersuchung zur Frage der beruflichen Lösungsmittelbelastung mit Aceton. Bericht über die 19. Jahrestagung der Deutschen Gesellschaft für Arbeitsmedizin, Münster, 1.–5. Mai 1979, K. Norpoth (ed.) Gentner Verlag, Stuttgart 1983, pp. 403–408
62. Elkins, H. B.: AMA Arch. Ind. Hyg. *9* (1954), 212–222
63. Dutkiewicz, T., Blochowicz, A.: Med. Pracy *18* (1981), 132–141

64. Tada, O. et al.: J. Science of Labour *50* (1974), 239–248
65. Angerer, J., Lehnert, G.: Acta Pharmacol. Toxicol. *41* (2) (1977), 551–556
66. Angerer, J. et al.: Arbeitshyg. Arbeitssch. Rehabil. *16* (7) (1981), 161–164
67. BG-Grundsatz: G 10, 1973. Herausgeber: Hauptverband der gewerblichen Berufsgenossenschaften e. V., Gentner Verlag, Stuttgart
68. Lauwerys, F.: Scand. J. Work Environ. Health *1* (1975), 139–172
69. Keeney, A. H., Mellinkoff, S. M.: Ann. Int. Med. *34* (1951), 331–338
70. Kahn, A., Blum, D.: J. Pediatrics *94* (1979) (5), 841–843
71. Naraqi, S. et al.: Aust. N. Z. J. Med. *9* (1) (1979), 65–68
72. Kane, R. W. et al.: Arch. Environ. Health *17* (1968), 119–129
73. Bennett, I. L. et al.: Medicine *32* (1953), 431–463

Author: W.-R. Delbrück
Approved by the Working Group: 10. 11. 1983

Nickel and sparingly soluble nickel compounds

(Nickel as nickel metal, nickel sulphide, sulphidic ores, nickel oxide, nickel carbonate)

EKA for exposure to nickel and sparingly soluble nickel compounds

The correlation between external and internal exposure yields the following data:

Air µg nickel/m^3	Urine µg nickel/l
100	15
300	30
500	45

Date of evaluation 1990

Chemical symbol Ni

Atomic weight 58.69

Melting point 1453 °C

Boiling point 2732 °C

MAK Carcinogenic substance: category IIIA1 of the List of MAK and BAT Values

A series of reviews and monographs have recently appeared on the occurrence, uptake, distribution and toxicity of nickel and its compounds (23, 25, 28, 30, 34, 39, 43, 46).

1 Metabolism and Kinetics

The gastro-intestinal and broncho-pulmonary systems are the main routes of absorption of nickel and its compounds. Uptake via the skin and also via parenteral routes (endoprostheses etc.) is of markedly less importance.

Essential BAT Value Documentations. DFG, Deutsche Forschungsgemeinschaft

ISBN 3-527-31477-6

In the non-occupational area by far the largest amount of nickel is taken up with food. Although individual foods, among other things due to their methods of preparation, contain extraordinarily different concentrations of this metal it can be assumed that an average adult takes in approx. 300 µg of nickel daily with food (46). Only a small amount of this, however, given at values between 1 % and 4 %, is absorbed and excreted via the kidneys. The rest is in the faeces. With a low-protein diet or under fasting conditions considerably more nickel can be absorbed.

Assuming that in urban areas the nickel concentrations in the air are on average 20 ng/m^3, then the daily uptake of this metal by inhalation is considerably less than the oral uptake.

At *workplaces exposed to nickel,* the relationship between the two routes of uptake is reversed. Here inhalation is of much greater importance than uptake via the gastro-intestinal tract, not only due to the amount but also due to the toxic effect. The site of deposition of the inhaled nickel dusts depends upon the size of the dust particles. With decreasing aerodynamic diameter (<10 µm) an increasing proportion of the dust particles reach the alveoli. The larger dust particles are deposited in the nose, throat, laryngeal area and tracheobronchial tree. Part of the deposited dust is exhaled again or is taken up via the gastrointestinal tract after clearance from the lung. The rest is absorbed in the lung. The rate of absorption depends on the physical-chemical properties of the nickel compound involved, in particular on the water solubility, the crystal form and size, the surface charge, etc. Readily soluble nickel compounds, such as nickel(II) chloride, are quickly absorbed and over 90 % is excreted via the kidneys (8, 13). The half-time of nickel elimination from the plasma and urine is 1–1.5 days, as was ascertained in the investigation of workers who were exposed to nickel in an electroplating works (44). Elimination half-times of this order of magnitude have also been described for stainless-steel welders (1). These authors have also demonstrated that in exposed welders, in addition to this relatively fast elimination, the nickel is excreted with a second considerably longer half-time. Even after a 4-week holiday these authors could determine significantly increased nickel concentrations in the urine of welders. With decreasing solubility of the nickel compounds these are absorbed from the lung more slowly and more incompletely. After occupational exposure to sparingly soluble nickel compounds, as for example in the smelting of nickel ores, half-times of nickel elimination of up to several years have been found. This means that sparingly soluble nickel compounds accumulate to a considerable extent in the bronchopulmonary system. Even in persons not occupationally exposed the nickel content of the lungs shows a marked increase with age (35, 36, 45).

Nickel is distributed very evenly in the human organs. Only in the lungs, thyroid gland and adrenal gland are there slightly higher values than for example in the kidneys, heart, liver, brain etc. (36). The nickel concentrations in lung tissue are quoted at values between 20 and 40 µg/kg wet weight (35, 45).

The nickel concentrations in the body fluids, blood and urine, described as normal values have shown a decreasing tendency over the last 10 years (2). This is mainly to be attributed to the increasing sophistication of the analytical methods and not, however, to a decreased uptake of nickel. It can be assumed that the nickel concentration in blood and plasma is normally below 1 µg/l. The upper normal limit for the nickel concentration of urine is about 3 µg/l (2, 17, 27). This value corresponds well with the concentrations to be expected from the uptake with food.

After occupational exposure to nickel, accumulation of the metal has not been observed in organs other than the bronchopulmonary system. However, the concentrations in blood and urine increase considerably.

The transport of nickel in the human body takes place mainly in plasma, seldom, however, in the cells of the blood such as, e.g., in the erythrocytes. In plasma the nickel is bound to two high-molecular fractions (albumin and α_2-macroglobulin) and a fraction which can be ultrafiltered.

2 Critical Toxicity

In the last ten years a series of reviews and monographs on the toxicology of nickel have been published (7, 15, 16, 28, 29, 31, 37, 40).

After occupational exposure to nickel and its compounds, from the point of view of occupational medicine the carcinogenic and allergic effects are the most important.

The toxic effects of nickel and its compounds depend greatly on the way in which they entered the body. While orally absorbed nickel shows no systemic toxicity, after inhalation of this metal and its compounds the carcinogenic effect on the respiratory tract is relevant.

2.1 Carcinogenicity

At the workplace the inhalation of this metal and its compounds is of the greatest importance. The proved or potential carcinogenic effect of the various nickel species is the most important toxicological aspect. The target organs of the carcinogenic effect are above all the nasal cavities and paranasal sinuses as well as the bronchial tract. In investigations of large collectives who were exposed in Norway, England and Canada during the hot-dip smelting of nickel ores and the subsequent refining, it was proved that certain work processes were associated with an excessive cancer risk of the localities named above (11, 12, 24, 32, 38). Sunderman (43) has discussed various hypotheses on the carcinogenic effects of nickel.

Occupational-medical experience complemented by data from animal experiments and experiments with cell cultures have caused the Commission for the Investigation of Health Hazards of Chemical Compounds in the Work Area to classify "nickel (in the form of inspirable dusts/aerosols of nickel metals, nickel sulphide and sulphidic ores, nickel oxide and nickel carbonate, as they can occur during production and processing)" in category A1 with substances which have been shown to induce malignant tumours in humans (10). For readily soluble nickel compounds there is to date no evidence of human carcinogenicity.

2.2 Nickel-Induced Allergenic Effects

So-called nickel scabies, contact dermatitis occurring after sensitisation, is the longest known occupational toxicological illness caused by nickel. The development of this allergy is – given endogenous reactivity – dependent on the exposure concentration of the substance. The syndrome in itself, once allergy has developed, is not dependent on concentration. The eczema occurs at the site of exposure so that its cause can usually be determined. In over 80 % of cases sensitisation has its origins in private life as a consequence of skin contact with the metal or its compounds, e.g. in the form of fashion accessories, buttons etc. It is assumed that there is a relationship between the clinical activity of nickel dermatitis and the level of the nickel concentration in blood and urine (21, 22).

An oversensitivity to nickel can also cause asthmatic illnesses, conjunctivitis and inflammatory reactions round implants and endoprostheses (43).

3 Selection of the Indicators

Above all in the selection of the indicators the determination of the nickel concentration in the urine and plasma should be discussed.

For many reasons, urine is the preferred medium for determination of indicators. The sampling of urine for routine monitoring is easier to carry out than the taking of blood. Furthermore, the sampling of urine causes less inconvenience for the test person. But above all, urine has in its favour that the nickel concentration in this medium is approx. 8–10 times higher than that in blood. Thus this parameter is diagnostically considerably more sensitive than the determination in blood or serum. In addition to the better diagnostic sensitivity of the urine level as a parameter, at present nickel can also be determined in urine with greater analytical sensitivity. With the extraction-enrichment processes usual today and atomic absorption spectrometry, nickel concentrations in the physiological and environmental range can be determined. With these methods, concentrations as low as 0.1 µg nickel per litre urine can be routinely determined (3, 27).

Furthermore, the database for the external nickel exposure and the resulting nickel excretion in the urine is very extensive. Compared to this there are only few data for the relationship between the nickel concentration in the air, on the one hand, and that in the serum, on the other.

Urine has disadvantages, however, compared to serum, where a different uptake of fluids greatly changes the nickel concentration in urine. Also the danger of exogenous contamination endangers the accuracy of the nickel findings in urine. In these cases, in particular when the confirmation of individual values is required, therefore, in addition to the nickel concentration in urine the metal concentration in serum should be determined. Whole blood seems less suitable as it is now known that nickel does not occur in the erythrocytes.

4 Methodology

For the determination of nickel the Working Group "Analysen in biologischem Material" ("Analyses of Hazardous Substances in Biological Materials") of the DFG Commission for the Investigation of Health Hazards of Chemical Compounds in the Work Area has published a tested analytical procedure (3, 4).

In the procedure for the determination of nickel in urine the metal is separated from the urine by means of a chelation/extraction step and at the same time concentrated. The quantitative determination takes place by atomic absorption spectrometry after electrothermal atomisation in the graphite furnace. The evaluation is carried out with aqueous standard solutions which are prepared and analysed in the same way. This procedure is simple and can be carried out in a large series. Therefore it is particularly suited for routine monitoring. The high sensitivity of the method combined with the low detection limit enables concentrations not only in the occupational medical range but also the general environmental concentration range to be determined accurately. The detection limit is approx. 0.1 µg nickel/l urine. As the total sample preparation can be carried out in a disposable container and requires only few procedural steps and small quantities of chemicals, the error due to losses and/or endogenous contamination can be reduced to a minimum. The low susceptibility to interference is reflected in high precision of the procedure. The specificity of the procedure is a result of the extraction step during sample preparation and the specificity of the atomic absorption spectrometric method. The procedure suggested by the IUPAC for the determination of nickel in the urine or serum (6) also uses a chelation/extraction step. Recent experience indicates that the mineralisation of the biological material stipulated there can be dispensed with.

For the determination of nickel in whole blood or serum an atomic absorption spectrometric procedure has proved suitable in which the biological material after eightfold dilution is analysed directly and without further sample preparation. The biological sample is subjected to a three-stage mineralisation programme in a graphite furnace before the atomisation takes place at 2650 °C. Evaluation takes place by means of the so-called standard addition procedure in which increasing, known amounts of nickel are added to the sample which is analysed each time.

Using this direct procedure the influence of the matrix on the analysis result is minimised, on the one hand, by dilution of the biological material, on the other, by the greatly differentiated mineralisation procedure. The detection of nickel can therefore take place very specifically. A minimum analytical background interference is eliminated without difficulty by the use of deuterium compensation or the Zeeman effect. Due to the dilution of the sample, the detection limit is between 1 and 2 µg/l so that physiological or environmentally-produced nickel concentrations in the blood or serum cannot be determined. The procedure is, however, suitable without restrictions for the occupational medical concentration range. The accuracy and precision of the method are good. Other procedures described in the literature for the determination of nickel in serum or whole blood which use de-proteinisation (41) or mineralisation (6) or in which oxygen (9) or a matrix modifier is used as a mineralisation aid, produce poorer results (18).

5 Relationship between External and Internal Nickel Exposure and Evaluation of Exposure Equivalents

In the following synopsis of the literature available on the question of a relationship between external and internal nickel exposure only those investigations are included in which humans are in contact with sparingly soluble nickel compounds. As already mentioned, these compounds are characterised by their carcinogenic effect. Furthermore, the kinetics of the uptake and excretion of all these compounds are similar. Biological monitoring can be carried out on this basis.

Table 1 shows a summary of the studies in which the external and internal nickel exposure at different workplaces have been reported. In all cases the exposure was to sparingly soluble forms of nickel. At the workplaces where nickel alloy steel is welded (1, 2, 14, 33, 47) it is to be assumed that the welding fumes contain nickel mostly in metallic and oxidised form. There is exposure to metallic nickel in the mechanical processing of nickel alloys by grinding and polishing (5). Also in flame spraying (5, 34) and the production of metal powders (26) the exposure to metallic nickel is foremost. On the other hand in the drying of metal oxides (26) or the roasting of metal sulphides (19) there is exposure to nickel oxides and sulphides.

A comparison of the results of the studies listed in table 1 makes clear that there is nothing that speaks against the view that these different nickel species are subject to comparable uptake and excretion kinetics. This view is supported by investigations by various authors who have succeeded in producing good correlations between the nickel concentration in the air at the workplace and the nickel concentration in the urine of the exposed persons (14, 33, 35, 42) (Tab. 2). In these studies the values measured in the ambient air are results of personal air sampling. The results by Emmerling et al. (14) whose relationship is based on the investigation of 176 welders seem to be particularly useful in this respect. Sunderman et al. (42) have succeeded in creating a relationship between the nickel concentration in air and that in urine on the basis of groups with different exposures. This correlation is based on results reported by Morgan and Rouge (26).

From these observations the exposure equivalents represented in table 3 for nickel concentrations in urine can be deduced. They refer firstly to urine as the assay material. This parameter is of the greatest importance for monitoring exposed collectives for the reasons mentioned above (see section 3). The orienting values given for the nickel concentration in plasma were calculated from the known relationship between nickel concentrations in plasma and urine; according to this the ratio of the nickel concentration in urine to that in the serum is about 8:1 (2, 5).

Tab. 1: Relationship between the concentration of sparingly soluble nickel compounds in the air at the workplace and the nickel concentration in the blood and urine of the exposed persons

$\bar{x}$: mean
s: standard deviation
m: median
–: no data
M: male
F: female

MAG: metal active gas welding
MMA: manual metal arc welding
TIG: tungsten inert gas welding

No.	Occupation	Test persons	Exposure concentration Air µg/m^3 $\bar{x}$ ± s; (range)	m	Plasma/serum µg/l $\bar{x}$ ± s; (range)	m	Urine µg/l $\bar{x}$ ± s; (range)	m	Authors
1	Polishers of aeroplane parts	6M 1F	26 ± 41; (0.05 – 129.0)	–			4.1 ± 3.2; (0.5 – 9.5)	–	Bernacki et al., 1978
	Grinders (nickel alloys)	7M 2F	1.6 ± 3.0; (0.02 – 9.5)	–			5.4 ± 2.4; (2.1 – 8.8)	–	
	Welders (MMA)	7M 3F	6.0 ± 14.3; (0.2 – 46.0)	–			6.3 ± 4.1; (1.6 – 14.0)	–	
	Aviation mechanics	4M 4F	52.0 ± 94.0; (0.01 – 252.0)	–			12.2 ± 13.6; (1.4 – 41.0)	–	
	Flame sprayers	4M 1F	2.4 ± 2.6; (0.04 – 6.5)	–			17.2 ± 9.8; (1.4 – 26.0)	–	
	Nickel refining								
2	Roasting, melting	24	860.0 ± 1200.0;	–	7.2 ± 2.8;	–	65.0 ± 58.0;	–	Høgetveit et al., 1978
	Other areas	13	420.0 ± 490.0;	–	6.4 ± 1.9;	–	45.0 ± 27;	–	
3	Nickel refining; (Exposure to in-soluble nickel compounds)		240.0;	–			31.7;		Høgetveit et al., 1980

* 68 %-range

Tab. 1: Continued

No.	Occupation	Test persons	Exposure concentration Air µg/m³ $\bar{x}$ ± s; m (range)	Plasma/serum µg/l $\bar{x}$ ± s; m (range)	Urine µg/l $\bar{x}$ ± s; m (range)	Authors
4	Welders (high alloyed stainless steel; up to 34 % Ni) (MMA)	10M	150.0; – (30.0 – 1780.0)	1.2(B); – (0.58 – 2.9)(B)	11.5*; – (7.8 – 26.5)	Rahkonen et al., 1983
5	Nickel catalyst production	73	(<200.0 – 5870.0)	8.0; – (2.0 – 41.0)	64.0; – (9.0 – 300.0)	Zwennis and Franssen, 1983
6	Stainless steel welders (TIG)	10M	–; 2.3 (0.7 – 9.0)		–; 4-6 (1.4 – 9.5)	Zober et al., 1984
	Smelting of ores containing nickel					
7	Drying of nickel oxides	67	310; – (10.0 – 5000)		24.0 ± 24.0; –	Morgan and Rouge, 1984
	Drying of nickel oxides	37		8.9 ± 5.9; –	37.0 ± 30.0; –	
	Production of nickel powder	48	310; – (90.0 – 1530)			
	Production of nickel powder	25		7.2 ± 4.8; –		
	Contact with sparingly soluble nickel compounds	15 7	1540; – (220 – 4180)	7.4 ± 5.1; –	39 ± 28; –	

8	Welding of high alloyed steel (75 % Ni)	11M	440; (70.0 – 1100)	–			18; (9.7 – 38.0)	–	Åkesson and Skerfing, 1985
9	Welders (stainless steel) (MMA)	41M	(95 % < 500)				–; (2.5 – 144.0)	23.8	Zober and Weltle, 1985
	Hollow glass industry-mould manufacturing + maintenance								
10	Mechanics	406	(18 – 3800)				7.4; (2.9 – 24.3)	–	Raithel et al., 1987
	Mechanics	140			0.9; (0.75 – 2.05)	–			
	Powder flame sprayers	114	(3 – 600)				25.3; (8.5 – 81.5)	–	
	Powder flame sprayers	40			1.95 (0.75 – 3.25)				
	Combined jobs	394	(300 – 410)				17.5 (4.9 – 53.9)		
	Combined jobs	108			1.65 (0.75 – 4.10)				
11	Stainless steel welders (MAG, MMA)	103M	93 ± 81.4; (<50 – 320)	60	4.9 ± 4.0; (<1.8 – 19.6)	3.9	18.5 ± 28.5; (0.1 – 209.4)	10.2	Angerer and Lehnert, 1989
	Stainless steel welders								
12	MMA	61	–; (7.4 – 52.7)*	24	–; (0.4 – 3.2)*	1.0	–; (3.4 – 20.1)*	10.1	Emmerling et al., 1989
	MAG	46	–; (22.1 – 238.7)*	68.6	–; (0.7 – 2.8)	1.5	–; (4.4 – 34.3)*	14.0	
	TIG	16	–; (2.1 – 20.3)*	8	–; (0.2 – 2.7)	1.1	–; (1.8 – 15.4)*	5.7	

Tab. 2: Correlation between the concentration of sparingly soluble nickel compounds in the air of the workplace and the metal concentration in the body fluids c_U, c_A: nickel concentration in the urine and air

Linear regressions		Number of pairs of value	Correlation coefficient	Authors
c_U (µmol/l)	$= 0.08 + 0.8\ c_A$(mg/l);	10	0.95	Rahkonen et al., 1983
c_U (µg/g creatinine)	$= 13.5 + 0.05\ c_A$(µg/m^3);	22	0.52	Raithel, 1987
c_U (µg/l)	$= 10.84 + 0.007\ c_A$(µg/m^3);	174	0.52	Emmerling et al., 1989
c_U (µg/l)	$= 8.49 + 56.88\ c_A$(mg/m^3);		0.86	Sunderman et al., 1986* according to data by Morgan and Rouge, 1984

* Correlation on the basis of groups exposed to different extents

Tab. 3: Exposure equivalents for nickel valid for exposures to sparingly soluble nickel compounds

Air µg nickel/m^3	Urine µg nickel/l	Plasma µg nickel/l
	(EKA values)	(supplementary values for purposes of orientation)
100	15	<2
300	30	4
500	45	6

6 Interpretation of the Data

The exposure equivalents evaluated in section 5 for nickel are only valid for the occupational medical surveillance of exposed persons who are exposed to sparingly soluble nickel compounds, such as nickel sulphide, nickel oxides or metallic nickel in powder form. This applies above all to activities which are connected with the mining of ores containing nickel, their smelting and refining, with the mechanical processing (e.g. grinding) of alloys containing nickel, with the welding of alloys containing nickel and with the so-called powder flame spraying.

The exposure equivalents do *not* apply for contact with readily soluble nickel salts, for exposure to nickel carbonyl or for the area of electrolysis of solutions containing nickel salts.

The kinetics of the uptake and elimination of nickel described in section 1 indicated that the sampling of biological material should take place at the end of the work period after several consecutive work shifts.

As is generally the case after exposure to heavy metals, exogenous contamination of biological material can lead to considerable errors in the values measured. Care must therefore be taken that sampling takes place in a contamination-free atmosphere. The test person should as far as possible be wearing ordinary clothes. As already mentioned, high *individual values* in the analysis of urine samples should be verified by additional determination of the nickel content of plasma samples, better still by the renewed investigation of a urine sample.

The different dilution of urine samples is taken into account most easily if the specific weight of the urine is used as an exclusion criterion. Urines with specific weights <1,010 are not included in the evaluation.

As already mentioned, the normal or ecologically-defined upper normal limits of the nickel concentration in urine or plasma lie at around 3 µg/l urine or under the detection limit of approx. 1 µg/l plasma. Higher concentrations of nickel indicate an occupational exposure.

In the case of nickel concentrations in urine which are less than 10 µg/l it can be assumed with great probability that the exposure of the person in question is permanently less than the currently valid TRK value (status 1990). The prerequisite is, however, that the urine is of normal concentration. The specific weight should be markedly greater than 1.01.

7 References

1. Åkesson, B., Skerfing, S.: Int. Arch. Occup. Environ. Health *56* (1985), 111–117
2. Angerer, J., Lehnert, G.: Int. Arch. Occup. Environ. Health *62* (1990), 7–10
3. Angerer, J., Schaller, K. H.: Analyses of Hazardous Substances in Biological Materials. Vol. 1. Deutsche Forschungsgemeinschaft. VCH Verlagsgesellschaft, Weinheim 1985
4. Angerer, J., Schaller, K. H.: Analyses of Hazardous Substances in Biological Materials. Vol. 3. Deutsche Forschungsgemeinschaft. VCH Verlagsgesellschaft, Weinheim 1990
5. Bernacki, E. J., Parsons, G. E., Roy, B. R., Mikac-Devic, M., Kennedy, C. D., Sunderman, F. W.: Ann. Clin. Lab. Sci. *8* (1978), 184–189
6. Brown, S. S., Nomoto, S., Stoeppler, M., Sunderman, F. W. jr.: Clin. Biochem. *14* (1981), 295–299
7. Brown, S. S., Sunderman, F. W. (eds.): Progress in nickel toxicology. Blackwell, Oxford 1985
8. Carvalho, S. M. M., Ziemer, P. L.: Arch. Environ. Contamin. Toxicol. *11* (1982), 245–248
9. Delves, H. T. et al.: Proceedings of the 2nd international workshop trace element analytical chemistry, Neuherberg, April 1982, Vol. 2. de Gruyter, Berlin 1983, pp. 1123–1127
10. Deutsche Forschungsgemeinschaft: Maximale Arbeitsplatzkonzentrationen und Biologische Arbeitsstofftoleranzwerte 1990. Mitteilung XXVI der Senatskommission zur Prüfung gesundheitsschädlicher Arbeitsstoffe. VCH Verlagsgesellschaft, Weinheim 1990
11. Doll, R., Morgan, L. G., Speizer, F. E.: Br. J. Cancer *24* (1970), 623–632
12. Doll, R., Mattheus, J. D., Morgan, L. G.: Br. J. Ind. Med. *34* (1977), 102–105
13. English, J. C., Parker, R. D.: Am. Ind. Hyg. Assoc. J. *42* (1989), 486–492
14. Emmerfing, G., Zschiesche, W., Schaller, K. H., Weltle, D., Valentin, H.: Arbeitsmedizinische Untersuchung von Chrom-Nickel-Stahlschweißern: Epidemiologische Querschnittsstudie zur Belastung sowie zur bronchopulmonalen und renalen Beanspruchung. DVS-Verlag, Düsseldorf 1989
15. Environmental Protection Agency (EPA): Relative carcinogenic potencies among 54 chemicals evaluated by the carcinogen assessment group as suspect human carcinogens 11-124-11-126
16. Grandjean, Ph., Selikoff, I. J., Shen, S. K., Sunderman, F. W.: Am. J. Ind. Med. *1* (1980), 181–189
17. Heinrich, R., Angerer, J. in: Bolt, H. M., Piekarski, C., Rutenfranz, J. (eds.): 25. Jahrestagung in Dortmund vom 22. bis 25. Mai 1985. Gentner Verlag, Stuttgart 1985
18. Heinrich-Ramm, R., Angerer, J.: Trace elements in human health and disease, in: WHO, CEC, EPA (eds.) Environmental Health *20* (1987), 70–73
19. Høgetveit, A. C., Barton, R. T., Kostal, C. O.: Ann. Occup. Hyg. *21* (1978), 113-120
20. Høgetveit, A. C., Barton, R. T., Andersen, J.: J. Occup. Med. *22* (1980), 597–600

21. Jongh, De, G. J., Spruit, D. et al.: Contact Dermatitis *4* (1978), 142–156
22. Kaaber, K., Veien, N.: Br. J. Dermatol. *98* (1978), 197–201
23. Leonard, A. et al.: Mutat. Res. *87* (1981), 1–15
24. Magnus, K., Andersen, A., Høgetveit, A. C.: Int. J. Cancer *30* (1982), 681–685
25. Mastromatteo, E.: Am. Ind. Hyg. Assoc. J. *47* (1986), 589–601
26. Morgan, L. G., Rouge, P. J. C. in: Sunderman, F. W. (ed.): Nickel in the human environment. IARC Lyon 1984, pp. 507–520
27. Mundt-Becker, W., Angerer, J.: Int. Arch. Occup. Environ. Health *49* (1981), 187–192
28. Nieboer, E., Rossetto, F. E., Menon, C. R., In: Sigel, H., Sigel, A. (eds.): Metal ions in biological systems, Vol. 23. Marcel Dekker, New York 1988
29. National Institute for Occupational Safety and Health (NIOSH): NIOSH Publication No. 77–164. US Government Printing Office, Washington DC 1977, pp. 1–282
30. Norseth, T., Piscator, M.: Nickel. In: Friberg, F., Nordberg, G. F., Vouk, V. B. (eds.): Handbook on the toxicology of metals. Elsevier, Amsterdam 1979
31. Nriagu, J. O. (ed.): Environ. Sci. Technol. Serv. Wiley and Sons, New York 1980
32. Pedersen, E., Høgetveit, A. C., Andersen, A.: Int. J. Cancer *12* (1973), 32–41
33. Rahkonen, E., Junttila, M.-L., Kalliomäki, P. L., Olkiroura, M., Koponen, M., Kalliomäki, K.: Int. Arch. Occup. Environ. Health *52* (1983), 243–255
34. Raithel, H. J., Ebner, G., Schaller, K. H., Schellmann, B., Valentin, H.: Am. J. Ind. Med. *12* (1987), 55–70
35. Raithel, H. J.: Arbeitsmed. Sozialmed. Präventivmed. *22* (1987), 268–274 and 301–310
36. Rezuki, W. N., Knight, J. A., Sunderman jr., F. W.: Am. J. Ind. Med. *11* (1987), 419
37. Rigaut, J. P.: Commission des Communautes Europeennes. Luxembourg Do CCE/LUX/V/E/24/83 (1983)
38. Shannon, H. S., Julian J. A., Roberts, R. S.: JNCI. *73* (1984), 1251–1258
39. Stockinger, H. E.: Nickel. In: Clayton, G. D., Clayton, F. E. (eds.): Patty's Industrial Hygiene and Toxicology, 3rd ed. Vol. 2. Wiley & Sons, New York 1981
40. Sunderman, F. W. (ed.): IARC Scientific Publications, No. 53, Lyon 1984
41. Sunderman, F. W. et al.: Annals of clinical and laboratory science *14* (1984), 232–241
42. Sunderman, F. W., Aitio, A., Morgan, L. G., Norseth, T.: Toxicol. Ind. Hlth. *2* (1986), 17–78
43. Sunderman, F. W. In: Seiler, H. G., Sigel, H., Sigel, A. (eds.): Handbook on toxicity of inorganic compounds. Marcel Dekker, New York 1988
44. Tossavainen, A., Nurminen, M., Mutanen, P., Tola, S.: Br. J. Ind. Med. *37* (1980), 285–291
45. Turhan, V., Wollburg, C., Angerer, J., Szadkowski, D.: Arbeitsmed. Sozialmed. Präventivmed. *20* (1985), 277–281
46. Zimmerli, B., Candrian, U., Schlatter, Ch.: Mitt. Gebiete Lebensm. Hyg. *78* (1987), 344–396
47. Zober, A., Schaller, K. H., Weltle, D.: Staub Reinh. Luft *44* (1984), 465–468
48. Zober, A., Weltle, D.: J. Soc. Occup. Med. *35* (1985), 79–84
49. Zwennis, W. C. M., Franssen, A. G.: Abs. Second Intern. Conf. Clin. Chem. Clin. Toxicol. Metals, Montreal (1983)

Author: J. Angerer
Approved by the Working Group: 28th March 1990

2-Propanol

BAT	Acetone 50 mg/l blood Acetone 50 mg/l urine Sampling time: end of exposure or end of shift
Date of evaluation	1990
Synonyms	Isopropanol Isopropyl alcohol
Formula	$(CH_3)_2CHOH$ $CH_3—CH(OH)—CH_3$
Molecular weight	60.10
Melting point	−88.5 °C
Boiling point	82.4 °C (760 torr)
Vapour pressure at 20 °C	44 hPa
MAK	400 ml/m^3 (ppm) 980 mg/m^3

2-Propanol is a colourless liquid under normal conditions of temperature and pressure. It is miscible with water in all proportions.

2-Propanol is used predominantly as an antifreeze, as a solvent, in cleaning agents also together with other organic solvents, for chemical syntheses, for the manufacture of cosmetics and in the pharmaceutical industry.

1 Metabolism and Kinetics

2-Propanol can be absorbed by humans via inhalation, perorally and percutaneously. After peroral application 2-propanol is quickly absorbed by the whole gastro-intestinal tract. More than 80 % of the dose is absorbed in this way within the first 30 minutes (37). With a distribution volume of 0.6−0.7 l per kg the substance is distributed after a maximum of two hours (25).

Essential BAT Value Documentations. DFG, Deutsche Forschungsgemeinschaft

ISBN 3-527-31477-6

Although 2-propanol can also be absorbed percutaneously (28) up until now no systemic effects could be observed on applying the alcohol to the skin. With occupational exposure to 2-propanol the uptake is predominantly by the lungs.

About 85 % of the 2-propanol is oxidised to acetone in the liver via the enzyme alcohol dehydrogenase. In vitro 500 times more of the enzyme was necessary to achieve a turnover rate similar to that with ethanol (22). The rest is excreted unchanged via the lungs and the kidneys. Furthermore, there is a resecretion in the gastric juice and saliva. Due to this reabsorption of the substance the duration of an intoxication can be considerably increased (see Fig. 1).

The further metabolism of the main metabolite acetone is dependant on the concentration in the serum. In high concentrations acetone is excreted almost unchanged via the lungs and kidneys as well as the skin, in low concentrations, however, it is oxidised mainly to carbon dioxide and water (see MAK documentation: acetone). Small quantities of formic acid, aceto-acetate and β-hydroxy butyrate can also be formed (4).

The elimination of 2-propanol and acetone takes place in patients with or without known ethanol abuse according to a simple exponential function (7, 27). The course of the acetone-plasma level after the application of 2-propanol can be described sufficiently exactly by the Bateman function (1, 30).

With regard to the elimination of 2-propanol in humans there are only data from cases of intoxication. As the blood level cannot be continuously checked and therapeutic measures such as dialysis, diuresis, infusions and artificial respiration can influence the elimination, the description of the elimination kinetics derived from this

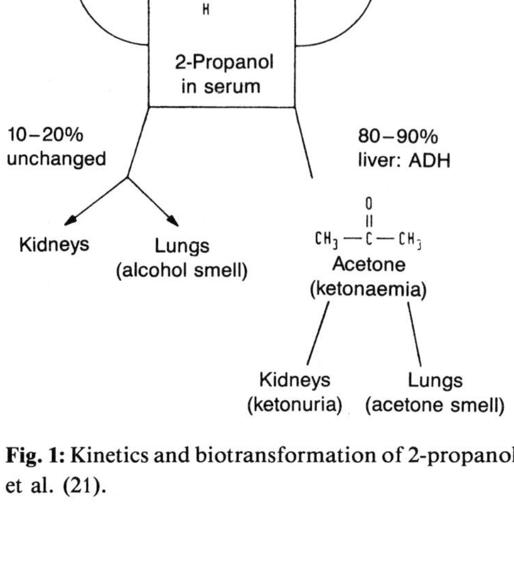

Fig. 1: Kinetics and biotransformation of 2-propanol in humans, modified diagram according to Lacouture et al. (21).

is of limited significance. According to Daniel et al. (7) as well as Bohn et al. (5), the elimination of 2-propanol is to be regarded as obeying first order kinetics with a half-life of 2.5 to 3 hours. Natowitz et al. (27) as well as Lacouture et al. (21) discuss 3 – 6.4 hours as the biological half-life. A case reported by Taylor et al. (32) in which in 6 hours the 2-propanol concentration in the blood decreased from 2.03 to 0.94 g/l and the acetone concentration of 2.43 increased to 3.58 g/l makes one, however, suspect kinetics of zero order with an hourly decrease of 0.18 g/l (17).

For the acetone concentration in the serum half-lives of 22.4 hours (27) and 24 hours (24) were ascertained after acute 2-propanol intoxication. Baumann and Angerer (4) give lower values for the excretion of acetone.

According to Thiess (33) acetone is reduced in the organism to a certain extent to 2-propanol. 2-Propanol is therefore to be regarded as a normal physiological product of metabolism whose blood concentration lies, however, below 0.1 mg/l (35) or 0.05 mg/l (19). 2-Propanol is comparable with ethanol in its pharmacological effects and its pharmacokinetic parameters such as distribution volumes, lipid solubility, break-down of ADH, as well as chemical and physical properties (16). The reports by Alexander et al. (3) make one suspect that the oxidation of 2-propanol to acetone is inhibited by ethanol. In controlled drinking experiments Iffland et al. were able to confirm this (17). With blood-ethanol concentrations, which were kept at a level of 0.5 g/l for several hours, the initially high turnover of 2-propanol is decreased by approx. 70%. Complete inhibition, however, does not take place. Evidently ethanol has no inhibiting effect if the concentrations in the blood have decreased to 0.1 g/l.

2 Critical Toxicity

The pharmacological features of 2-propanol are similar to those of ethanol, the intoxicating effect lasts, however, longer. This difference is to be attributed to the metabolism of 2-propanol. The metabolic end product is acetone (see also section Metabolism and Kinetics).

Intoxications with 2-propanol are in comparison with ethanol intoxications only sparsely documented (12, 17, 20, 21).

After ingestion, generally intestinal symptoms occur first of all and later central nervous symptoms. Then, cardiovascular disturbances can arise (31).

Iffland et al. (17) describe the case of a man who had drunk ethanol and 2-propanol in large quantities. The unconscious patient showed at the time of admittance to the clinic the following blood levels: ethanol 2.23 g/l, 2-propanol 0.99 g/l and acetone 0.47 g/l. The patient recovered fully under therapy.

In animal-experimental investigations it was deduced that the neurotoxic effects of 2-propanol on the central nervous system are approx. twice as pronounced as those of ethanol (26). The reason for this could be the greater lipid solubility of 2-propanol which can also pass the blood-brain barrier more quickly.

The acetone produced in metabolism has been held responsible for the longer states of coma observed with intoxication. It is known that acetone has a depressive effect on the central nervous system and intensifies the effects of 2-propanol (7).

With comatose patients with a 2-propanol intoxication cardiac irregularities in the form of arrhythmia, bradycardia and hypotension with diastolic blood pressure values of < 40 mmHg are described as cardial complications (13, 21). In general there is a severe intoxication present with blood or serum concentrations of more than 4000 mg/l (21). According to the data from Lacouture et al. (21) the greatest serum concentration that was survived was 5600 mg/l.

According to the reports available it can be assumed that 2-propanol shows no great hepatotoxicity or nephrotoxicity (13, 21).

With a fatal 2-propanol intoxication a renal tubule necrosis was found by autopsy (2).

In another case rhabdomyolysis, myopathy and haemolytic anaemia were observed (18). Retrobulbar neuritis as with methanol poisoning is not known with 2-propanol (11). There are also no reports of other visual disorders in connection with 2-propanol intoxication (36).

Severe intoxications after inhalation of 2-propanol fumes at the workplace are, after consultation of the relevant literature, so far not known (10).

For the evaluation of health impairment after chronic 2-propanol exposure, four animal-experimental studies have to be referred to, as systematic investigations with humans are still lacking. An exception is the investigation by Wilz (38) who, after a daily uptake of 2.6 to 6.4 mg 2-propanol per kg body weight by healthy test persons over a period of 6 weeks, could not discover any adverse effects on health.

Within the framework of an occupational-medical study with women occupationally exposed to 2-propanol, Triebig et al. (35) found no effects on health nor haematological, clinical-chemical or psychological parameters. The women had been employed in this area on average for 34 months (2 – 204 months). At the time of the investigation the mean 2-propanol exposure amounted to 106 ppm (1 – 227 ppm).

It is important to mention at this point the investigation by Folland et al. (9), who observed liver and kidney damage in workers exposed simultaneously to 2-propanol and carbon tetrachloride. Corresponding to animal-experimental studies it can be deduced that simultaneous exposure to halogenated hydrocarbons can have an intensifying effect on 2-propanol (34). Probably the acetone produced in metabolism also plays a pathophysiological role here.

Pure 2-propanol is not carcinogenic for humans (15). The increase in tumours of the respiratory passages observed with workers with the "Starksäureverfahren" (strong acid procedure) – propylene gas is brought to reaction in concentrated sulphuric acid – for the production of 2-propanol is probably to be attributed to isopropyl oil. The carcinogenic substance(s) have so far not been defined (8).

3 Exposure and Effect

According to experience with severe acute and chronic 2-propanol intoxication, the liver, kidneys, central nervous system and haematopoietic system can be damaged in humans. In an occupational-medical cross-sectional study on 60 women exposed to 2-propanol specific anamnesis, neurological and psychological test examinations were carried out. The employees had been exposed on average for 34 months (range: 2–204 months) and at the time of the investigation to a mean 2-propanol concentration in the ambient air of 106 ppm (range: 1- 227 ppm). The exposure levels were thus considerably under the valid MAK value of 400 ppm. In this study there were no findings or signs of possible 2-propanol induced health effects. The investigations on the internal exposure revealed 2-propanol concentrations in the blood of 1.7 mg/l and in the urine of 2.2 mg/l after an 8-hour exposure. After 16 exposure-free hours, in about 75% of cases both the blood and the urine level of 2-propanol had decreased to under the detection limit of 0.1 mg/l again and thus corresponded to the values found in the control group. The acetone concentration in the blood amounted to a median 16.3 mg/l (range: 3.2–39.6 mg/l) in the post-shift samples. After a 16-hour work pause a concentration of 3.4 mg/l was measured, in the control persons approx. 3 mg/l. The renal acetone elimination showed a median post-shift value of 14.5 mg/l. After a 16-hour exposure-free interval the values lay within the normal range (35). Brugnone et al. (6) also carried out investigations on the relationship between external and internal 2-propanol exposure with workers from a printing shop. The external exposure of 3 to 264 ppm corresponded to 2-propanol concentrations in blood and urine of less than 1 mg/l, corresponding to the analytical detection limit. The acetone-blood concentrations varied during the shift from 0.76–15.6 mg/l blood. The renal acetone excretion reached values during the shift of between 0.9–18.2 mg/l, while the urine samples which were collected between the end of the shift and the beginning of the next shift showed acetone levels between 0.85 and 35.0 mg/l urine.

4 Selection of the Indicators

According to current data there are merely exposure parameters available for the monitoring of persons exposed to 2-propanol. Both 2-propanol concentrations and acetone concentrations in the blood and urine samples can be considered as indicators. Only the post-shift samples are suitable as investigation materials.

Occupational-medical examinations of persons exposed to 2-propanol showed significant correlations between the 2-propanol concentration in the workplace air and the 2-propanol and acetone concentrations in blood and urine (6, 35). Triebig. et al. (35) found only a slight increase in the 2-propanol concentration in the blood and urine on comparing the pre-shift and post-shift values. Brugnone et al. (6), due to the insensitivity of the methods used, could also find no 2-propanol in the post-shift samples. This is to be attributed to the rapid metabolism of 2-propanol to acetone. The determination of 2-propanol in the blood and urine is therefore not a suitable indicator for the estimation of internal 2-propanol exposure.

This was also confirmed in investigations by Kawai et al. (19) who, with persons exposed to 2-propanol despite external exposure and increased acetone levels, could only find a measurable 2-propanol excretion with 30 of the 99 test persons.

On the other hand there were more marked increases for the acetone measurements between the pre-shift and post-shift samples. The biological half-life of acetone in the human organism makes this parameter suitable for biological monitoring. According to Litovitz (24) the acetone level is a direct measure of the 2-propanol turnover since the metabolite is itself hardly metabolised. Kawai et al. (19) conclude from a study on 99 persons occupationally exposed to 2-propanol that the acetone excretion in the urine is a valuable indicator for biological monitoring. This parameter is also suitable for the determination of low level exposure to 2-propanol in the range up to 70 ppm.

Although Brugnone et al. (6) were able to show in their investigations that there is a significant correlation between the 2-propanol concentrations in the ambient and the alveolar air as well as between the concentration of 2-propanol in the alveolar air and the blood concentration, this parameter is, due to great variations depending on the time of sampling as well as practical considerations, not suitable for routine biological monitoring at the present state of the art.

With persons not occupationally exposed to 2-propanol, no measurable level of the solvent can be detected with the common analytical procedures. The values lie below the detection limit of 0.1 mg/l. On the other hand in blood and urine samples from not occupationally exposed persons, acetone can be determined as a physiological product of metabolism. According to Triebig et al. (35) the median acetone concentration in blood amounts to 2.9 mg/l (range: $< 0.1 - 4.7$ mg/l), the renal excretion 3.4 mg/l (range $1 - 14.7$ mg/l). The "normal values" of Baumann and Angerer (4) and Brugnone et al. (6) are of the same order of magnitude. Kawai et al. (19) quote $<0.05 - 1.6$ mg/l ($<0.05 - 3.6$ mg/g creat.) as the normal acetone excretion.

It is known that after acetone exposure there is an increased formic acid excretion (4). Measurements of formic acid excretion with persons exposed occupationally to 2-propanol are not known. According to Litovitz (24) the metabolite acetone is hardly metabolised. The determination of the formic acid excretion in the urine thus does not seem to be a suitable parameter for the biological monitoring of persons exposed to 2-propanol. The usefulness of the formic acid excretion is further limited by the fact that it is an unspecific parameter. Increased formic acid excretions have been observed as the result of a methanol exposure and also alimentary influences. The normal formic acid excretion is to a certain extent subject to considerable inter-individual and intraindividual fluctuations (see also BAT value documentation "Methanol").

5 Methodology

For the quantitative determination of 2-propanol and acetone in whole blood or urine today only head space gas chromatography is used. The DFG Commission for the Investigation of Health Hazards of Chemical Compounds in the Work Area have published a reliable method in their loose-leaf collection "Analysen in biologischem Material" ("Analyses of Hazardous Substances in Biological Materials") (head space gas chromatography). Both 2-propanol and acetone are highly volatile substances. The samples must therefore be transferred to head space vials immediately after sampling. These containers are suitable both for transport and also for the storage of the samples. The analytical determination is performed directly by head space gas chromatography.

6 Evaluation of the BAT Value

Due to the occupational health and safety and hygienic conditions prevailing mostly today the concentrations of hazardous substances which occur at the workplace are increasingly departing from the values at which negative effects on the health of the employees can be observed. Particularly in large enterprises, due to measures of occupational hygiene, concentrations mostly fall greatly below the MAK values valid today. This is particularly true for the solvent 2-propanol. Thus there is at present no chance of evaluating threshold limit values in biological material for 2-propanol on the basis of a sufficiently large collective by means of a correlation between the exposure parameter and the health effects. The exposure and effect study carried out by Triebig et al. (35) took place with external exposure values of 106 ppm (range: 1 – 227 ppm). These values are thus considerably below the presently valid MAK value of 400 ppm.

This also applies to the study by Brugnone et al. (6) in which 12 workers at a printing shop were exposed to 3 – 264 ppm 2-propanol. The 2-propanol exposure levels for 99 workers at a printing shop were even lower in an investigation by Kawai et al. (19). Determined with personal air sampling they varied between 1 and 66 ppm. At the same time there was exposure to toluene (1 – 233 ppm), xylenes (up to 69 ppm) as well as to methyl ethyl ketone (17 – 76 ppm) and acetic acid ester (26 – 183 ppm).

Investigations on parameters of internal medicine and neurology, as well as haematology, clinical chemistry and psychology came to no findings or signs of health effects induced by 2-propanol at these exposure levels (35).

A BAT value evaluation on the basis of an extrapolation from acute intoxications with 2-propanol is also not possible. Due to the lack of these opportunities of evaluating a BAT value today on the basis of clinical-epidemiological investigations, in analogy with the procedure used for other solvents such as e. g. toluene, a procedure must be used which allows one, via the estimation of the external exposure with the establishment of a solvent concentration in the blood or urine, to refer to the clinical experiences which form the basis of the MAK values. The MAK value is usually based on scientific knowledge of the relationship between the concentrations of the hazardous substance occurring at the workplace and the observed health effects. This knowledge comes from a time in which, due to the limited possibilities for occupational hygiene, ambient air concentrations often led to health impairment. The BAT values evaluated for 2-propanol are thus based on an analysis of the correlation between the external and internal exposure. The conditions under which this kind of evaluation is valid are presented in detail in the BAT value documentation "Toluene" (39).

In the study by Kawai et al. (19) the external 2-propanol exposure of 99 workers in a printing shop was measured by personal air sampling (2 – 66 ppm) as well as the 2-propanol and acetone excretion in the urine. The urine sampling took place at the end of the work shift. 2-Propanol was only detectable in the urine of those persons with a greater exposure (>5 ppm), for the renal acetone elimination there was, however, over the whole exposure range a good correlation between external and internal exposure ($r = 0.84$). From the regression equation $y = 1.488 + 0.269\,x$, for the MAK value of 400 ppm a corresponding acetone excretion of 108 mg/l can be calculated. The limitations of this evaluation are that the extrapolation is based on very low external 2-propanol exposures and that there was a considerable coexposure to other solvents such as toluene.

The BAT values derived for 2-propanol are based predominantly on the investigations of Triebig et al. (35). In this study significant correlations between the 2-propanol-air concentrations and the acetone levels in the blood and urine sampled at the end of exposure could be established. In the examination of 60 persons exposed to 2-propanol there were Spearman correlation coefficients of 0.7 for the relation of 2-propanol in the ambient air to the acetone excretion in the urine (see Fig. 2). The acetone concentration in the whole blood and urine was determined in samples which were taken immediately after the end of the work period. Taking as a basis the results of the occupational-medical investigations and a linear relationship between external and internal exposure for a 2-propanol-air concentration of 400 ppm the following BAT values result:

50 mg acetone/l whole blood

50 mg acetone/l urine

The study carried out by Brugnone et al. (6) on the relationship between external exposure and the acetone concentration in the blood and urine led to slightly lower biological values than in the study by Triebig et al. (35). Acetone concentrations of 0.76–15.6 mg/l blood (during the shift) or acetone excretion between 0.85 and 35 mg/l (sampling from the end of the shift to the beginning of the next shift) corresponded to an external exposure of 3–264 ppm. The BAT values evaluated on the basis of the data by Triebig et al. (35) thus represent a good compromise between the three relevant studies.

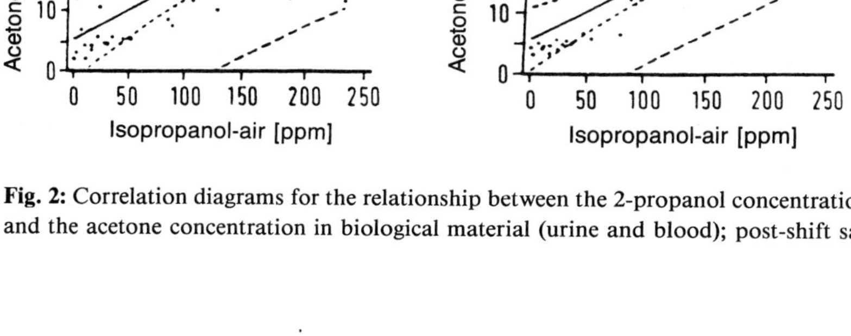

Fig. 2: Correlation diagrams for the relationship between the 2-propanol concentration in the ambient air and the acetone concentration in biological material (urine and blood); post-shift sampling (35).

7 Interpretation of the Data

2-Propanol has much in common with ethanol in its pharmacological effects and its pharmacokinetic parameters such as distribution volumes, lipid solubility, metabolic capacity of ADH, as well as chemical and physical properties (16). The reports by Alexander et al. (3) indicate that the oxidation of 2-propanol to acetone is inhibited by ethanol. In controlled drinking experiments Iffland et al. (17) were able to confirm this. The blood-ethanol concentrations, which were kept at a level of 0.5 g/l, decreased the initially high turnover of 2-propanol by approx. 70 %. There are thus considerably lower acetone concentrations in the blood and urine than expected for the external exposure. A complete inhibition does, however, not take place. Ethanol obviously no longer inhibits when the concentration in the blood has been reduced to 0.1 g/l.

Statements on the level of the internal 2-propanol exposure of the organism and the adherence to the BAT values require blood and urine analyses in examination materials which were taken at the end of the work shift. A "berufsgenossenschaftlicher Grundsatz" (guideline issued by the Employers' Liability Insurance Association) or recommendations on the carrying out of occupational health surveillance with persons exposed to 2-propanol at present do not exist in the Federal Republic of Germany.

8 References

1. Abshagen, U., Rietbrock, N.: Kinetik der Elimination von 2-Propanol und seines Metaboliten Aceton bei Hund und Ratte. Naunyn-Schmiedebergs Arch. Pharmak. *264* (1969), 110–118
2. Adelson, L: Fatal intoxication with isopropyl alcohol (rubbing alcohol). Amer. J. Clin. Path. *38* (1962), 144–151
3. Alexander, C. B., McBay, A. J., Hudson R. P.: Isopropanol and Isopropanol Deaths – Ten Years' Experience. J. For. Sci. *27* (1982), 541–548
4. Baumann, K., Angerer, J.: Untersuchungen zur Frage der beruflichen Lösungsmittelbelastung mit Aceton. In: K. Norpoth (ed.): Verhandlungen der Deutschen Gesellschaft für Arbeitsmedizin e. V., 19. Jahrestagung Münster 1979. Gentner Verlag, Stuttgart 1979
5. Bohn, G., Ullrich, K., Jorch, G: Spontanelimination von Propanol-2 bei einem Kleinkind. Toxichem. Krim.-Techn. *50* (1987), 10–12
6. Brugnone, F., Perbelli, L., Apostoli, P., Bellomi, M., Caretta, D.: Isopropanol exposure: environmental and biological monitoring in a priniting works. Brit. J. Ind. Med. *40* (1983) 160–168
7. Daniel, D. R., McAnalley, B. H., Garriott, J. C.: Isopropyl Alcohol Metabolism After Acute Intoxication in Humans. J. Anal. Toxicol. *5* (1981), 110–112
8. Henschler, D. (ed.) Propylalkohol/Isopropylalkohol. In: Gesundheitsschädliche Arbeitsstoffe. Toxikologisch-arbeitsmedizinische Begründung von MAK-Werten. 6. Lieferung, VCH Verlagsgesellschaft, Weinheim 1971
9. Folland, D. et al.: Carbon tetrachloride toxicity potentiated by isopropyl alcohol. J. Amer. Med. Assoc. *236* (1976), 1853–1856
10. Fritz, M. C.: Arbeitsmedizinische Untersuchungen von beruflich 2-Propanol-exponierten Personen, Inaugural-Dissertation am Institut für Arbeits- und Sozialmedizin der Universität Erlangen-Nürnberg 1989
11. Fuller, H. C., Hunter, A. M.: Isopropyl alcohol – an investigation of its physiologic properties. J. Lab. Clin. Med. *12* (1927), 326
12. Garrison, R. F.: Acute poisoning from use of isopropyl alcohol in tepid sponging. J. Amer. Med. Assoc. *152/4* (1953), 317–318

13. Gosselin, R. E. et al. (eds.): Isopropyl Alcohol. In: Clinical Toxicology of Commercial Products, 4th Ed. Williams and Wilkins Co., Baltimore, MD 1976, pp. 185–187
14. Hawley, P. C., Falko, J. M.: "Pseudo" renal failure after isopropyl alcohol intoxication. South Med. J. *75* (1981), 630–631
15. Henschler, D. (ed.): Gesundheitsschädliche Arbeitsstoffe. Toxikologisch-arbeitsmedizinische Begründung von MAK-Werten. 5. Lieferung, VCH Verlagsgesellschaft, Weinheim 1977
16. Iffland, R., Kost, H.-G., Staak, M.: Intoxikation durch Äthanol und Isopropanol. Med. Klinik *84* (1989), 224–336
17. Iffland, R., Staak, M., Lieder, F.: Äthanol- und Isopropanolkonsum. Beiträge zur gerichtl. Medizin *XLVII* (1989), 369–378
18. Juncos, L., Tiguchi, J. T.: Isopropyl alcohol intoxication: Report of a case associated with myopathy, renal failure and hemolytic anemia. J. Amer. Med Assoc. *204* (1968), 732–734
19. Kawai, R., Yasugi, T., Horiguchi, S., et al.: Biological monitoring of occupational exposure to isopropyl alcohol vapor by urinalysis for acetone. Int. Arch. Occup. Environ. Health *62* (1990), 409–413
20. Kelner, M. and Bailey, D. N.: Isopropanol ingestion: interpretation of blood concentrations and clinical findings. J. Toxicol.-Clin. Toxicol. *20* (1983), 497–507
21. Lacouture, P. G. et al.: Acute ispropyl alcohol intoxication diagnosis and management. Am J. Med. *75* (1983), 680–686
22. Laham, S.: Studies on inhalation toxicity of 2-Propanol. Drug and Chem. Toxicol *3* (1980), 343–360
23. Lehmann, A. J., Schwerma, H., Rickards, E.: Isopropylalcohol: Acquired tolerance in dogs, rate of disappearence from the blood stream in various species. J. Pharmac. Exp. Ther. *85* (1945), 61–69
24. Litovitz, T.: The Alcohols: Ethanol, Methanol, Isopropanol, Ethylene Glycol. Ped. Clin. North Am. *33* (1986), 311–323
25. Mecikalski, M. B.: Peritoneal dialysis for Isopropanol intoxication. West J. Med. *137* (1982), 322–325
26. Morris, H. J., Lightbody, H. D.: The toxicity of isopropanol. J. Ind. Hyg. Toxicol *20* (1934), 428–434
27. Natowitz, M. et al.: Pharmacokinetic analysis of a case of isopropanol intoxication. Clin. Chem. *31* (1985), 326–328
28. Rom, W. N. (ed.): Environmental and occupational medicine. Little, Brown & Co., Boston 1983, pp. 524–525
29. Savolainen, H.: Neurochemical and behavioral effects of extended exposure to isopropanol vapour with simultaneous ethanol intake. Chem. Biol. Interact. *28* (1979), 237–248
30. Siebert, H., Siebert, G., Bohn, G.: Tierexperimentelle Untersuchungen zum Stoffwechsel von Propan-2-ol. Dtsch. Apoth. Ztg. *112* (1972), 1040–1041
31. Smith, M. S.: Solvent Toxicity: 2-Propanol, Methanol, and Ethylen Glycol. Ear, Nose and Throat J. *62* (1983), 126–135
32. Taylor, C. D., Conwart, C. O., Ryan, N. T.: Isopropanol Intoxication: Managing the Coma. Hosp. Practice *20* (1985), 173–175
33. Tiess, D.: Zur Biotransformation Aceton (Propan-2-on)/Isopropanol (Propan-2-ol) in der Leber. Z. Ges. Hyg. *31* (1985), 530–531
34. Traiger, G. J., Plaa: Chlorinated hydrocarbon toxicity. Potentiation by isopropyl alcohol and acetone. Arch. Environ Health *28* (1974), 276–278
35. Triebig, G., Fritz, M., Schaller, K. H., Helbing, F., Bünte, E. M., Kufner, G., Weltle, D.: Arbeitsmedizinische Untersuchungen bei beruflich Iso-Propanol-exponierten Frauen. Arbeitsmed. Sozialmed. Präventivmed. *24* (1989), 27–31
36. Vermeulen, R.: Isopropyl alcohol and diabetes. Penn. Med. J. *69* (1966), 53–54
37. Wax, J., Ellis, F. W., Lehmann, A. J.: Absorption and distribution of isopropyl alcohol. J. Pharm. Exp. Ther. *97* (1949), 229–237
38. Wilz, J. H.: Effects on man of daily ingestion of small doses of isopropyl alcohol. Toxicol. Appl. Pharmacol. *15* (1969), 560–565
39. Greim, H., Lehnert, G. (eds.): Biological Exposure Values for Occupational Toxicants and Carcinogens. Volume 2 (in preparation), VCH Verlagsgesellschaft, Weinheim

Authors: K. H. Schaller, G. Triebig
Approved by the Working Group: 28th March 1990

Styrene

BAT	600 mg mandelic acid and phenylglyoxylic acid/g creatinine Sampling time: end of exposure or end of shift after several previous shifts
Date of evaluation	1996
CAS No.	100-42-5
Synonyms	Cinnamene Phenylethylene Vinylbenzene Ethenylbenzene Cinnamol Styrol Styrolene
Formula	C_8H_8

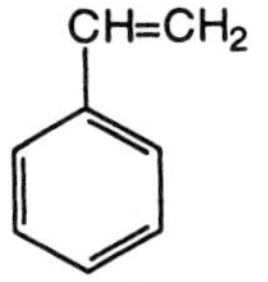

Molecular weight	104.14
Melting point	–33 °C
Boiling point	146 °C
Vapour pressure at 20 °C	6.4 hPa
MAK [last established: 1987]	20 ml/m^3 (ppm) 85 mg/m^3

1 Metabolism and Kinetics

Comprehensive literature on the biotransformation and toxicokinetics of styrene in the human organism can be found for example in the WHO Environmental Health Criteria Document of Styrene (1) and in Härkönen (2).

Styrene is mainly absorbed by the lungs and to a small extent also through the skin. Experimental studies have shown that absorption takes place rapidly. The specified rate of absorption via inhalation differs from study to study and can vary from 66 % (3) to

Essential BAT Value Documentations. DFG, Deutsche Forschungsgemeinschaft

ISBN 3-527-31477-6

82 % or 93 % (4). Styrene is distributed rapidly in the human organism. *Bio-accumulation* in special organ and fat depots is thought to play a role. This supposition is supported in particular by elimination kinetics which fit a two-compartment model (5, 6). The data gained in experiments by Engström *et al.* (7, 8) yielded a half-life for styrene in subcutaneous adipose tissue of 2.2 and 4 days.

Biotransformation takes place mainly in the liver. The first known metabolite of styrene is styrene oxide, which is hydrolysed to styrene glycol. This compound is oxidised to mandelic acid and then phenylglyoxylic acid.

The biotransformation of styrene is represented in Figure 1.

Mandelic acid and phenylglyoxylic acid are excreted mainly in the urine, while styrene glycol could not be detected in human urine to date. Much smaller amounts (about 5 %) of hippuric acid are also formed.

If a linear pharmacokinetic two-compartment model is assumed, there is a fast and a slow clearance phase for the styrene in blood. The half-lives of styrene for these clearance phases were calculated to be 0.6 and 13 hours (6).

According to Ramsey *et al.* (6) at least 97 % of the absorbed styrene is metabolised and about 86 % is transformed into the metabolites mandelic acid and phenylglyoxylic acid. Mandelic acid makes up about 57 % and phenylglyoxylic acid 33 %, only 2.6 % of the absorbed styrene is exhaled unchanged (9). The half-times for mandelic acid and phenylglyoxylic acid stated in the literature are shown in Table 1. As already mentioned, the absorption, distribution, metabolism and elimination of styrene can best be described by a two-compartment model.

Renal elimination of the metabolites is probably two-phase. The maximum of the renal excretion of mandelic acid and phenylglyoxylic acid must therefore be shortly after the end of exposure.

Exogenous factors can influence the absorption, metabolism and excretion of styrene. The most important of these are increased physical activity and the accompanying increase in the respiratory minute volume (10). This effect is also seen as one of the reasons for the wide range of interindividual and intraindividual variation in the levels measured in blood and urine of persons exposed to styrene. In addition, possible percutaneous absorption of styrene at the workplace must be borne in mind. Overall, however, the amount percutaneously absorbed can be considered insignificant for the total exposure. Wilson *et al.* (11) demonstrated that alcohol influences the kinetics of mandelic acid excretion in man. Ethanol inhibits the biotransformation of styrene so that the maximum of the excretion of mandelic acid is postponed by about 3 hours. This effect is already seen after "tolerable" amounts of alcohol (about 25 g alcohol/70 kg body weight). This aspect is relevant particularly during sample collection.

It must also be borne in mind that some solvents that can occur at the workplace are also metabolised to mandelic acid and phenylglyoxylic acid. Mandelic acid and phenylglyoxylic acid are the metabolites of ethylbenzene and phenylglycol (12). Interference can also occur from other substances such as medicines. It is known that some common analgesics and spasmolytics (e.g. Spalt®, Melabon®) contain derivatives of mandelic acid and that with medicines such as the psychopharmaceutical Pemolin (Tardon®) and the muscle relaxant Phenyramidol (Cabral®) mandelic acid can occur as a product of metabolism (13).

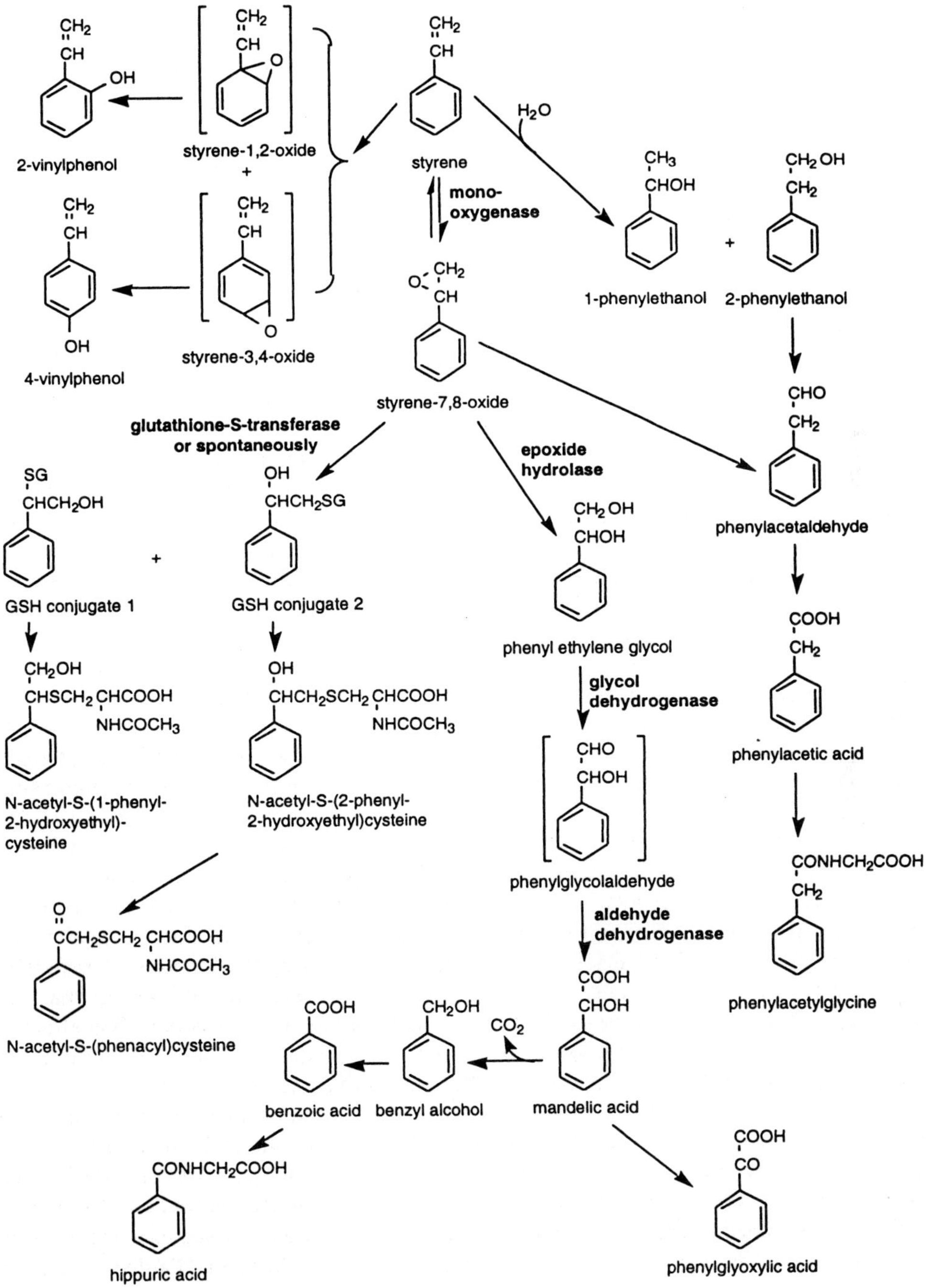

Fig. 1: Biotransformation of styrene in man (39)

Tab. 1: Half-times for renal excretion of mandelic acid and phenylglyoxylic acid after exposure to styrene

Exposure conditions Exposure (ml/m^3)	 Time (hours)	Half-time for mandelic acid (hours)	Half-time for phenylglyoxylic acid (hours)	Observation period after exposure (hours)	Type of elimination kinetics	Authors
50	8	4–7	–	–	single phase	Bardodej 1964 (12)
50–200	2.5	7.8 ± 1.9 (7)	8.5 ± 2.4 (7)	0–80	single phase	Ikeda *et al.* 1974 (35)
103 206	8 8	22.9 26.5	21.5 26.7	20–200 20–200	single phase	Caperos 1978 (36)
23	8	9.4 (7.1–11.9) 16.6 (9.8–56.0)	– –	0–18 19–64	two-phase	Engström *et al.* 1976 (37)
248 (155–291)	8	6.4 (4.7–7.6)	–	0–15		
50–200	4.8	3.9 ± 0.9 (21) 24.7 ± 10.3 (13)	– 10.5 ± 1.4 (19)	0–20 30–60	two-phase	Guillemin *et al.* 1979 (9)

2 Critical Toxicity

There are numerous national and international reports of experimental studies and field studies with occupationally exposed workers (14, 15).

For the setting of a BAT value, long-term exposure to styrene is more important than short-term exposure in the evaluation of the critical toxicity of styrene. After long-term exposure to styrene the effects on the following organs or organ systems are of particular relevance:

I. Skin and mucous membranes
II. Liver
III. Central and peripheral nervous system

The mutagenic properties of styrene and styrene oxide should also be mentioned (16, 17, 18, 19). There are also various reports of an increase in the incidence of chromosomal aberrations in leukocytes with styrene workers (20, 21). According to the IARC (22), no carcinogenic risk for man, however, can be deduced from the data available so far.

3 Exposure and Effect

The concept of exposure and effect treated in the relevant occupational-medical and toxicological literature is discussed below.

3.1 Skin and Mucous Membranes

Irritative effects on the mucous membranes resulting from exposure to styrene are described in several studies (2, 14). Visible irritation can occur from concentrations of 100 ml/m^3 (23). Habituation seems to play a role, as mainly workers with no previous exposure to styrene complained of mucous membrane irritation (14). According to one investigation there was no relationship between the extent of mucous membrane irritation and the level of exposure (24). Repeated exposure of the skin to liquid styrene can sometimes lead to toxic dermatosis (25, 26). The allergenic potential of styrene seems to be low (26, 27).

While mucosal irritation is of importance for the setting of MAK values, in the case of substances causing local irritation, due to the conditions prevailing at the workplace, e.g. increased physical activity, no direct conclusions can be drawn about the level of internal exposure because of possible percutaneous absorption or different metabolic and excretion behaviour. It follows that irritation of the mucous membranes need not represent the decisive effect for the evaluation of the BAT value. It must be remembered that observance of the BAT value is no acquittal from the responsibility of monitoring the concentration of the substance in the air.

3.2 Liver

Lorimer *et al.* (1976) (14), who investigated 471 workers with low and high exposure to styrene, found no pathological changes in the liver parameters γ-GT[1], ALT[2], AST[3] and AP[4]. Details on the level of exposure to styrene, however, are lacking.

Thiess and Friedheim (28) found no statistically significant increase in the incidence of pathological liver values (γ-GT, AST, ALT) in their study with 84 workers exposed to styrene concentrations of 50–300 ml/m^3. No increase in the incidence of abnormal liver values was detected in the course of long-term exposure.

According to a study by Hotz *et al.* (29) increased liver values (γ-GT, OCT[5], ALT and AST) were conspicuously frequent in 57 workers exposed to styrene with workplace concentrations of over 50 ml/m^3. The authors emphasise, however, that

1. only a few of the enzyme activities were in the pathological range
2. on the basis of their results, the question of possible hepatotoxic effects of styrene cannot be answered.

Triebig *et al.* (30) investigated the parameters γ-GT, AST, ALT and GLDH[6] in 29 workers exposed to styrene. Under the prevailing exposure conditions (styrene 20–200 ml/m^3 $\bar{x}$ = 120 ml/m^3, mandelic acid (end of shift) 180–1880 mg/g creatinine, phenylglyoxylic acid (end of shift) 43–110 mg/g creatinine) no hepatotoxic effects could be objectified. Also Härkönen *et al.* (54) found no increased incidence of altered liver enzyme values (γ-GT, AST, ALT) in 34 workers exposed to styrene (average concentration in air 30–40 ml/m^3) relative to that in a control group.

3.3 Nervous System

For the following evaluation only those studies were included which allowed statements to be made about relationships between internal exposure to styrene and the occurrence of adverse effects in man.

Several current publications also contribute to the estimation of health effects attributed to styrene (45, 46, 48, 51, 58, 59). Due to the lack of sufficient data on internal exposure to styrene these findings, however, could not be used for the re-evaluation of the BAT value.

In addition to the neurotoxic effects already mentioned, recent findings from neuroendocrinology are also taken into account.

---

[1] γ-Glutamyl transpeptidase
[2] Alanine aminotransferase (= GPT)
[3] Aspartate aminotransferase (= GOT)
[4] Alkaline phosphatase
[5] Ornithine carbamoyltransferase
[6] Glutamate dehydrogenase

3.3.1 Neurotoxicity

Murata *et al.* (53) reported significantly delayed nerve conduction velocities and evidence of dysfunction of the autonomous nerve system in laminating workers after long-term exposure to styrene. The differences relative to a control group occurred after average excretion of mandelic acid and phenylglyoxylic acid in post-shift samples of 446 mg per gram creatinine (range: 60 to 1270 mg per gram creatinine).

The published findings confirm some of the results of other studies (45, 59). On the other hand, in a longitudinal study with 29 laminating workers exposed to styrene, Triebig *et al.* (57) were not able to detect any significant reductions in nerve conduction velocity or dose-response relationships.

The method of measurement used by Murata *et al.* (53) with determination of the distribution of the nerve conduction velocities in the nerve fibres did lead to an increase in sensitivity, but the delayed nerve conduction velocities determined in the persons exposed to styrene were within the physiological range. In addition, the low number of test persons of only 11 exposed workers and the lack of dose-response relationships considerably limits the usefulness of these findings.

The determination of somatosensory evoked potentials in laminating workers exposed for many years revealed prolonged latency periods, which indicate functional disturbances in the peripheral and central nervous system (55). The amount of mandelic acid excreted in urine sampled at the end of the shift was between 270 mg and 1880 mg per gram creatinine. With increasing exposure duration abnormal findings were more frequent. The lack of data concerning confounding factors is to be criticised, which together with the relatively small number of persons (n = 20) limits any conclusions.

Gobba *et al.* (49) reported dyschromatopsia in 75 men and women exposed to styrene. The Colour Confusion Index (CCI) measured according to Lanthony's method correlated with the styrene excreted in urine, but not with mandelic acid. The mandelic acid concentrations in the post-shift urine samples of the exposed persons were between 15 mg and 3000 mg per litre with a mean value of 343 mg per litre. Significantly increased CCI values were described for those persons externally exposed to an average level during the shift of more than 50 ppm (this corresponds to about 1000 mg mandelic acid per litre urine in the post-shift sample). No data was given on the level of internal exposure. The study has various shortcomings. Alcohol consumption, for example, was not taken into consideration as a possible confounding factor. The values measured have a large range of scatter and there is a large difference in the number of test persons with low exposure (n = 55) and high exposure (n = 14). In addition, the pathogenesis of dyschromatopsia related to exposure to styrene is unclear. These findings must first of all be verified by further investigations. Yokoyama *et al.* (60) carried out psychological investigations with 12 persons exposed to styrene. The test results were significantly worse than those found with a control group. The average level of mandelic acid excreted in the post-shift samples of the exposed persons was 511 ± 418 mg per gram creatinine. The small number of test persons, the lack of dose-response relationships and the fact that only one test variable was significantly different, considerably limit the meaningfulness of this study.

Jégaden *et al.* (50) reported that the results obtained in psychological tests with laminating workers exposed to styrene were significantly worse than those for a control group. During the investigations the sum of mandelic acid and phenylglyoxylic acid in post-shift samples for the group of exposed persons was on average 575 mg per gram creatinine with a range of 90 mg to 2180 mg per gram creatinine. External exposure was on average 23 ppm (range 4 to 55 ppm). The authors also report the results of 254 urinary analyses which were carried out over a period of 43 weeks. The mean value was 722 mg mandelic acid plus phenylglyoxylic acid per gram creatinine with a range of 610 mg to 833 mg per gram creatinine. If the extensive data on exposure are taken into consideration, the lack of dose-response relationships is an important deficit in this study. This applies both for acute and chronic effects.

Neurological investigations, including quantitative EEG analysis, with 99 laminating workers exposed to styrene demonstrated that symptoms and abnormal EEG findings were found more frequently in exposed persons with an average level of mandelic acid excreted of 560 mg per litre in the post-shift samples (standard deviation 1120 mg/l) (52). The authors refer to an exposure-effect relationship, but quantitative evaluation of the relationship between EEG parameters and the exposure index is lacking. No threshold dose is defined.

3.3.2 Neuroendocrinological and Biochemical Findings

The research group around Franchini and Mutti reported in 1987 and 1990 prolactin measurements in the serum of women exposed to styrene (40, 47). The prolactin serum concentrations increased significantly in 16 women before and after stimulation with tyrosine releasing hormone (TRH) relative to control values. The increase also correlated with the level of mandelic acid and phenylglyoxylic acid excreted in urine. The metabolite concentrations were given as 200 mg and 171 mg per gram creatinine with sampling 15 hours after the end of exposure. In this respect the data cannot be directly compared with the results of other studies. The concentrations of styrene in air were between 5 ppm and 143 ppm (median 25 ppm).

The authors argue that the findings are in harmony with the hypothesis that styrene reduces dopaminergic modulation of pituitary secretion. It should, however, be noted that four points in the publication were commented on by the editor of the journal (42). He described the conclusions of the authors that "the observed health complaints can therefore be explained biochemically" as "risky" (42).

Checkoway *et al.* (43, 44) reported reduced activity of monoamine oxidase B in thrombocytes with increasing exposure to styrene. This finding is interpreted by the authors as evidence that monoamine oxidase B is a biomarker for the neurotoxicity of styrene. A significant effect can be deduced for the higher styrene concentration in blood from 5 µg per litre (43). There are no data available on urinary excretion of mandelic acid and phenylglyoxylic acid. The results of the study must be interpreted as provisional as they have not yet been confirmed by other research groups.

3.4 Genotoxicity

Tomanin *et al.* (56) reported on genotoxic effects after exposure to styrene with an average level of mandelic acid excreted of 725 mg per gram creatinine (post-shift samples). The results of this investigation agree more or less with the general evaluation of the genotoxicity of styrene. Barale (41) concludes on the basis of literature research that the threshold dose for chromosomal aberrations is about 50 ppm. This average air concentration during the shift corresponded with an average level of mandelic acid excreted of about 1000 mg/l in urine samples collected after the shift.

Walles *et al.* (58) reported on the determination of single strand breaks in 17 plastics workers exposed to styrene. The genotoxic effect was observed with an average level of mandelic acid excreted in post-shift samples of 70 mg per gram creatinine (range: detection limit up to 261 mg per gram creatinine). The authors were able to demonstrate that these were reversible effects which were no longer detectable the following morning.

4 Selection of the Indicators

There are various parameters of exposure available for objectifying and quantifying occupational exposure to styrene. Styrene itself can be measured in alveolar air, whole blood and urine. The styrene metabolites mandelic acid and phenylglyoxylic acid can be used as parameters for the internal exposure to styrene. The haemoglobin adduct of styrene-7,8-oxide can be determined by measuring the modified *N*-terminal valine as a parameter of effect. This assay has to date only been implemented in scientific studies and with relatively high external exposure to styrene (71, 62). This also applies to the detection of styrene-7,8-oxide in blood (67). Korn *et al.* (68) determined styrene-7,8-oxide concentrations of 0.9–4.1 µg/l in the blood of 13 persons exposed to styrene (10–73 ppm). The styrene-7,8-oxide concentration in blood calculated from a linear correlation for external exposure to 20 ppm was 1 µg/l.

Table 2 shows the advantages and disadvantages of the various biological monitoring parameters. It also contains information on the analytical methods.

The determination of styrene in whole blood or alveolar air has to date been little used in practice. The reasons for this are the limited practicability of alveolar air analysis and the necessity of strictly adhering to the sampling time, due to the relatively short biological half-life and analytical problems (69). Italian research groups have suggested measuring the styrene excreted in urine as a parameter of biological monitoring (64, 65). There is, however, little practical experience of this parameter in occupational medicine and the database is at present insufficient to be able to evaluate a BAT value.

To date the styrene metabolites mandelic acid and phenylglyoxylic acid are still thought to be the most suitable parameters for biological monitoring. Experience with these parameters is extensive. There are good correlations with external exposure and the total amount of metabolites excreted corresponds to about 90 % of the absorbed styrene. The sensitivity, specificity and validity of these parameters have been found to be very high both in simulations and in field studies (10, 69). Ethylbenzene, phenylglycol and some medicines (analgesics and spasmolytics), which contain mandelic acid derivatives, can, however, also be metabolised to mandelic acid and phenylglyoxylic acid and thus limit the specificity of the metabolite analysis (13).

This applies both for the excretion of mandelic acid and the total metabolites, with sampling at the end of the shift or the next morning prior to the shift. There is, however, only extensive experience with postshift samples. In addition, the analyte concentrations in the postshift samples are higher than those in the preshift samples and therefore yield more reliable analytical results.

Recent studies have shown that the relationship between the excretion of mandelic acid and phenylglyoxylic acid is not constant and is influenced by numerous factors, in particular the level of exposure and sampling time. The fact that the biological half-life of phenylglyoxylic acid is longer than that of mandelic acid is important as it means that in the course of a working week phenylglyoxylic acid accumulates (54).

Using the results from two field studies as an example, Table 3 shows how the relationship between the levels of mandelic acid and phenylglyoxylic acid excreted can vary. Quotients of between 4 and 0.66 are found depending on the level of exposure and sampling time. The total level of excreted metabolites depends less on these factors and is therefore better suited for monitoring persons exposed to styrene. In addition, the total level of excreted metabolites usually correlates better with external exposure than the data for single metabolites (69). In other studies comparable correlations were found for the elimination of mandelic acid (66, 65). The values for phenylglyoxylic acid, however, did not correlate as well. The correlation coefficients between external exposure and creatinine-related metabolite values are better than for litre-related values.

Evaluation of a BAT value should therefore be based on the total metabolites excreted related to creatinine. Sampling should be carried out at the end of exposure after several previous shifts.

5 Methodology

To date methods are available for the analysis of mandelic acid and phenylglyoxylic acid from the fields of photometry, isotachophoresis and chromatography. In recent years gas chromatography and high-pressure liquid chromatography have been found to be particularly practicable and reliable techniques.

With gas chromatographic methods, a derivatisation step must be carried out, which is particularly problematical with phenylglyoxylic acid (32). Guillemin and Bauer (33) therefore suggested determining phenylglyoxylic acid using gas chromatography after reduction to mandelic acid. The derivatives can be formed by silylation or methylation.

Tab. 2: Biological monitoring parameters for determining occupational exposure to styrene – advantages, disadvantages and analytical methods

Parameter	Advantages	Disadvantages	Method	References
Styrene in alveolar air	specific, sensitive, non-invasive	limited practicability, immediate analysis necessary, high variation, influenced by sampling time	adsorption tubes GC-FID	Wilson 1986 (72) Ong *et al.* 1994 (69)
Styrene in blood	specific, sensitive	invasive, influenced by sampling time	GC-FID GC-MS	Bartolucci *et al.* 1986 (61) Ong *et al.* 1994 (69)
Styrene in urine	specific, sensitive, non-invasive	little experience	GC-MS	Gobba *et al.* 1993 (65) Gobba *et al.* 1995 (64)
Styrene-7,8-oxide in whole blood	specific, correlation with exposure	invasive, method time-consuming, low concentration, short half-time	GC-FID	Korn *et al.* 1994 (68)
Styrene-7,8-oxide in haemoglobin	specific, parameter of effect	invasive, method time-consuming, not sufficiently sensitive	GC-MS detection of *N*-terminal valine	Severi *et al.* 1994 (71) Christakopoulos *et al.* 1993 (62)
Mandelic acid in postshift urine	non-invasive, extensive experience, main metabolite, basis for threshold evaluation	not absolutely specific	HPLC quality control possible	BAT documentation 1996 (63)
Phenylglyoxylic acid in postshift urine	specific, non-invasive	little experience, low concentration	HPLC quality control possible	BAT documentation 1996 (63)
Mandelic acid + phenylglyoxylic acid in postshift urine	good correlation with external exposure, corresponds to 90 % of the styrene absorbed	not absolutely specific	HPLC quality control possible	BAT documentation 1996 (63)
Styrene metabolites preshift (MA, PGA and MA + PGA)	good correlation with external exposure	little experience, low concentrations	HPLC quality control possible	Ong *et al.* 1994 (69)

Tab. 3: Ratio of mandelic acid and phenylglyoxylic acid levels in urine with regard to sampling time and the level of internal exposure as found in two cross-sectional studies

MA postshift mg/l	PGA postshift mg/l	Relationship MA:PGA	MA postshift mg/g creat.	PGA postshift mg/g creat.	Relationship MA:PGA	MA preshift mg/g creat.	PGA preshift mg/g creat.	Relationship MA:PGA	References
867	219	4	758	272	2.8	76.5	116.5	0.66	Ong *et al.* 1994 (69)
475	234	2	360	172	2.1	151	104	1.5	Schaller *et al.* 1997 (70)

MA = mandelic acid

PGA = phenylglyoxylic acid

High-pressure liquid chromatography has proved particularly suitable for determination of mandelic acid and phenylglyoxylic acid. Using the reverse phase separation principle and a particle size of 5 µm, the two metabolites can be determined directly in the urine. Parallel to this, other aromatic carbonic acids such as hippuric acid, methylhippuric acid etc. can be determined. A recommended method can be found in the loose-leaf collection "Analyses of Hazardous Substances in Biological Materials" (31).

During sample collection and storage, Guillemin and Bauer (9) observed decomposition of phenylglyoxylic acid under acid conditions. The sample material should therefore be stored at –20 °C after collection. Further information on the preanalytical phase can be found in Angerer *et al.* (34).

Analytical determination of mandelic acid and phenylglyoxylic acid in urine must be carried out according to TRgA 410 of the Hazardous Substances Ordinance under the conditions of statistical quality control according to the regulations of the German Federal Medical Council.

6 Evaluation of a BAT Value

The evaluation of the BAT values is based on recent data for the relationship between internal exposure and effects. Some studies used improved methods compared with those used in earlier studies and this increased the sensitivity of the detection of neurotoxic effects. Even if the meaningfulness of some studies is limited due to a relatively small number of test persons, the great range of scatter of metabolite concentrations in urine and the lack of dose-response relationships, synoptic evaluation of all the results leads to more or less consistent findings. Effects associated with styrene apparently occur more frequently in exposed persons when the average urinary concentration is 500 mg mandelic acid plus phenylglyoxylic acid per gram creatinine (or higher). The extent of internal exposure correlates well with that determined from the relationship between external exposure and internal exposure. The current MAK value and the suggested BAT values both therefore correspond to a fifth of the former threshold limit values in air and urine.

Also pharmacokinetic models confirm that excretion of mandelic acid and phenylglyoxylic acid at a level of about 500 mg per litre or 500 mg per gram creatinine with sampling at the end of the shift correspond to an external exposure to styrene of 20 ppm (10, 54). On this basis, the following BAT values have been set:

500 mg mandelic acid and phenylglyoxylic acid per gram creatinine
400 mg mandelic acid per gram creatinine.

Sampling should be carried out at the end of exposure or the end of the shift.

7 References

1. WHO: Environmental Health Criteria Document of Styrene (1982/83)
2. Härkönen, H.: Scand. J. Work Environ. Health *4* (1978), 104–113
3. Fiserova-Bergova, V., Teisinger, J.: Ind. Med. Surg. *34* (1965), 620–622
4. Fernandéz, J., Caperos, J.: Int. Arch. Occup. Environ. Health *40* (1977), 1–12
5. Ramsey, J. C., Young, J. D.: Scand. J. Work Environ. Health *4* (1978), 84–91
6. Ramsey, J. C., Young, J. D., Karbowski, R. J., Chenoweth, M. B., McCarthy, L. P., Braun, W. H.: Toxicol. Appl. Pharmacol. *53* (1980), 54–63
7. Engström, J., Bjurström, R., Åstrand, I., Ovrum, P.: Scand. J. Work Environ. Health *4* (1978), 315–323
8. Engström, J., Åstrand, I., Wigaeus, E.: Scand. J. Work Environ. Health *4* (1978), 324–329
9. Guillemin, M., Bauer, D.: Int. Arch. Occup. Environ. Health *44* (1979), 249–263
10. Droz, P. O., Guillemin, M. P.: Human Styrene Exposure. V. Development of a Model for Biological Monitoring, Int. Arch. Occup. Environ. Health *53* (1983), 19–36
11. Wilson, H. K., Robertson, S. M., Woldron, H. A., Gompertz, D.: Brit. J. Ind. Med. *40* (1983), 75–80
12. Bardodej, Z.: Cesk. Hyg. *9* (1964), 223–239
13. Schaller, K. H., Goßler, K., Bost, H. P., Valentin, H.: ASP *11* (1976), 24–26
14. Lorimer, W. V., Lilis, R., Nicholson, W. J., Anderson, H., Fischbein, A., Daum, S., Rom, W., Rice, L., Selikoff, I. J.: Environ. Health Perspect. *17* (1976), 171–181
15. Härkönen, H., Lindström, K., Seppäläinen, A. M., Asp, S., Hernberg, S.: Scand. J. Work Environ. Health *4* (1978), 53–59
16. Vainio, H., Pääkkönen, R., Rönnholm, K., Raunio, V., Pelkonen, O.: Scand. J. Work Environ. Health *3* (1976), 147–151
17. deMeester, C., Poncelet, F., Roberfroid, M., Rondelet, J., Mercier, M.: Mutat. Res. *56* (1977), 147–152
18. Loprieno, N., et al.: Mutat. Res. *40* (1976), 317–324
19. Milvy, P., Garro, A. J.: Mutat. Res. *40* (1976), 15–18
20. Meretoja, T., Järventaus, H., Sorsa, M., Vainio, H.: Scand. J. Work Environ. Health *4*, Suppl. *2* (1978), 259–264
21. Fleig, J., Thiess, A. M.: Scand. J. Work Environ. Health *4*, Suppl. *2* (1978), 254–258
22. IARC (Lyon): Monographs on the Evaluation of the Carcinogenic Risk of Chemicals to Humans *19* (1979), 231–259; Suppl. *4* (1982), 229–233
23. Stewart, R. D., Dodd, H. C., Baretta, E. D., Schaffer, A. W.: Arch. Environ. Health *16* (1968), 656–662
24. Härkönen, H.: Int. Arch. Occup. Environ. Health *40* (1977), 231–239
25. Wilson, R. H.: J. Am. Med. Assoc. *124* (1944), 701–703
26. Bourne, L. B., Milner, F. J. M.: Brit. J. Ind. Med. *20* (1963), 100–109
27. Meneghini, C., Rantuccio, F.: Berufsdermatosen *11* (1963), 181–202
28. Thiess, A. M., Friedheim, M.: Scand. J. Work Environ. Health *4* (1978), 203–214
29. Hotz, Ph., Guillemin, M. P., Lob, M.: Scand. J. Work Environ. Health *6* (1980), 206–215
30. Triebig, G., Schaller, K. H., Kentner, M., Hartung, M.: Verhandlungen der Deutschen Gesellschaft für Arbeitsmedizin e.V., 23. Jahrestagung in Göttingen vom 4–7. Mai 1983. Ed.: K. Stalder, Gentner Verlag, Stuttgart 1983
31. Angerer, J., Schaller, K. H. (Eds.): Analyses of Hazardous Substances in Biological Materials, Vol. 2, pp 47–66, VCH-Verlagsgesellschaft, Weinheim (1988)
32. Bauer, D., Guillemin, M. P.: Int. Arch. Occup. Environ. Health *37* (1976), 47–55
33. Guillemin, M., Bauer, D.: Int. Arch. Occup. Environ. Health *37* (1976), 57–64
34. Angerer, J., Schaller, K. H., Seiler, H.: Trends in Analytical Chemistry *2* (1983), 257–261
35. Ikeda, M., Imamura, T., Hayashi, M., Tabuchi, T., Hara, I.: Int. Arch. Arbeitsmed. *32* (1974), 93–101

36. Caperos, J. R.: Etudes experimentale sur des sujets humains de l'absorption, du métabolisme et de l'elimination du styrene, du m-xylène et du toluène. Thèse de doctorat 1978, Neuchâtel
37. Engström, K., Härkönen, H., Kalliokoski, P., Ratanen, J.: Scand. J. Work Environ. Health *2* (1976), 12–16
38. Härkönen, H., Lentniemi, A., Aitio, A.: Scand. J. Work Environ. Health *10* (1984), 59–61
39. Summer, S. J., Fenell, T. R.: Review of the Metabolic Fate of Styrene, Critical Reviews in Toxicology *24* (1994), 11–33
40. Arfini, G., Mutti, A., Vescovi, P., Ferroni, C., Ferrari, M., Giaroli, C. et al.: Impaired Dopaminergic Modulation of Pituitary Secretion in Workers Occupational Exposed to Styrene: Further Evidence from PRL Response to TRH Stimulation, J. Occup. Med. *29* (1987), 826–830
41. Barale, R.: The genetic toxicology of styrene and styrene oxide, Mut. Res. *257* (1991), 107–126
42. Beidleman, B.: Editorial Comment, J. Occup. Med. *29* (1987), 826
43. Checkoway, H., Costa, L. G., Camp, J., Coccini, J., Daniell, W. E. et al.: Peripheral markers of neurochemical function among workers exposed to styrene, Brit. J. Ind. Med. *49* (1992), 560–565
44. Checkoway, H., Echeverria, D., Moon, J.-D., Heyer, N., Costa, L. G.: Platelet monoamine oxidase B activity in workers exposed to styrene, Int. Arch. Occup. Environ. Health *66* (1994), 359–362
45. Cherry, N., Gautrin, D.: Neurotoxic effects of styrene: further evidence, Brit. J. Ind. Med. *47* (1990), 29–37
46. Edling, Ch., Anundi, H., Johanson, G., Nilsson, K.: Increase in neuropsychiatric symptoms after occupational exposure to low levels of styrene, Brit. J. Ind. Med. *50* (1993), 843–850
47. Franchini, I., Ferroni, C., Selis, C., Folli, D., Gamberale, F., Iregren, A., Mutti, A.: A Cross-Sectional Reappraisal of the Neurobehavioral and Neuroendocrine Changes in Styrene-Exposed Workers, 23rd International Congress on Occupational Health, Montreal, Canada, 22nd–28th September 1990
48. Geuskens, R. B., van der Klaauw, M. M., van der Tuin, J., et al.: Exposure to Styrene and Health Complaints in the Dutch Glass-Reinforced Plastics Industry, Ann. Occup. Hyg. *36* (1992), 47–57
49. Gobba, F., Galassi, C., Imbriani, M., Ghittori, S., Candela, S., Cavalleri, A.: Acquired Dyschromatopsia among Styrene-Exposed Workers, J. Occup. Med. *33* (1991), 761–765
50. Jégaden, D., Amann, D., Simon, J. F., Habault, M., Legoux, B. et al.: Study of the neurobehavioural toxicity of styrene at low levels of exposure, Int. Arch. Occup. Environ. Health *64* (1993), 527–531
51. Letz, R., Mahoney, F. C., Hershman, D. L., Woskie, S., Smith, T.J.: Neurobehavioral Effects of Acute Styrene Exposure in Fiberglass Boatbuilders, Neurotoxicol. Teratol. *12* (1990), 665–668
52. Matikainen, E., Forsman-Grönholm, L., Pfäffli, P., Juntunen, J.: Nervous System Effects of Occupational Exposure to Styrene: A Clinical and Neurophysiological Study, Environm. Res. *61* (1993), 84–92
53. Murata, K., Arakiö, S., Yokoyama, K.: Assessment of the Peripheral, Central, and Autonomic Nervous System Function in Styrene Workers, Am. J. Ind. Med. *20* (1991), 775–784
54. Perbellini, L., Mozzo, P., Turri, P. V., Zedde, A., Brugnone, F.: Biological exposure index of styrene suggested by a physiologico-mathematical model, Int. Arch. Occup. Environ. Health *60* (1988), 187–193
55. Stetkárová, I., Urban, P., Procházka, B., Lukás, E.: Somatosensory evoked potentials in workers exposed to toluene and styrene, Brit. J. Ind. Med. *50* (1993), 520–527
56. Tomanin, R., Ballarin, C., Bartolucci, G. B., De Rosa, E., Sessa, G. et al.: Chromosome aberrations and micronuclei in lymphocytes of workers exposed to low and medium levels of styrene, Int. Arch. Occup. Environ. Health *64* (1992), 209–215

57. Triebig, G., Schaller, K. H., Valentin, H.: Investigations on neurotoxicity of chemical substances at the workplace, VII. Longitudinal study with determination of nerve conduction velocities in persons occupationally exposed to styrene, Int. Arch. Occup. Environ. Health *56* (1985), 239–247
58. Walles, S. A. S. Edling, Ch., Anundi, H., Johanson, G.: Exposure dependent increase in DNA single strand breaks in leucocytes from workers exposed to low concentrations of styrene, Brit. J. Ind. Med. *50* (1993), 570–574
59. Yokoyama, K., Murata, K., Araki, S.: Psychological Performance and Peripheral Nerve Conduction Velocities in Workers Exposed to Low Level of Styrene, 23rd International Congress on Occupational Health, Montreal, Canada, 22nd–28th September 1990
60. Yokoyama, K., Araki, S., Murata, K.: Effects of Low Level Styrene Exposure on Psychological Performance in FRP Boat Laminating Workers, Neurotoxicol. *13* (1992), 551–556
61. Bartolucci, G.B., De Rosa, E., Gori, G.P., Corona., Perbellini, L., Brugnone, F.: Biomonitoring of occupational exposure to low styrene levels, Appl. Ind. Hyg. *1* (1986), 125–131
62. Christakopoulos, A., Bergmark, E., Zorcec, V., Norppa, H., Mäki-Paakkanen, J.: Monitoring of occupational exposure to styrene from hemoglobin adducts and metabolites in blood, Scand. J. Work. Environ. Health *19* (1993), 255–263
63. Greim, H., Lehnert, G. (Eds.): Biologische Arbeitsstoff-Toleranz-Werte (BAT-Werte) und Expositionsäquivalente für krebserzeugende Arbeitsstoffe (EKA), VCH-Verlagsgesellschaft, Weinheim (1996)
64. Gobba, F. et al.: Letter to the editor: Biomonitoring of low levels of exposure to styrene, Am. J. Ind. Med. *28* (1995), 142–146
65. Gobba, F., Galassi, C., Ghittori, S., Imbriani, M., Pugliese, F., Cavalleri, A.: Urinary styrene in the biological monitoring of styrene exposure, Scand. J. Work. Environ. Health *19* (1993), 175–182
66. Guillemin, M.P., Berode, D.: Biological monitoring of styrene: A review, Am. Ind. Hyg. Assoc. J. *49 (10)* (1988), 497–505
67. Kessler, W., Jian, X.-L., Filser, J.G.: Empfindlicher, direkter Nachweis von Styrol-7,8-oxid im Blut, in: A. Meyer-Falcke, G. Jansen (Eds.): Bericht über die 29. Jahrestagung der Deutschen Gesellschaft für Arbeitsmedizin e.V. Gentner Verlag, Stuttgart (1989), 521–522
68. Korn, M., Gfrörer, W., Filser, J.G., Kessler, W.: Styrene-7,8-oxide in blood of workers exposed to styrene, Arch. Toxicol. *68* (1994), 524–527
69. Ong., C.N., Shi, C.Y., Chia, S.E., Chua, S.C., Ong, H.Y., Lee, B.L., Ng, T.P., Teramoto, K.: Biological monitoring of exposure to low concentrations of styrene, Am. J. Ind. Med. *25* (1994), 719–730
70. Schaller, K.H., Angerer, J., Weltle, D.: Querschnittsstudie zur Styrol-Belastung und Arbeitsplätzen in Laminierbetrieben – Konsequenzen für eine BAT-Wert-Evaluierung, Arbeitsmed. Sozialmed. Präventivmed. 1997 (in press)
71. Severi, M., Pauwels, W., van Hummelen, P., Roosels, D., Kirsch-Volders, M., Veulemans, H.: Urinary mandelic acid and hemoglobin adducts in fiberglass-reinforced plastics workers exposed to styrene, Scand. J. Work. Environ. Health *20* (1994), 451–458
72. Wilson, H.K.: Breath analysis: Physiological basis and sampling techniques, Scand. J. Work. Environ. Health *12* (1986), 174–192

Authors: K. H. Schaller, G. Triebig
Approved by the Working Group: 18th April 1995

Addendum to Styrene

8 Re-evaluation of the BAT Value

The BAT values for occupational exposure to styrene were last set in 1995. They were 400 mg mandelic acid per gram creatinine and 500 mg mandelic acid plus phenylglyoxylic acid per gram creatinine. The BAT values were based on the relationship between internal exposure and the effects. The effects were evaluated from neurotoxic and neuroendocrinological findings. The studies on which the evaluation is based are discussed in detail in the documentation to styrene from 1996. The BAT value for the sum of the styrene metabolites is still based on the relationship between mandelic acid and phenylglyoxylic acid postulated in the literature. This relationship was found in older studies with styrene exposures greatly above the named BAT values.

The use of two BAT values of comparable meaning for the occupational-medical–toxicological evaluation of occupational exposure to styrene caused problems in everyday use. There were cases when the BAT value for mandelic acid was adhered to while the value for the sum of the styrene metabolites was exceeded. This happened particularly with exposure to styrene over a working week and sampling at the end of the week. Investigations have shown that preshift urine samples already contain levels of excreted metabolites above the normal level and that the amount of phenylglyoxylic acid is disproportionately high. This is due to the longer biological half-life of phenylglyoxylic acid of about ten hours compared to about two to four hours for mandelic acid (15, 6, 2). In view of all this it was necessary to reconsider the choice of monitoring parameters and to re-evaluate the BAT value for the parameters selected.

8.1 Recent Field Studies with Persons Occupationally Exposed to Styrene

The results of older field studies are contained in the BAT value documentation for styrene from 1983 (2). The new literature on field studies investigating the relationship between internal exposure and the effects was presented in the addendum to this documentation (3). These studies were used for the evaluation of the BAT value of 400 mg mandelic acid per gram creatinine and 500 mg mandelic acid plus phenylglyoxylic acid per gram creatinine based on exposure/effect reactions.

In the meantime, further studies have appeared which demonstrate the relationship between external and internal exposure to styrene. They can be used to evaluate a new BAT value for the total metabolites excreted in urine.

These investigations were carried out in companies producing products reinforced with glass-fibre mainly using a manual laminating procedure. Difficulties adhering to the MAK value occur in these factories in particular when single items are made and powerful exhaust systems cannot generally be installed (4, 10, 8, 13).

Essential BAT Value Documentations. DFG, Deutsche Forschungsgemeinschaft

ISBN 3-527-31477-6

Dornow *et al.* (4) investigated 18 laminators exposed to styrene. The styrene concentrations in blood and the metabolites excreted in urine were determined. The external exposure was not measured, but was deduced on the basis of the styrene concentrations determined in blood. Values equivalent to the MAK value of 20 ppm are, according to these studies, 290 mg/g creatinine for mandelic acid and 410 mg/g creatinine for mandelic acid plus phenylglyoxylic acid.

In a boat factory in Singapore where glass-fibre reinforced polyester resins were used, the styrene levels in the alveolar air, blood and urine, and metabolites in the urine of 39 male workers were investigated. The external exposure was determined during the whole 8-hour workshift using passive monitoring. The geometric mean for the external exposure to styrene was 10.4 ppm (about 43 mg/m^3), the range varied from 0.2 to 32.3 ppm. Significant relationships were found between external and internal exposure and between the parameters of biological monitoring. The correlation coefficients for the creatinine-related metabolites in the postshift sample and the styrene levels in the air were 0.83 for mandelic acid, 0.84 for phenylglyoxylic acid and 0.86 for the sum of both metabolites. A level of mandelic acid excreted in urine of 758 mg/g creatinine corresponded to an external exposure of 50 ppm, while for phenylglyoxylic acid a level of 272 mg/g creatinine was found and for mandelic acid plus phenylglyoxylic acid a level of 1012 mg/g creatinine (10, 11). The correlation coefficients for the relationship between the excretion of mandelic acid and phenylglyoxylic acid and the total metabolites were calculated as 0.98 and 0.92. The results also showed that relating the urinary metabolites to creatinine led to an improvement in the correlations.

Koch *et al.* (8) determined the styrene concentrations in alveolar air and blood and the mandelic acid concentrations in urine of 99 employees in 16 laminating factories. The external exposure to styrene was measured using personal air sampling. The mean of all ambient air samples was 255.6 mg/m^3, the range varied from 3.0 to 1837 mg/m^3. The average level of mandelic acid excreted was 567 mg/l (range 7.0–3416 mg/l). Unlike in other studies, no correlations were found between the styrene concentration in ambient air and the concentration of styrene metabolites in urine. This applies both for mandelic acid and the combined value for mandelic acid and phenylglyoxylic acid. For this reason and because neither the phenylglyoxylic acid values nor those for the total metabolites are given, this study cannot be used for a re-evaluation of the BAT value for the total metabolites excreted.

A cross-sectional study was carried out in 1994 and 1995 to determine the current external and internal exposure to styrene at laminating workplaces (13). 121 persons from 19 laminating factories took part. The external exposure to styrene was determined using personal air sampling. In the urine samples taken at the end of the shift the styrene metabolites were detected using gas chromatography. Determination of styrene in the air yielded values of 3 mg/m^3 to 968 mg/m^3. The average exposure was 127 mg/m^3, the median 81 mg/m^3. In 52 % of cases the MAK value was exceeded by 85 mg/m^3. The creatinine-related median excretion of mandelic acid was 265 mg/g creatinine, that of phenylglyoxylic acid 150 mg/g creatinine and for the sum of the metabolites there was a median of 528 mg/g creatinine.

Table 4 shows the levels of excreted styrene metabolites compared to the styrene concentration in the air. Taking the BAT value for mandelic acid in urine of 400 mg/g creatinine as a basis, the BAT value is exceeded in 42 % of those investigated in the total collective. If the total metabolites excreted are considered, this is true of 51 %. If the ambient exposure is considered with a MAK value for styrene of 85 mg/m^3, then levels of mandelic acid above the BAT value but adhering to the MAK value were only found in 5 % of those investigated. This plausible finding cannot be confirmed for the sum of the styrene metabolites mandelic acid and phenylglyoxylic acid. Despite adherence to the MAK value, the BAT value is exceeded in 22 % of cases. This indicates that the BAT value for the sum of the styrene metabolites excreted is too low. Analytical evaluation of the correlations yielded significant relationships between the styrene concentration in air and creatinine-related metabolite excretion. The correlation coefficients were 0.815 for mandelic acid and 0.806 for mandelic acid plus phenylglyoxylic acid. Mandelic acid levels of 475 mg/l or 360 mg/g creatinine corresponded to the MAK value of 85 mg/m^3. The corresponding value for the sum of the metabolites was 711 mg/l or 531 mg/g creatinine.

9 Evaluation of the BAT Value

The BAT values of 400 mg mandelic acid per gram creatinine and 500 mg mandelic acid plus phenylglyoxylic acid per gram creatinine for occupational exposure to styrene were based on recent data for the relationship between internal exposure and the effects. The effects were evaluated from neurotoxic and neuroendocrinological findings. For the reasons mentioned above and wishes expressed in everyday practice it was necessary to re-evaluate the BAT values. The aim of this re-evaluation was to establish **one** BAT value. The sum of the renally excreted styrene metabolites, mandelic acid and phenylglyoxylic acid, was chosen. The BAT value is creatinine-related and is valid for urine sampled at the end of exposure or the end of the shift after several previous shifts. In accordance with the BAT value concept, the evaluated value must meet the requirements of disease prevention in the individual. It can be deduced from the data collected in field studies that external exposure to styrene at a level of 20 ppm (85 mg/m^3) corresponds with a total level of excreted metabolites of 500 to 600 mg/m^3. This is supported by observations that effects associated with styrene apparently occur more often when urinary concentrations of mandelic acid exceed an average of 400 mg/g creatinine. If this value is taken as the basis for the calculation of the total metabolites excreted, the three studies discussed yield the total metabolite levels shown in Table 5.

A level of 600 mg/g creatinine for the total metabolites excreted corresponds to a mandelic acid level excreted in urine of 400 mg/g creatinine. This applies more or less for the litre-related metabolite concentrations too. Calculation of the total level of renally eliminated metabolites equivalent to the amount of mandelic acid excreted is based on the average metabolite level in urine. According to definition, the BAT value is the maximum permissible quantity of a chemical substance in biological materials which, even when it is attained, does not affect the health of the employee adversely. This requirement is fulfilled in the present case.

Tab. 4: Level of urinary styrene metabolites compared to the styrene concentration in the air

	Styrene concentration in the air (mg/m³)		Mandelic acid in urine (mg/g creatinine)				Mandelic acid + phenylglyoxylic acid (mg/g creatinine)		
Exposure range	Median	95th percentile	N	Median	95th percentile	N above BAT	Median	95th percentile	N above BAT
Total	81	407	121	265	1136	51 (42 %)	528	2426	61 (51 %)
1–85 mg/m³	41	84	60	152	466	3 (5 %)	258	759	13 (22 %)
> 85 mg/m³	160	724	49	739	1587	36 (74 %)	1019	2095	37 (76 %)

Tab. 5: Metabolite levels excreted in urine

Mean styrene conc. in air (mg/m^3)	Mean excretion of MA (mg/g creat.)	Mean excretion of MA + PGA (mg/g creat.)	MA + PGA excreted equivalent to 400 mg MA/g creat.	References
–	290	410	570	Dornow *et al.* 1992 (4)
212	758 867 (mg/l)	1012 1127 (mg/l)	550 520 (mg/l)	Ong. *et al.* 1994 (10)
85	360 475 (mg/l)	531 711 (mg/l)	590 600 (mg/l)	Schaller *et al.* 1997 (13)

MA = mandelic acid
PGA = phenylglyoxylic acid

A BAT value has therefore been set of:

600 mg mandelic acid plus phenylglyoxylic acid per gram creatinine.

This value also corresponds more or less with the correlates for metabolite excretion evaluated from field studies and pharmacokinetic modelling on the basis of the relationship between external and internal exposure (12, 11).

Sampling should be carried out at the end of exposure or the end of the shift after several previous days of exposure.

10 Interpretation of the Data

Urine sampling must be carried out at the end of the shift or the end of exposure after several previous shifts. This is when the maximum level of metabolites is excreted. The consumption of alcohol can lead to inhibition of styrene metabolism and the time at which the maximum amount of mandelic acid is excreted can be delayed by several hours (16, 1, 7). This aspect must be taken into consideration in the evaluation of the results of biological monitoring with persons exposed to styrene.

Effects of co-exposure with acetone have not been observed with either short-term or long-term exposure (15, 9).

Another relevant influence on metabolite excretion is the level of physical activity at the workplace (5, 7).

As already mentioned, the measurement of the styrene metabolites mandelic acid and phenylglyoxylic acid in urine is not a specific test. Mandelic acid is also excreted as a metabolite of ethylbenzene and phenylglycol. This also applies to some medicines (analgesics and spasmolytics), which can contain mandelic acid derivatives (14).

There are no problems due to contamination or losses during the preanalytical phase.

10 References

1. Berode, M., Droz, P.O., Boillat, M.A., Guillemin, M., P.: Effect of alcohol on the kinetics of styrene and 1st metabolites in volunteers and in workers, Appl. Ind. Hyg. *1* (1986), 25–28
2. Henschler, D., Lehnert, G. (Eds.): Biologische Arbeitsstoff-Toleranz-Werte (BAT-Werte) und Expositionsäquivalente für krebserzeugende Arbeitsstoffe (EKA), VCH-Verlagsgesellschaft, Weinheim (1983)
3. Greim, H., Lehnert, G. (Eds.): Biologische Arbeitsstoff-Toleranz-Werte (BAT-Werte) und Expositionsäquivalente für krebserzeugende Arbeitsstoffe (EKA), VCH-Verlagsgesellschaft, Weinheim (1996)
4. Dornow, R., Knecht, U., Woitowitz, H.J.: Zur Validität des Biomonitoring bei styrolexponierten Arbeitnehmern, in: Bericht über die 32. Jahrestagung der Deutschen Gesellschaft für Arbeitsmedizin, Gentner Verlag Stuttgart (1992), pp 473–476
5. Droz, P.O., Guillemin, M.P.: Human Styrene Exposure, Int. Arch. Occup. Environ. Health *53* (1983), 19–36
6. Guillemin, M.P., Bauer, D.: Human exposure to styrene: III. Elimination kinetics of urinary mandelic and phenylglyoxylic acids after single experimental exposure, Int. Arch. Occup. Environ. Health *44* (1979), 249–263
7. Guillemin, M.P., Berode, D.: Biological monitoring of styrene: A review, Am. Ind. Hyg. Assoc. J. *49 (10)* (1988), 497–505
8. Koch, K.-D., Wehrle, G., Bittighofer, P.M., Schwarzbach, E.: Aspekte des Gesundheitsschutzes bei der Verarbeitung von Styrol im Handlaminierverfahren, Zbl. Arbeitsmed. *46* (1996), 111–118
9. Mizunuma, K., Yasugi, T. et al.: Exposure-excretion relationship of styrene and acetone in factory workers: A comparison of a lipophilic solvent and a hydrophilic solvent, Arch. Environ. Contam. Toxicol. *25* (1993), 129–133
10. Ong., C.N., Shi, C.Y., Chia, S.E., Chua, S.C., Ong, H.Y., Lee, B.L., Ng, T.P., Teramoto, K.: Biological monitoring of exposure to low concentrations of styrene, Am. J. Ind. Med. *25* (1994), 719–730
11. Ong., C.N.: Letter to the editor: Biomarkers for monitoring of styrene exposure, Am. J. Ind. Med. *28* (1995), 147–149
12. Perbellini, L., Mozzo, P., Turri, P.V., Zedde, A., Brugnone, F.: Biological exposure index of styrene suggested by a physiologico-mathematical model, Int. Arch. Occup. Environ. Health *60* (1988), 187–193
13. Schaller, K.H., Angerer, J., Weltle, D.: Querschnittsstudie zur Styrol-Belastung und Arbeitsplätzen in Laminierbetrieben – Konsequenzen für eine BAT-Wert-Evaluierung, (1997), unpublished report, available from the commission
14. Schaller, K. H., Goßler, K., Bost, H. P., Valentin, H.: Arbeitsmed. Sozialmed. Präventivmed. *11* (1976), 24–26
15. Shi, C.Y., Chua, S.C., Lee, B.L., Ong, H.Y., Jeyaratnam, J., Ong, C.N.: Kinetics of styrene urinary metabolites: a study in a low-level occupational exposure setting in Singapore, Int. Arch. Occup. Environ. Health *65* (1994), 319–323
16. Wigaeus, E., Lof, A., Byfalt Nordqvist, M.: Uptake, distribution, metabolism and elimination of styrene in man. A comparison between single exposure and co-exposure with acetone, Br. J. Ind. Med. *41* (1984), 539–546

Authors: K. H. Schaller, G. Triebig
Approved by the Working Group: 21st November 1996

Tetrachloroethene

BAT	9.5 ppm (64 mg/m^3) tetrachloroethene in the alveolar air 1000 µg tetrachloroethene/l blood Sampling time: approx. 16 hours after end of exposure
Date of evaluation	1982
Synonyms	Perchloroethylene
Formula	C_2Cl_2 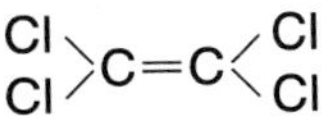
Molecular weight	165.83
Melting point	−23.5 °C
Boiling point	121.1 °C
Vapour pressure at 20 °C	18.6 hPa
MAK	50 ml/m^3 (ppm), 345 mg/m^3

1 Metabolism and Kinetics

Since the establishment of the MAK documentation for tetrachloroethene (perchloroethylene) (1) in 1974 relevant more recent studies on the metabolism and kinetics of this substance have appeared. Tetrachloroethene differs considerably from trichloroethene (2) in its distribution behaviour and the speed of its metabolism.

1.1 Metabolism

Tetrachloroethene is oxidised by microsomal mono-oxygenases to the epoxide (tetrachlorooxirane) which is transformed spontaneously to trichloroacetyl chloride (see 1, 3–6). These reactive intermediates can bind covalently to proteins (3–6); no binding to DNA was found (7). The transformation product, trichloroacetic acid, is

Essential BAT Value Documentations. DFG, Deutsche Forschungsgemeinschaft

ISBN 3-527-31477-6

excreted in the urine. In rats oxalic acid was recently described as a further urinary metabolite of tetrachloroethene (5).

Whereas earlier several investigators (using the colorimetric Fujiwara method) reported excretion of trichloroethanol after tetrachloroethene exposure (1, 8 – 10) this could not be confirmed in more recent studies. It was suggested that a possible explanation for this (11) is that earlier samples of tetrachloroethene used for investigation may have been contaminated with 5 – 10 % trichloroethene. The metabolism of tetrachloroethene is presented in figure 1.

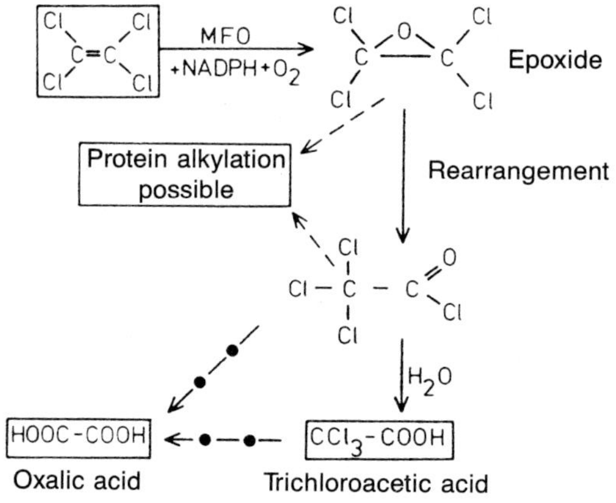

Fig. 1: Metabolism of tetrachloroethene (6). Detected urine metabolites are trichloroacetic acid and (with rats) oxalic acid.
MFO = Microsomal monooxygenase.

Animal-experimental investigations on rats (5) and mice (6) have shown that the rate of metabolism of tetrachloroethene shows saturation characteristics. This confirms earlier investigations on man (12) according to which the excretion of trichloroacetic acid with exposure to tetrachloroethene levels above 50 to 100 ppm did not increase proportionately any longer. These non-linear kinetics of the metabolism and the long half-life of the trichloroacetic acid in the organism (see 2) are probably the reason that occupational medical studies on the quantification of the trichloroacetic acid excretion after tetrachloroethene exposure led to the conclusion that there was no strict correlation between the metabolite excretion and exposure (13, 14).

1.2 Kinetics

The pharmacokinetics of tetrachloroethene have been investigated in volunteers by various working groups. In its behaviour in the organism tetrachloroethene shows two great differences from the chemically related trichloroethene (see BAT value documentation for trichloroethene (2)): the accumulation in the organism (in particular in the adipose tissue) is greater due to its physical properties (lipophilic, low volatility) (15) and the speed of the metabolic transformation (see Fig. 1) is considerably slower (1) than in the case of trichloroethene. As only a very small part of the absorbed tetrachloroethene is metabolised (approx. 1 % appears within 70 hours as trichloroacetic acid in the urine (16, 17)) after the end of exposure tetrachloroethene is exhaled again almost completely in the unchanged form (1, 16). For this reason the studies available on the kinetics of tetrachloroethene in volunteers (10, 11, 14, 16, 18–23) concentrate mostly on the investigation of the non-metabolised substance in the blood and/or expired air. Simulations with computer models have also been published (22).

It is well-documented (21, 22) that the distribution of tetrachloroethene in the organism takes place in various compartments from which the mobilisation after the end of exposure occurs with very different speeds. Thus, the distribution compartments may be differentiated as (22): 1. Organs well supplied with blood, e. g. brain, heart, hepatoportal system, kidneys, glandular tissue; 2. muscles; 3. adipose tissue; 4. tissues badly supplied with blood, e. g. bones, cartilage, ligaments etc.

All investigations carried out agree that an initial fast decrease in the tetrachloroethene concentration in the exhaled air which is observed within the first 30 minutes after exposure is to be attributed to a "wash-out effect" of the tetrachloroethene present in the central lung compartment. Afterwards the course of the concentration curves in blood and exhaled air run parallel. During the elimination of the substance from various "deep" compartments different successive half-lives in the blood or exhaled air are observed (16, 22, 23). As an example figure 2 shows the course of the

Tetrachloroethene in the alveolar air after a single 8-hour exposure

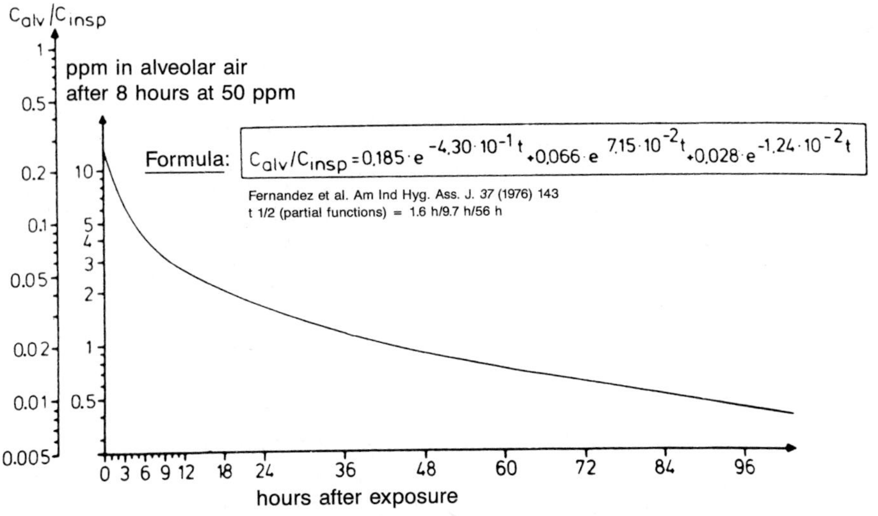

Fig. 2: Course of the tetrachloroethene concentration in the alveolar air after a single 8-hour exposure according to the equation by Fernandez et al. (23). That the curve is composed of several exponential functions indicates that tetrachloroethene is distributed in several compartments.

function of the concentration of tetrachloroethene in the alveolar air after 8-hour experimental exposure quoted by Fernandez et al. (23); this function consists of three partly exponential functions whose half-lives are given in figure 2. Very similar curves were also described by other investigators (10, 16).

Under the conditions of daily repeated tetrachloroethene exposure for several hours the kinetics diverge markedly from those for a single exposure (20): apparently longer half-lives are observed. This can probably be attributed to the fact that under the conditions of multiple exposure the deeper compartments are increasingly filled so that the slow elimination process after the end of the exposure series is more noticeable. It must be criticised here that it was not taken into account in all experiments (22, 23) that multiple exposures had been carried out.

Figure 3 shows the tetrachloroethene concentration in the alveolar air after the end of exposure of 5 volunteers (median values and individual extreme values) who had inhaled 100 ppm tetrachloroethene for 5 days (7 hours/day) at rest (21). The cumulative effect is shown clearly in the difference between figures 2 and 3. Figure 3 also shows that it is possible for practical reasons to describe the course of the exhalation curve in the interval between 15 and 71 hours after the end of a multiple exposure, as discussed in section 6, with sufficient exactness by a single exponential function. This consideration is a fundamental basis for the method of establishment of a BAT value for tetrachloroethene as carried out here.

For further details on the pharmacokinetics of tetrachloroethene in the blood and exhaled air reference is made to section 4.

Tetrachloroethene in the alveolar air after multiple exposure (5 days; 7 hours/day)

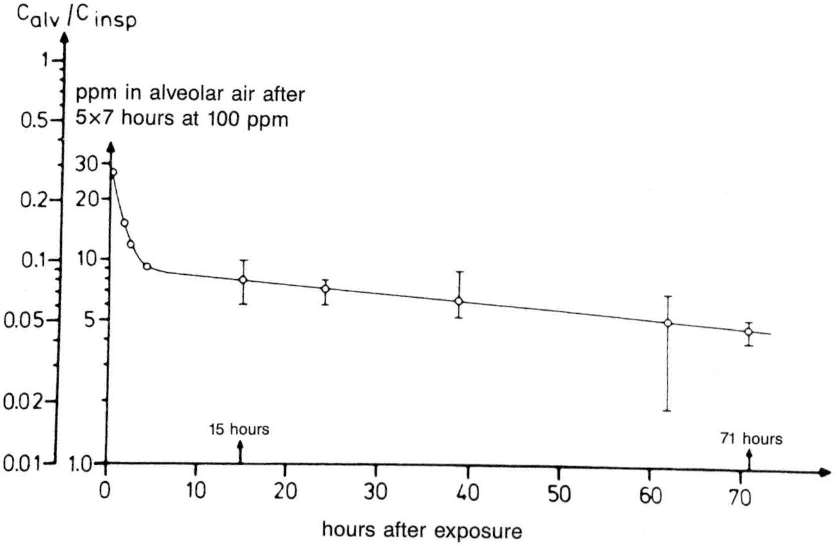

Fig. 3: Decrease of the tetrachloroethene concentration in the alveolar air after exposure of test persons for 5 days (7 hours/day) to 100 ppm tetrachloroethene. Median values and individual extreme values according to Stewart et al. (21).

1.3 Conditions of Exposure at the Workplace

Various conditions of exposure at the workplace can result in quantitative changes in the relationships found in laboratory experiments. The effect of physical work has been investigated (16): it could be shown that corresponding to the increased respiratory minute volumes during physical work also the uptake of tetrachloroethene is increased. This should be taken into account when extrapolating laboratory data to the conditions at the workplace.

2 Critical Toxicity

The most important findings on the toxicology of this substance have been compiled in the documentation of the MAK value for tetrachloroethene (1).

As with other halogenated hydrocarbons a sensibilisation of the heart to catecholamines has also been observed with tetrachloroethene (24). In analogy to the animal-experimental investigations with trichloroethene (25) it seems probable that this effect is caused by the chlorinated hydrocarbon itself and not by one of its metabolites.

Damaging effects of tetrachloroethene on liver and kidney have been described from time to time in animal-experimental investigations, mostly after a high acute dose or also after repeated exposure (26–28). The data in the literature for the damage of parenchymatous organs by tetrachloroethene are, however, partly contradictory and difficult to evaluate. Such an effect could possibly be associated with alkylation of proteins (4) by the metabolites of tetrachloroethene (see section 1.1).

The documentation of the MAK value (1) defines the central nervous effects of tetrachloroethene as the "critical toxicity" for the setting of the threshold limit value. Repeated experimental exposures of volunteers (5 days, daily 7 hours) to concentrations as low as the formerly valid MAK value of 100 ppm tetrachloroethene resulted in slight CNS effects (21) as mentioned in section 6. As, unlike the situation with trichloroethene (see 14) no metabolites of tetrachloroethene come into question as being responsible for the CNS-depressive effects, it can be assumed that these effects are caused by the unchanged tetrachloroethene and represent the first signs of the narcotic effect observed with higher concentrations of tetrachloroethene. This view is supported by the cumulation in particular of tetrachloroethene in "deep compartments" of the organism (see section 1.2).

3 Exposure and Effects

The basis of the critical discussion of exposure and effects should be occupational medical field studies (29). Such investigations are, however, lacking so far. For this reason merely the following general definition based on the discussions in the preceding section can be given here as an aid.

Exposure: If one assumes that the central nervous effects should be regarded as the "critical toxicity" and that these are caused by unmetabolised tetrachloroethene then the "internal exposure" is given by the concentration of the tetrachloroethene in the brain. Appropriate parameters of internal exposure may be provided by determination of the tetrachloroethene in biological media which allow conclusions to be drawn on the tissue concentration in the brain which cannot be determined directly. As the brain, as an organ well supplied with blood, equilibrates relatively quickly with the blood with respect to the concentration of tetrachloroethene and is thus regarded as part of the "central compartment" of organs well supplied with blood (22, see section 1.2), the determination of tetrachloroethene in the blood is an indicator of the "internal exposure".

Effects: The central nervous effects caused by tetrachloroethene can be regarded as "strain reaction" (1).

4 Selection of the Indicators

For the biological monitoring of persons exposed to tetrachloroethene indicators of effect have so far not been developed or suggested. The determination of tetrachloroethene in the expired air and/or blood as well as of trichloroacetic acid in the urine have been discussed (11) as indicators of exposure. Due to the pharmacokinetic properties already discussed (low metabolic rate, long half-life of trichloroacetic acid) the urinary excretion of these metabolites is generally seen as an unsuitable indicator of exposure to tetrachloroethene (13, 14).

In the previous section it was explained that on the basis of the concept of exposure and effect the determination of the content of unchanged *tetrachloroethene in the blood* is a suitable parameter of "internal exposure". On the other hand it is known that after the end of the initial "wash-out phase", which immediately follows exposure (see section 1.2), the concentration of tetrachloroethene in the expired air bears a strict and numerically defined relation, defined by the distribution coefficient, to the concentration in the blood (11, 16, 22, 23). Investigations of these relationships (11, 16) have shown that in the (mixed) expired air the tetrachloroethene concentration is about 23 times (23 ± 4) lower than in the blood; if measurements are carried out in the expired alveolar air (for methodology see (23)) the results differ to those obtained with the (mixed) expired air by a factor of 1.4 (16): the concentration of *tetrachloroethene in the alveolar* air is 16 times lower than in the blood. This applies for the time *after* exposure subsequent to the "wash-out phase", which lasts about 30 min.

For these reasons the measurement of tetrachloroethene in the alveolar air, carried out exactly according to the method, has the same meaning as determination in the blood.

Therefore, the determination of tetrachloroethene in these two biological media are chosen as alternative indicators; the BAT values must differ by a factor of 16 due to the above-mentioned relationships.

5 Methodology

The DFG Commission for the Investigation of Health Hazards of Chemical Compounds in the Work Area in the loose-leaf collection "Analysen im biologischen Material" ("Analyses of Hazardous Substances in Biological Materials") (30) have conceived a reliable method (head-space gas chromatography) for the investigation of the concentration of *tetrachloroethene in the blood.*

A corresponding standardised procedure for the determination of *tetrachloroethene in the expired air (alveolar air)* has so far not been devised; such development research is, however, under way at present. Difficulties occur with the determination in the alveolar air under the conditions found in practice mainly in sampling, transport of the samples and storage of the samples. In laboratory investigations in which these difficulties can be avoided (11, 21–23) it has been shown that the investigation of tetrachloroethene in the alveolar air is practically equivalent to the investigation in blood as long as (for pharamacokinetic reasons, see section 4) the investigation is carried out at least 30 min *after* the end of exposure. The investigation in the alveolar air has the advantage that it is a non-invasive procedure.

The BAT value for tetrachloroethene is set either as a threshold limit value in the blood or in the alveolar air; these bear a numerical relation to one another. As at present there is no practical standardised method available for the investigation of the alveolar air, the investigation of blood samples will for the time being remain most important. Decisive for the investigation and evaluation of the results with regard to the BAT value given here is, for pharmacokinetic reasons, the correct adherence to the time of sampling (see section 7).

6 Evaluation of the BAT Value

The central nervous symptoms occurring under exposure conditions should be regarded as the "critical toxicity" (see section 2) of tetrachloroethene. The central nervous effects of tetrachloroethene were also the starting point for the lowering of the MAK value in 1982 from 100 ppm to 50 ppm. Resetting of the threshold limit value for tetrachloroethene in the air at the workplace was carried out in the USA (TLV: 50 ppm) and in the Netherlands (MAC: 35 ppm).

Occupational medical field studies which could be included for the consideration of a threshold limit value with regard to a BAT value are lacking at the moment. Therefore, the available experimental laboratory investigations must be used instead.

6.1 Tetrachloroethene in the Alveolar Air

Stewart et al. (21) subjected healthy volunteers both to a single tetrachloroethene exposure for 7 hours and to exposure for 5 days (each day for 7 hours) at a concentration of 100 ppm. Both with the single and repeated exposures with a few test persons slight subjective effects occurred (e.g. slight headache, slight irritation of the conjunctiva and the mucous membranes of the upper respiratory tract). With single exposure it is also reported that individual test persons complained of a "slight drowsiness". These data were substantiated by an "abnormally modified Romberg Test" during the first 3 hours of the laboratory exposure; other tests (Crawford, Flannegan, as well as neurological tests and lung function tests) were normal. Obviously the sensitivity of different individuals to the CNS effects of tetrachloroethene is developed to a very differing extent.

In the investigations of Stewart et al. (21) at the same time very well documented determinations of tetrachloroethene in the alveolar air were carried out subsequent to exposure; they can be used for the setting of a BAT value. The data relevant for the BAT value documentation are presented in figure 3. The level of the BAT value can be oriented on the symptoms described above which can be regarded as the beginning of a central nervous effect of tetrachloroethene. If one takes into account that the laboratory exposures of Stewart et al. (21) were carried out under resting conditions at 100 ppm and also the effects of light to medium physical work, which were investigated in more detail later (16), then a laboratory exposure of 100 ppm corresponds in its order of magnitude to exposure at the workplace at the MAK of 50 ppm (see section 6.1).

Due to the kinetic processes (c. f. Fig. 3) a BAT value for tetrachloroethene can only be set for a defined sampling time. As sufficient kinetic data are at present available only for the time period after the end of exposure, a time after the end of exposure must be selected; due to the "wash-out phase" from the central lung compartment after the end of exposure an interval of at least 30 minutes must have passed before sampling (see section 1.2). For practical reasons the following alternatives have been suggested (11):

a) Sampling during the working week before the start of the shift (= approx. 16 hours after the end of the last exposure).
b) Sampling at the beginning of the working week (normally on Mondays before the start of the shift, i.e. about 64 hours after the end of exposure).

For the setting of a BAT value the former sampling time (approx. 16 hours after the end of exposure) is selected.

Assuming a uniform exposure profile, there is a measurable accumulation of tetrachloroethene during the working week (16, 21, 22). For pharmacokinetic reasons, with measurements taken at the beginning of different days of the working week, theoretically at least, in the first half of the working week different BAT values would have to be defined. For this reason it is a prerequisite that the sampling of blood or alveolar air must have been preceded by at least 3 consecutive work shifts. Normally, therefore, sampling takes place on a Thursday or Friday of a working week (*before* the beginning of exposure).

In the investigation by Stewart et al. (21) the exposure conditions were such that with some of the test persons it led to the first slight CNS effects. With these test persons 15 hours after the end of the last (fifth) seven-hour exposure an alveolar tetrachloroethene concentration between 6.0 and 9.7 ppm was measured (c.f. Fig. 3). Thus the BAT value for this sampling time (*15–16 hours after the end of exposure*) is set at

9.5 ppm (= 64 mg/m³) tetrachloroethene in the alveolar air.

For other sampling times (between 15 and 71 hours after the end of exposure) the appropriate biological threshold limit value to be used can be deduced in the following manner:

Stewart et al. (21) found with the same test persons 71 hours after the end of the multiple exposures alveolar tetrachloroethene concentrations between 3.9 and 5.1 (c.f. Fig. 3). A threshold limit value for this sampling time (*71 hours after the end of exposure*) should therefore be set at

5 ppm (= 33 mg/m³) tetrachloroethene in the alveolar air.

As explained in detail in section 1.2 for practical reasons a logarithmic interpolation between these two time intervals is permissible. The interpolation (see Fig. 4) produces a BAT value for any time interval required, which, however, must lie between 15 and 71 hours after the end of exposure. Thus, the necessity of being able to carry out biological monitoring even after a weekend pause is taken into account.

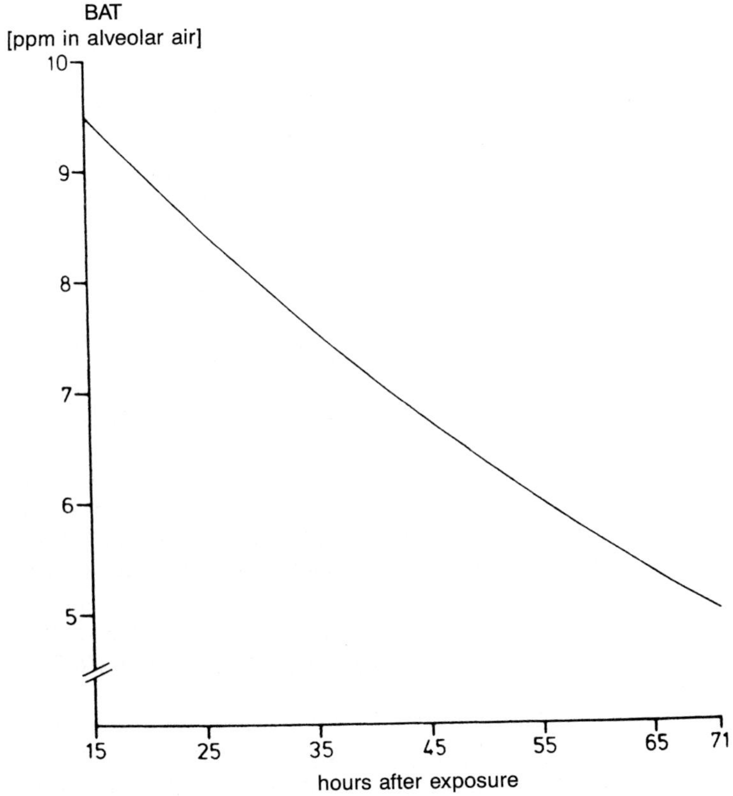

Fig. 4: Interpolation curve between 15 and 71 hours after the end of exposure for the BAT value for tetrachloroethene in the alveolar air (see also Tab. 1).

In each case the measurement must be carried out *before* the beginning of the new exposure (before the beginning of the shift).

The individual time-dependent threshold limit values to be used (see Fig. 3) can be calculated from the general formula

$$\textbf{BAT (ppm in alveolar air)} = \mathbf{11.28 \times e^{-0.01146 \times t}} \text{ or}$$

$$\textbf{BAT (mg/m}^3\textbf{ in alveolar air)} = \mathbf{75.59 \times e^{-0.01146 \times t}}$$

where 14 hours < t < 71 hours.

The values calculated have been compiled in table 1 (in ppm and in mg/m³).

Tab. 1: Biological threshold limit values for tetrachloroethene in alveolar air and in blood at different times after the end of exposure.

Time (t) after end of exposure – hours	Threshold limit values – alveolar air		Threshold limit values – blood
	ppm	mg/m³	mg/l
15 to 16	9.5	64	1.0
18	9.2	62	0.98
20	9.0	60	0.96
22	8.8	59	0.94
24	8.6	57	0.92
28	8.2	55	0.88
32	7.8	52	0.84
36	7.5	50	0.80
40	7.1	48	0.77
44	6.8	46	0.73
48	6.5	44	0.70
52	6.2	42	0.67
56	6.0	40	0.64
60	5.7	38	0.61
64	5.4	36	0.58
68	5.2	35	0.56
71	5.0	34	0.54

The values calculated have been rounded up or down to 2 decimal places for the table.
Intermediate values not listed can for practical purposes be calculated by linear interpolation.

6.2 Tetrachloroethene in the Blood

As at present there are no data present which could be included for the setting of threshold limit values for tetrachloroethene in the blood at a time immediately after the end of exposure, the BAT values in the blood are set provisionally in analogy to those in the alveolar air for the time interval discussed in section 6.1 (15–71 hours after exposure). The tetrachloroethene concentration in the blood runs completely parallel to that in the alveolar air during this time interval; the difference in concentration between the two biological media is described by the distribution factor of 16 explained in section 4. For the time t = 71 hours after exposure a threshold limit value of 0.54 mg/l is thus calculated; *for the time t = 15 hours there is a threshold limit value of 1 mg/l.* The general expression for the BAT value in the blood is:

$$\textbf{BAT (mg/l blood)} = \mathbf{1.209 \times e^{-0.01146 \times t}}$$

The individual values for different sampling times can be taken from table 1.

As there are not yet any sufficient occupational medical pharmacokinetic field studies on the question of biological threshold limit values the BAT values set here for tetrachloroethene should be regarded as provisional.

This documentation should be amended or changed upon the availability of appropriate data.

6.3 Relationship of the BAT Value to the MAK Value

As there are no occupational medical field studies available the existing pharmacokinetic laboratory investigations must be used to obtain the relationship of the BAT value to the MAK value of 50 ppm.

Compared to the single exposure, as shown in figure 2, after experimental multiple exposures (5 × 7 or 5 × 8 hours) at a time interval of 64–66 hours after the end of the last exposure, values around 5% of the given exposure concentration are measured in the alveolar air (21); this agrees with model calculations (22).

Accordingly under laboratory conditions an ambient air concentration of 50 ppm in the middle of the week would correspond to a concentration in the alveolar air after 64–66 hours of 2.5 ppm. If one takes into consideration the effect of physical work on the pharmacokinetics, physical stress of 100 W for 2 × 0.5 hours increased the tetrachloroethene uptake by 40% (compared with that found at rest (16, 18) and a (slight) cumulative effect was also observed over the working week) then it is apparent that at the workplace even with continuous adherence to the MAK value, in rare individual cases the BAT value can be reached and even exceeded. Very provisional scanty data from workplaces (11) seem to confirm these assumptions. In this context reference is made to the theoretical basis of the BAT values concept ((29); section "Relationship between BAT and MAK Values").

7 Interpretation of the Data

From the explanations above it can be clearly seen that the sampling of blood (or alveolar air) for the purpose of using the BAT concept should take place *before* the beginning of renewed exposure. If samples are taken at times other than the 15–71 hours after the end of work, particularly during the shift, higher values will be found for which the BAT value may under no circumstances be used.

Occupational medical health surveillance of persons exposed to tetrachloroethene should otherwise be carried out in the Federal Republic of Germany according to the "Berufsgenossenschaftlicher Grundsatz" G 17 (guideline issued by the Employers' Liability Insurance Association). Here time intervals for follow-up investigations are given. With borderline findings more frequent control investigations may be appropriate.

The BAT value is to be understood as an individual ceiling value (29) which should not be exceeded in individual cases.

8 Summary

For the biological monitoring of persons exposed to tetrachloroethene the concentration of unmetabolised tetrachloroethene in the expired air (alveolar air) and in the blood can be used. The BAT values were evaluated for the time interval between 15 and 71 hours *after* exposure.

For a sampling time 15 – 16 hours after the last exposure

9.5 ppm (64 mg/m^3) tetrachloroethene in the alveolar air as well as
1000 µg/l tetrachloroethene in the whole blood

have been evaluated as BAT values.

The corresponding threshold limit values for other sampling times (up to 71 hours after the end of exposure) are, due to the kinetic processes taking place, dependent on the time interval that has passed since the end of exposure. These values can be seen in table form (c. f. Tab. 1).

As sufficient occupational medical field studies are still lacking these BAT values are to be regarded as provisional.

9 References

1. Henschler, D. (ed.): Tetrachlorethen. Gesundheitsschädliche Arbeitsstoffe. Toxikologisch-arbeitsmedizinische Begründung von MAK-Werten. 1. Lieferung, VCH Verlagsgesellschaft, Weinheim 1974
2. Bolt, H. M.: ASP *16* (1981), 116
3. Costa, A. K., Ivanetich, K. M.: Biochem. Pharmacol. *29* (1980), 2863
4. Bonse, G., Urban, Th., Reichert, D., Henschler, D.: Biochem. Pharmacol. *24* (1975), 1829
5. Pegg, D. G., Zempel, J. A., Braun, W. H., Watanabe, P. G.: Toxicol. Appl. Pharmacol. *51* (1979), 465
6. Bolt, H. M., Link, B.: Verh. Dtsch. Ges. Arbeitsmed. *20* (1980), 463
7. Schumann, A. M., Quast, J. F., Watanabe, P. G.: Toxicol. Appl. Pharmacol. *55* (1980), 207
8. Ikeda, M., Ohtsuji, H.: Brit. J. Ind. Med. *29* (1972), 99
9. Ikeda, M., Imamura, T.: Int. Arch. Arbeitsmed. *31* (1973), 209
10. Ikeda, M.: Environ. Health Perspect. *21* (1977), 239
11. Monster, A. C.: Kinetics of chlorinated hydrocarbon solvents. Studies in volunteers exposed to trichloroethene, 1,1,1-trichloroethane and tetrachloroethene. Dissertation, University Amsterdam 1978

12. Ikeda, M., Ohtsuji, H., Imamura, T., Komoike, Y.: Brit. J. Industr. Med. *29* (1972), 328
13. Kündig, S., Högger, D.: Int. Arch. Arbeitsmed. *26* (1970), 306
14. Essing, H. G., Schäcke, G., Schaller, K. H., Valentin, H.: Med. Welt *24* (1973), 242
15. Filser, J. G., Bolt, H. M.: Arch. Toxicol. *42* (1979), 123
16. Monster, A. C., Boersma, G., Steenwag, H.: Int. Arch. Occup. Environ. Health *42* (1979), 303
17. Ogata, M., Takatsuka, Y., Tomokuni, K.: Br. J. Ind. Med. *28* (1971), 386
18. Monster, A. C.: Int. Arch. Occup. Environ. Health *42* (1979), 311
19. Monster, A. C., Houtkooper, J. M.: Int. Arch. Occup. Environ. Health *42* (1979), 319
20. Stewart, R. D., Gay, H. H., Erley, D. S., Hake, C. L., Schaffer, A. W.: Arch. Environ. Health *2* (1961), 40
21. Stewart, R. D., Baretta, E. D., Dodd, H. C., Torkelson, T. R.: Arch. Environ. Health *20* (1970), 224
22. Guberan, E., Fernandez, J.: Brit. J. Indust. Med. *31* (1974), 159
23. Fernandez, J., Guberan, E., Caperos, J.: Amer. Ind. Hyg. Ass. J. *37* (1976), 143
24. Johnson, H. E., Shanor, S. P.: Toxicol. Appl. Pharmacol. *12* (1968), 297
25. White, J. F., Calson, G. P.: Toxicol. Appl. Pharmacol. *47* (1979), 515
26. Kylin, B., Reichard, H., Sümegi, E., Yllner, S.: Nature *193* (1962), 395
27. Ogata, M., Tomokuni, K., Watanabe, W.: Industr. Health. *6* (1968), 116
28. Kylin, B., Sümegi, I., Yllner, S.: Acta pharmacol. *22* (1965), 379
29. Lehnert, G.: ASP *15* (1980), 266
30. Angerer, J. in: D. Henschler (ed.) Analytische Methoden zur Prüfung gesundheitsschädlicher Arbeitsstoffe. Band 2: Analysen in biologischem Material. 6. Lieferung, VCH Verlagsgesellschaft, Weinheim 1982

Author: H. M. Bolt
Approved by the Working Group: 5. 2. 1982

Tetrachloroethene, Addendum

EKA

The correlations between external and internal exposure yield the following data:

Air Tetrachloroethene (ml/m^3)	Air Tetrachloroethene (mg/m^3)	Whole blood Tetrachloroethene (mg/l)
10	69	0.2
20	138	0.4
30	206	0.6
50	344	1.0

Sampling time: about 16 hours after end of shift

Date of evaluation 2001

The toxicity of tetrachloroethene was reviewed in Volume 1 of the present series (Henschler and Lehnert 1994). After reclassification of tetrachloroethene in Carcinogen category 3B and withdrawal of the MAK value, the previous BAT value for tetrachloroethene of 1 mg/l blood (sampling 16 hours after the end of the shift) was reviewed. The substance has been reclassified as experiments yielded evidence that tetrachloroethene may cause cancer of the kidneys (Greim 1998).

1 Withdrawal of the BAT Value for Alveolar Air

The BAT values for tetrachloroethene evaluated in 1982 were given for both whole blood and alveolar air. In both cases sampling was recommended 16 hours after the end of exposure.

The quantitative determination of the tetrachloroethene concentration in whole blood sampled before exposure after several working days has proved reliable in practice, and the evaluated BAT value has been accepted both at a scientific level and by occupational physicians. Taking into consideration an external occupational exposure to tetrachloroethene of 50 ppm and the sampling conditions given above, the evaluated BAT value is in agreement with the American BEI.

A somewhat higher value of 1.6 mg/l blood was evaluated under the same conditions in a Korean study (Jang *et al.* 1993). The reason for this difference was thought to be e.g. ethnic differences (Jang *et al.* 1997).

Essential BAT Value Documentations. DFG, Deutsche Forschungsgemeinschaft

ISBN 3-527-31477-6

The results of tetrachloroethene determinations in blood sampled before the shift for monitoring occupationally exposed persons, can therefore be reliably evaluated with the existing BAT value.

The determination of tetrachloroethene in alveolar air, however, has not become established in practical occupational medicine. This state of affairs is not substance-specific, but applies for determinations in alveolar air in general. This is mainly due to the fact that there are no practical and reliable sampling systems commercially available. Also the great influence on the values determined of the sampling time, the co-operation of the test person and analytical difficulties explain the rejection of this material for occupational-medical investigations. In view of this, the BAT value for the tetrachloroethene concentration in alveolar air has been withdrawn from the *List of MAK and BAT Values*.

2 Evaluation of the Biological Exposure Equivalents

As described in the chapter on tetrachloroethene in Volume 1 of this series (Henschler and Lehnert 1994), after absorption the substance is exhaled mainly unchanged in man. The metabolized amount is transformed mainly oxidatively into trichloroacetic acid, which is excreted in the urine. A quantitatively less important metabolic pathway, which, however, is associated with the occurrence of kidney tumours, takes place via the conjugation of tetrachloroethene with glutathione and transformation into the nephrotoxic metabolites via the "beta-lyase" of the kidneys (Völkel *et al.* 1998). Studies of the toxicokinetics and metabolism of tetrachloroethene led to the creation of new toxicokinetic models ("Physiologically Based Pharmacokinetics" (PBPK) and population models; Bois *et al.* 1996, Reitz *et al.* 1996).

The relationships between external exposure to tetrachloroethene and the levels of tetrachloroethene in blood are very well documented and supported by different independent studies (see the chapter on tetrachloroethene in Volume 1 of this series (Henschler and Lehnert 1994)). The preference of the tetrachloroethene level in blood for the biological monitoring of tetrachloroethene was particularly emphasised (Skender *et al.* 1991).

On the basis of the data for the previous BAT value, the following correlations between external exposure to tetrachloroethene and the levels of tetrachloroethene in blood can be established:

Air Tetrachloroethene		Blood Tetrachloroethene
(ml/m³)	(mg/m³)	(mg/l)
10	69	0.2
20	138	0.4
30	206	0.6
50	344	1.0

Sampling: about 16 hours after the end of the shift.

Otherwise, the information in the earlier chapter applies.

3 References

Bois FY, Gelman A, Jiang J, Maszle DR, Zeise L, Alexeef G (1996) Population toxicokinetics of tetrachloroethylene. Arch Toxicol 70: 347–355

Greim H (Ed.) (1998) Tetrachloroethylene. in: Occupational toxicants, Vol. 3, VCH, Weinheim

Henschler D, Lehnert G (Eds) (1994) Tetrachloroethene. in: Biological exposure values for occupational toxicants and carcinogens – Critical data evaluation for BAT and EKA values, Vol. 1, VCH, Weinheim, pp. 139–151

Jang J-Y, Kuang S-K, Chung HK (1993) Biological exposure indices of organic solvents of Korean workers. Int Arch Occup Environ Health 65, 219–222

Jang J-Y, Droz PO, Berode M (1997) Ethnic differences in biological monitoring of several organic solvents. I. Human exposure experiment. Int Arch Occup Environ Health 69, 343–349

Reitz RH, Gargas ML, Mendrala AL, Schumann AM (1996) *In vivo* and *in vitro* studies of perchloroethylene metabolism for physiologically based pharmacokinetic modeling in rats, mice and humans. Toxicol Appl Pharmacol 136: 289–306

Skender LJ, Karacic V, Prpic-Majic D (1991) A comparative study of human levels of trichloroethylene and tetrachloroethylene after occupational exposure. Arch Environ Health 46: 174–178

Völkel W, Friedewald M, Lederer E, Pahler J, Parker J, Dekant W (1998) Biotransformation of perchloroethene: dose-dependent excretion of trichloroacetic acid, dichloroacetic acid and N-acetyl-S-(trichlorovinyl)-L-cysteine in rats and humans after inhalation. Toxicol Appl Pharmacol 153: 20–27

Authors: K.H. Schaller, H.M. Bolt

Approved by the Working Group: 08.07.1997 and 20.02.2001

Vinyl chloride

EKA The correlation between external and internal exposure yields the following data:

Air Vinyl chloride (ml/m³)	(mg/m³)	Urine Thiodiglycolic acid (mg/24 h)
1	2.6	1.8
2	5.2	2.4
4	10	4.5
8	21	8.2
16	41	10.6

Sampling: 24 hours after the beginning of the shift

Date of evaluation 1986

Synonyms Chloroethylene
VCM

Formula C_2H_3Cl

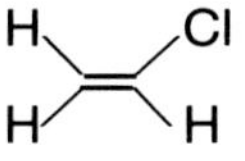

Molecular weight 62.50

Melting point –159.7 °C

Boiling point –13.9 °C

MAK [last established: 1977] Carcinogenic substance: category IIIA1 of the List of MAK and BAT Values

Essential BAT Value Documentations. DFG, Deutsche Forschungsgemeinschaft

ISBN 3-527-31477-6

1 Metabolism and Kinetics

1.1 Metabolism

Vinyl chloride (VCM) is, after uptake into the mammalian organism, either exhaled unchanged or converted after oxidative biotransformation into metabolites which are excreted renally. In figure 1 the metabolism is shown according to the currently available data (12, 23, 28).

In animal experiments carboxymethylcysteine, thiodiglycolic acid (thiodiacetic acid) and hydroxyethylmercapturic acid can be detected as degradation products. The metabolic pathway which leads to thiodiglycolic acid can be regarded as certain, while for the formation of hydroxyethylmercapturic acid various pathways are possible. Which of these pathways are followed can at present not be decided. Investigations on employees exposed to VCM show that thiodiglycolic acid is quantitatively the most important metabolite (22). Carboxymethylcysteine is an intermediate which is degraded

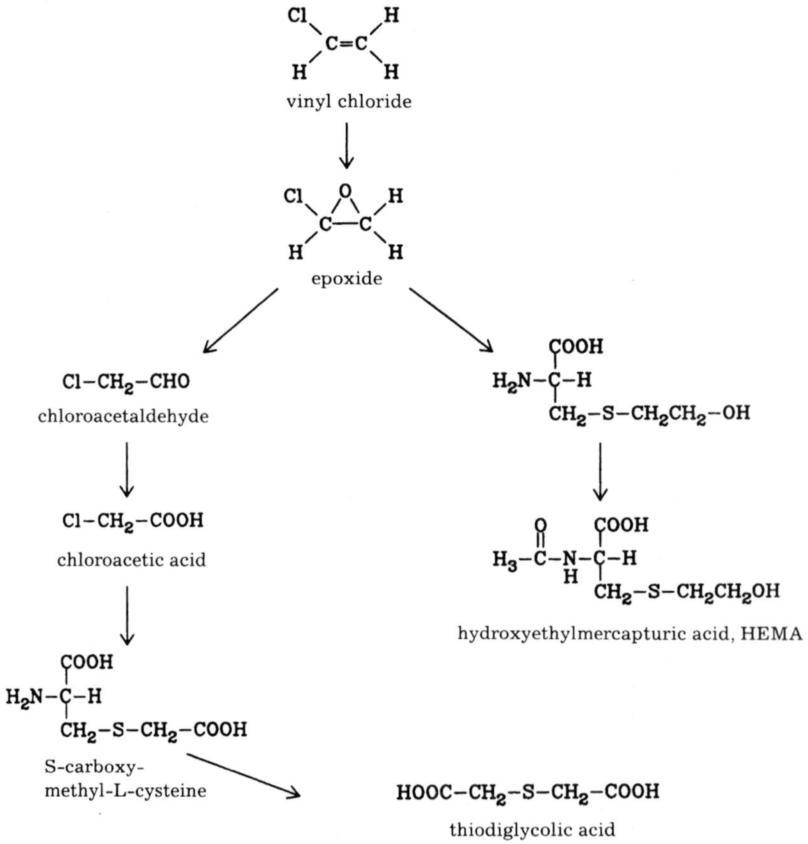

Fig. 1: Simplified diagram of the metabolism of vinyl chloride

to thiodiglycolic acid while the hydroxyethylmercapturic acid is only formed and excreted in small amounts, possibly because the enzyme activity of the microsomal glutathionyl transferases in the human liver is one tenth of that in rat liver (5).

1.2 Kinetics

Vinyl chloride is absorbed from the air relatively rapidly. With constant level exposure an equilibrium develops after approximately 30 minutes between the VCM concentration in the air and the VCM concentration in the body. Under these conditions approximately 25 % of the VCM amount inhaled is degraded by the organism through metabolism (6). The equilibrium constant for the steady state between the concentrations of VCM in the air and the body in persons of normal weight is 0.8 and increases in overweight persons as a consequence of the increased amount of adipose tissue to 1.2 (14). According to this the VCM concentration in the body can be calculated as follows:

body VCM concentration =

$$\left(\frac{0.8 \times \%\ \text{non-adipose tissue} + 0.8 \times \%\ \text{adipose tissue}}{100}\right) \cdot \text{air VCM concentration.}$$

The amount of VCM taken up and metabolised fluctuates and is dependent upon the changes in exposure profile with time. Thus, continuous low-level exposure leads to a higher internal exposure of the organism than comparable short-term peak exposures. This has been shown in model calculations (4, 9) and also in investigations of employees exposed to VCM (14).

2 Critical Toxicity

The symptoms of disease attributed to exposure to vinyl chloride in man are grouped together and called "vinyl chloride disease" (18). Originally acro-osteolysis, Raynaud phenomena, scleroderma-like changes of the skin, restrictive lung function disorders and liver function disorders were included in this syndrome. Further symptoms are thrombocytopenia, endocrine changes (hyperthyroidism, sexual disorders), immunological changes (hyper-immunoglobulinaemia with increased IgE, cryoglobulinaemia) (11). Also neurological symptoms were reported in workers exposed to vinyl chloride (17). The intensity of scleroderma-like changes induced by VCM seems to be associated with an accumulation of HLA-antigens (2). The changes mentioned are understood as direct tissue toxicity of vinyl chloride or its metabolites and as secondary changes due to vascular and/or immunological processes (11, 17). The actual critical effects of vinyl chloride are its human carcinogenic effects. The target organs of the carcinogenic effects include the liver, brain, lungs, hematopoietic and lymphatic systems (16). An increased incidence of tumours for liver angiosarcoma could be verified in many epidemiological investigations (3, 10, 13, 26, 27). For the development of liver angiosarcomas a latency period of between 5 and 40 years is given. Moreover, an increased incidence of brain tumours in workers exposed to vinyl chloride (20, 26, 29) and an increased incidence of lung tumours (7, 13, 15, 20, 26, 29) has been reported. Recently and for the first time a slightly increased incidence of malignant melanomas and thyroid gland carcinomas (15) has been detected. These findings must be clarified. In rats the formation of liver angiosarcomas, hepatomas, carcinoma of the Zymbal gland, nephroblastomas, neuroblastomas, mammary gland adenocarcinomas, forestomach papillomas and acanthomas and extrahepatic angiosarcomas could be shown (19). Tumour development after exposure to concentrations below 5 ppm or 0.03 mg/kg vinyl chloride was not detected.

Results for DNA alkylation by reactive VCM metabolites in several tissues (1) are in accordance with the report of a multipotent carcinogenic effect of vinyl chloride. It has become known that the introduction of etheno groups into DNA bases causes miscoding (30). Causal relationships between DNA binding of VCM metabolites and carcinogenesis, however, have yet to be clarified.

3 Exposure and Effects

Data from a study on the relationship between the exposure to the toxic substance (determined by personal air sampling) and the thiodiglycolic acid excretion (14) are available. The analysis of the data shows that it is not possible as a matter of course to deduce relationships between the VCM concentrations in the air and the concentration of the thiodiglycolic acid in the urine as individual variables, for example, the body weight, have considerable influence on the excretion of the metabolites. If, however, with the help of a kinetic model, one calculates the VCM concentrations in the

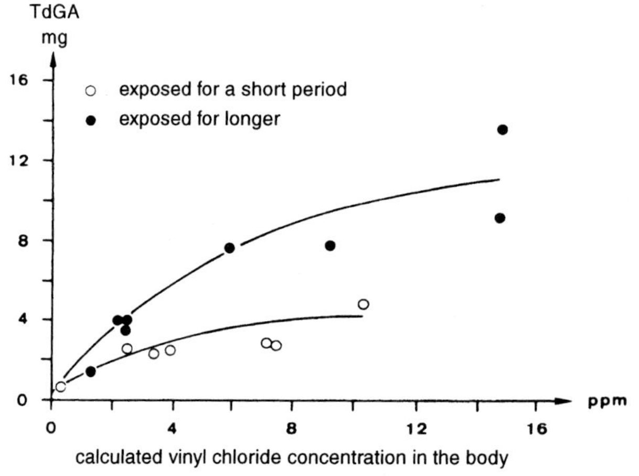

Fig. 2: Increase in the amount of thiodiglycolic acid (TdGA) in the urine of persons exposed to vinyl chloride (VCM), collected in the 24-hour period after the beginning of the shift, plotted against the effective concentration of VCM in the body calculated on the basis of the VCM concentrations in air determined by personal air monitoring (12-hour average value)

body which build up after uptake of the substance (14) and determines the relationship between the values obtained and the data for the thiodiglycolic acid excretion in the urine then plausible functions result for persons exposed for long periods and persons exposed for short periods at the same level of exposure (Fig. 2).

4 Selection of the Indicators

The only parameter available at present for the evaluation of the risk for persons exposed to VCM is thiodiglycolic acid in urine. For other urinary metabolites such as for example hydroxyethylmercapturic acid (22) and carboxymethylcysteine (21), dependence on the VCM uptake which would prove their validity as monitoring parameters, has not been demonstrated.

5 Methodology

5.1 Thiodiglycolic Acid in Urine

The determination of the thiodiglycolic acid in urine takes place by gas chromatography/mass spectrometry of the methyl ester (mass 146) after derivatisation with diazomethane and with the standard addition method (21). The method of determination of the thiodiglycolic acid as trimethylsilylester described by Draminski and Trojanowska (8) does not fulfil the validity criteria required for persons exposed to VCM due to its detection limit of 10 mg thiodiglycolic acid/l of urine.

5.2 Normal Values of Thiodiglycolic Acid

Normal values of thiodiglycolic acid can at present only be determined using the GC/MS-technique. For men these amount to 0.67 ± 0.32 mg/l and for women 0.51 ± 0.20 mg/l (24). It can be deduced from these investigations that a differentiation between exposed persons and non-exposed persons is possible when the 99 % tolerance level of 1.82 mg /l for men and 1.43 mg/l for women is exceeded.

Substances which also lead to the excretion of thiodiglycolic acid are listed in Tab. 1. These are workplace substances or drugs from which in the course of biotransformation chloroacetaldehyde can be produced or which have structures so similar to that of VCM that they yield the same end product (e.g. acrylonitrile) (25).

Tab. 1: Workplace substances and drugs which, like vinyl chloride, are transformed to the urinary metabolite, thiodiglycolic acid

Workplace substances	Drugs
Acrylonitrile	BCNU (Carmustine)
2,2´-Bis(chloroethyl)ether	CCNU (Lomustine)
Bromoethanol	Cyclophosphamide
Chloroethanol	Dibenamine
1,2-Dibromoethane	Dibenzyline
1,2-Dichloroethane	Distraneurin®
1,1,2-Trichloroethane	Iphosphamide
Vinyl bromide	Mannomustine

6 Evaluation of the Biological Exposure Equivalents for Carcinogenic Substances (EKA)

For a medium body weight of 75 kg relationships can be deduced from the data published between the VCM concentration in air and the thiodiglycolic acid excretion over 24 hours after the beginning of the shift. This correlation between the external exposure and the excretion of the metabolite is given in the following table.

Air Vinyl chloride (ml/m^3)	Urine Thiodiglycolic acid (mg/24 h)
1	1.8
2	2.4
4	4.5
8	8.2
16	10.6

7 Interpretation of the Data

The metabolism of vinyl chloride is subject to considerable individual fluctuations. Influencing factors include the degree of physical work and the body weight (see section 1.2). The thiodiglycolic acid excretion is influenced by drugs and other substances which are also transformed into this metabolite (see Tab. 1). To date little is known about the significance of individual differences in the activity of the microsomal oxidation systems.

The monitoring of persons exposed to VCM on the basis of the determination of thiodiglycolic acid in the urine requires the collection of all urine samples in the period of 24 hours from the beginning of the workshift. Single samples taken at the end of the shift cannot be recommended for investigation as the excretion of the metabolites in such samples is subject to excessive fluctuation relative to the VCM concentrations in air. Also the determination of concentrations in the urine cannot be recommended at present as only for the amount of metabolite excreted in 24 hours is the relationship to the VCM concentration in air known with sufficient certainty.

8 References

1. Bergman, K.: Arch. Toxicol. *49* (1982), 117–129
2. Black, C. M., Walker, A. E., Catoggio, T. J., Welsh, K. I., Bernstein, R. M., McGregor, A. R., Lloyd Jones, J. K.: Lancet *I* (1983), 53–55
3. Block, J. B.: JAMA *229* (1974), 53–54
4. Bolt, H. M., Filser, J. G., Buchter, A.: Arch. Toxicol. *48* (1981), 213–228
5. Bolt, H. M., Filser, J. G., Oesch, F., Guenthner, T. M., Friedberg, T., Bolt, M. In: Verhandlungen der Deutschen Gesellschaft für Arbeitsmedizin, 18. Jahrestagung. Gentner, Stuttgart 1981, pp. 507–509
6. Buchter, A., Bolt, H. M., Filser, J., Goergens, H. W., Laib, R. J., Bolt, W. In: Verhandlungen der Deutschen Gesellschaft für Arbeitsmedizin, 18. Jahrestagung. Gentner, Stuttgart 1978, pp. 111–124
7. Buffler, P. A., Wood, S., Eifler, C., Suarez, L., Kilian, D. J.: J. Occup. Med. *21* (1979), 195–202
8. Draminski, W., Trojanowska, B.: Arch. Toxicol. *48* (1981), 289–291
9. Filser, J. G., Bolt, H. M.: In: Verhandlungen der Deutschen Gesellschaft für Arbeitsmedizin. 22. Jahrestagung. Gentner, Stuttgart 1982, pp. 631–635
10. Fox, A. J., Collier, P. E.: Br. J. Ind. Med. *34* (1977), 1–10
11. Granger, R. G., Walker, A. E., Ward, A. M. In: Preger, L. (ed.): Drug, Irradiation, Occupation. Grune & Stratton 1979, pp. 191–124
12. Green, T., Hathway, D. E.: Chem. Biol. Interactions *II* (1975), 545–562
13. Greiser, E., Reinl, W., Weber, H.: Zentralbl. Arbeitsmed. *32* (1982), 44–62
14. Heger, M., Müller, G., Norpoth, K.: Int. Arch. Occup. Environ. Health *50* (1982), 187–196
15. Heldaas, S. S., Langard, S. L., Anderen, A.: Br. J. Ind. Med. *41* (1984), 25–30
16. International Agency for Research on Cancer (IARC): The evaluation of the carcinogenic risk of chemicals to humans. Chemicals, industrial processes and industries associated with cancer in humans, IARC Monographs Suppl. 4. IARC, Lyon 1982
17. Langauer-Lewowicka, H., Kurzbauer, H., Byczkowska, Z., Wocka-Marek, T.: Int. Arch. Occup. Environ. Health *52* (1983), 151–157
18. Lange, C. E., Jühe, S., Stein, G., Veltman, G.: Int. Arch. Occup. Health *32* (1974), 1–32
19. Maltoni, C., Lefemine, G., Ciliberti, A., Cotti, G., Carretti, D.: Environ. Health Persp. *41* (1981), 3–29
20. Monson, R. R., Peters, J. M., Johnson, M. N.: Lancet *II* (1974), 397–398
21. Müller, G., Brzezinka, H.: Thiodiessigsäure (Bis-(carboxymethyl)sulfid). In: Henschler, D. (ed.): Analytische Methoden zur Prüfung gesundheitsschädlicher Arbeitsstoffe. Bd. 2: Analysen in biologischem Material. VCH Verlagsgesellschaft, Weinheim 1982
22. Müller, G., Heger, M., Norpoth, K. In: Verhandlungen der Deutschen Gesellschaft für Arbeitsmedizin. 20. Jahrestagung. Gentner, Stuttgart 1980, pp. 533–536
23. Müller, G., Norpoth, K. In: Verhandlungen der Deutschen Gesellschaft für Arbeitsmedizin. 17. Jahrestagung. Gentner, Stuttgart 1977, pp. 237–241
24. Müller, G., Norpoth, K., Wickramasinghe, R. H.: Int. Arch. Occup. Environ. Health *44* (1979), 185–191
25. Müller, G., Verkoyen, C., Soton, N., Norpoth, K.: Arch. Toxicol. *60* (1987), 464–466
26. Tabershaw, I. R., Gaffey, W. R.: J. Occup. Med. *16* (1974), 509–518
27. Thériault, G., Allard, P.: J. Occup. Med. *23* (1981), 671–676
28. Watanabe, P. G., McGrowan, G. R.: Toxicol. Appl. Pharmacol. *36* (1976), 339–352
29. Waxweiler, R. J., Stringer, W., Wagoner, J. K., Jones, J., Falk, H., Carter, C.: Ann. N. Y. Acad. Sci. *271* (1976), 40–48
30. Zajdela, F., Croisy, A., Barbin, A., Malaville, C., Tomatis, L., Bartsch, H.: Cancer Res. *40* (1980), 352–356

Authors: G. Müller, K. Norpoth

Approved by the Working Group: 21st February 1986

Xylenes

BAT	2 g toluric acid/l urine 1.5 mg xylene/l blood Sampling time: end of exposure	
Date of evaluation	1984	
Synonyms	Dimethylbenzene	
Formula	$C_6H_4(CH_3)_2$	

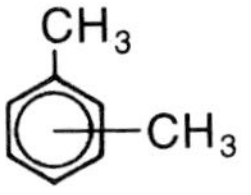

Molecular weight	106.2	
Melting point	–25 °C (*o*-xylene) –48 °C (*m*-xylene) 13 °C (*p*-xylene)	no data (tech. xylene)
Boiling point	144 °C (*o*-xylene) 139 °C (*m*-xylene) 138 °C (*p*-xylene)	137 °C–140 °C (tech. xylene)
Vapour pressure at 20 °C	6.7 mbar (*o*-xylene) 8 mbar (*m*-xylene) 8.2 mbar (*p*-xylene)	7–9 mbar (tech. xylene)
MAK [last established: 1983]	100 ml/m^3 (ppm) 440 mg/m^3	

1 Metabolism and Kinetics

Due to their high vapour pressure even at room temperature *o*-xylene, *m*-xylene and *p*-xylene are taken up at the workplace predominantly by inhalation. The amount of the toxic substance retained in the body is quoted in the literature as between 60 % and 70 % (1–5). The isomers do not seem to differ in this respect.

Liquid xylene can be absorbed via the intact skin approximately to the same extent as via inhalation during external exposure to 100 ml/m^3 (MAK). Thus, in the literature absorption rates for *m*-xylene of 2 µg and 2.5 µg (cm^2 · min)$^{-1}$ are reported (6,

Essential BAT Value Documentations. DFG, Deutsche Forschungsgemeinschaft

ISBN 3-527-31477-6

43). Considerable interindividual fluctuations have been observed (43). On the other hand xylene vapour is absorbed only to a minor extent via the skin (7).

Under workplace conditions the xylene concentration in the blood reaches equilibrium at the latest four hours after the beginning of exposure, which is a feature common to benzene, toluene and xylene aromatics (BTX aromatics) (8). After the end of exposure the concentration of the toxic substance in the blood decreases quickly (3, 9). The half-time for the first elimination phase is given as 30 min. Afterwards the xylene concentration decreases more slowly so that aromatics can be detected in the blood even 16 hours after the end of exposure.

The course of the changes in concentration of the xylenes in the alveolar air with time is more or less parallel to that in blood. After the end of exposure xylene is eliminated in the alveolar air in three elimination phases for which the half-times are given as 0–3 hours, 4–6 hours and >17 hours (9). Following exposure, altogether between 3.5 % and 5.8 % of the retained xylene is eliminated via the lungs (1, 3, 9).

By far the greatest part of the retained xylenes (almost 95 %) is transformed by oxidation of a methyl group into methylated benzoic acids and excreted after conjugation with glycine as methylhippuric acids (toluric acids) in the urine.

Šedivec (1) was able to disprove former assumptions and show that not only the aliphatic side chains of xylenes are oxidised but also the aromatic ring. Approx. 2 % of retained xylenes are excreted in the urine as glucuronides of the corresponding dimethylphenols (xylenols).

The amounts and the concentrations of the toluric acids excreted in the urine increase during exposure and reach their highest values at the end of an 8-hour working period (8). Under workplace conditions the proportion of the total amount of toluric acids excreted which was eliminated during the last two hours of the work shift was between 16 % and 47 % (10). Under experimental conditions in the laboratory this amount varies within narrower limits.

Šedivec and Flek (2) report the amount of toluric acid excreted at the end of the exposure period (8 hours) to be 23 % to 32 %.

2 Critical Toxicity

The literature on the toxicity of the xylenes has recently been summarised and critically reviewed (11–14). The following statements are therefore limited to those effects on health which were observed under exposure conditions within the range of the MAK values. Conditions under which the acute narcotic effects of xylenes occur are not discussed here; instead the reader is referred to the appropriate text books and handbooks of occupational medicine and industrial toxicology (15–18). The present discussion is limited, as far as possible, to observations in humans. Where animal experiments are taken into consideration this is expressly stated. There is no differentiation of the isomeric xylenes as experience of differing toxicity of the individual xylenes in humans is not available and because the results from animal experiments are contradictory on this point.

2.1 Eyes, Skin and Mucous Membranes

Xylene vapours, which can be clearly identified from the smell at concentrations of at least 40 ml/m^3 in the ambient air, begin to irritate the eyes, nose and throat depending upon individual sensitivity between 100 and 200 ml/m^3 (19, 20).

As a consequence of its defatting effect on the intact skin, contact with liquid xylene can lead to dermatitis.

2.2 Central Nervous System

Under conditions of chronic occupational exposure to xylene vegetative-nervous disturbances have been observed more frequently (21–23). According to these reports some of the exposed persons are said to have suffered from vegetative dystonia, headaches, insomnia, irritability, palpitations and digestive disturbances at ambient air concentrations as low as 12 ml/m^3. These studies, accused of having many shortcomings, (13) also suffer from the disadvantage that the complaints described above are neither specific to the substance nor objectifiable with medical scientific methods of investigation.

Recently Finnish authors have attempted to make the characteristic but unspecific health effects of organic solvents on the central nervous system accessible to scientific methods of measurement. Under the defined conditions of exposure possible in laboratory experiments, they subjected up to 22 male test persons to xylene concentrations between 90 and 460 ml/m^3. The test persons were exposed for up to eight days during six hours per day to xylene vapours. The parameters measured included the function of the vestibular organ and other neurophysiological parameters such as reaction time, flicker fusion threshold and manual dexterity. As little as four hours exposure to xylene at a level of 145 ml/m^3 was sufficient to produce impairment of vestibulary function. After a daily six-hour exposure to a xylene concentration of 100 ml/m^3 a decrease in the reaction time was found. After continuous exposure to xylene for only 70 minutes at the same level (100 ml/m^3) Gamberale (24) observed nausea and headaches in some test persons.

2.3 Haematopoietic System

The idea that xylenes, like benzene, cause changes in the blood count has been repeatedly discussed in the literature and is also to be found in text books on the subject (15, 16, 25). This observation was attributed to the presence of benzene which, as little as 25 years ago, was always found as a contaminant of xylene. This description of the differing metabolic behaviour of benzene and its alkyl derivatives was thought to explain the differing effects of these aromatics on the health of human beings. However, more recent reports also indicate that xylene has effects on the blood count (21–23, 26–28). These reports are, however, insufficiently documented (13).

In particular, the more recent finding that also xylenes are oxidised on the aromatic ring, although to a smaller extent than benzene itself, indicate that this question should be given more consideration in future.

Reports of functional disturbances in the liver and kidneys under conditions tolerated at the workplace today are not available. Nor have carcinogenic or teratogenic effects been reported. Animal experiments indicating possible teratogenicity (29–32) suggest that appropriate epidemiological investigations should be carried out on humans (33).

3 Exposure and Effects

As already explained in the section on critical toxicity, above all eyes and mucous membranes, the central nervous system, and possibly the haematopoietic system are the target organs of exposure to xylene.

Under laboratory conditions adverse effects on psychophysiological parameters and on the vestibular organ were found at xylene ambient air concentrations at the level of the currently valid MAK value (100 ml/m^3). For the evaluation of (chronic) occupational exposure, these acute functional disturbances are, however, of limited significance. Even during short-term exposure to substances in laboratory experiments habituation effects were identified. More serious is the suspicion that changes in the blood count occur under workplace conditions at xylene concentrations considerably below the MAK value (21–23).

The expected relationship between the xylene concentrations in the ambient air and the toluric acid excretion in the urine has been observed under laboratory experimental conditions and in field studies. In table 1A the results described in the literature have been listed. Extrapolation to an ambient air concentration of 100 ml/m^3 yields toluric acid concentrations in the urine expected at this concentration of between 0.9 and 3.3 g/l. It should be borne in mind that this is the average value for groups of persons exposed under the same conditions. This averaging conceals the extreme values of the toluric acid concentrations which have been seen in individual samples. Šedivec et al. (2) quote for the individual toluric acid concentration in the urine samples voided at the end of exposure a confidence interval between 1054 and 4018 mg/l. Under workplace conditions this range can be assumed to be even greater (34).

The reasons for this wide range include the differing respiratory minute volumes that occur under workplace conditions (34, 35) and at rest (39). For the same reasons under identical conditions of exposure between 20 % and 25 % less xylene is taken up and toluric acid excreted by women than by men (4). Naturally the fluctuation of the toluric acid concentration in the urine samples collected at the end of exposure is greater than that in the 24-hour urine which, however, cannot be collected under workplace conditions. Different amounts of fluid drunk and excreted also influence the toluric acid concentration in the urine.

It seems to be important that at a toluric acid concentration in the urine of as little as 3.1 g/l in a laboratory experiment a tendency towards a decrease in the systolic blood pressure was found (36).

In table 1B xylene levels in the blood which were measured in different groups of persons after differing exposure have been listed. It is surprising that after the same or supposedly the same external conditions of exposure to the toxic substance, the xylene concentration in the blood fluctuates very widely. If the blood concentrations presented in table 1B are recalculated for an ambient air concentration of 100 ml/m^3 then blood xylene concentrations between 0.09 and 5.8 mg/l result! Elimination of values over 5 mg/l, which are possibly caused by the greatly fluctuating exposure concentrations in these experiments, the great physical stress and the short exposure times, results in values mostly between 0.9 and 2.5 mg/l.

This still great range of deviation is caused by various factors. The research group of Savolainen and Riihimäki were able to show that at the same average ambient air concentration the blood xylene levels are higher the more the exposure concentration fluctuates (37, 38). To a great extent the xylene concentration in the blood is dependent on physical activity. In persons carrying out physical work Savolainen et al. (38) found that the blood xylene concentrations were more than twice those in persons at rest.

As the majority of the investigations described in the literature to date were carried out under laboratory experimental conditions, an investigation by members of the Commission on 35 painters in two factories and altogether six different workplaces is of particular importance (41). This is particularly true as the investigations made use of personal air sampling. According to these results, obtained under workplace conditions with an average concentration of the toxic substance in the ambient air at the level of the MAK value, blood xylene concentrations between 0.9 and 1.9 mg/l are to be expected.

Of great importance are the results of Savolainen who observed disturbances in the vestibular function at blood xylene concentrations of as little as 1.0 mg/l (37, 38).

4 Selection of the Indicators

For the biological monitoring of persons exposed to xylene the following parameters are available:

- determination of the xylene concentration in the alveolar air
- determination of the xylene concentration in the blood
- determination of the toluric acid excretion in the urine
- determination of the dimethylphenol excretion in the urine

Fundamentally the concentration of organic solvent in the alveolar air represents a diagnostic and sensitive parameter for objectifying the exposure to the toxic substance. Although recently there has been progress in the development of methods, this procedure cannot yet be applied as there is insufficient data for the establishment of a BAT value.

The xylene concentration in the blood represents an analytically and diagnostically satisfactory parameter for evaluating the individual xylene exposure (c.f. also BAT value toluene) and therefore seems suitable for biological monitoring especially since the toxic effect of this substance on the CNS is caused by the unchanged molecule. The necessity for blood sampling and the rapid decrease in the blood concentration of xylene after the end of exposure are the disadvantages of this method. If possible, the sampling of blood must therefore take place directly at the workplace.

The concentration of toluric acid in the urine represents, despite the great range of scatter of the results due to the differing dilution of the urine, a very suitable parameter for biological monitoring. The patient is hardly inconvenienced by the sampling of urine. Furthermore, since toluric acid is not excreted in the urine physiologically its occurrence is a diagnostically specific parameter of xylene exposure.

The determination of dimethylphenols in the urine also seems to be desirable. The suspicion that xylene can cause a disturbance in the function of the haematopoietic system has so far not been dispelled. The metabolic precursors of the xylenols are possibly closer to the active principle responsible for this disturbance than xylene itself or its main products of metabolism, the toluric acids. Due to the lack of data, at present the establishment of a biological threshold value for the dimethylphenol excretion in the urine does not seem to be possible.

5 Methodology

For the determination of toluric acids in urine above all gas chromatographic and high pressure liquid chromatographic methods are suitable. The working group "Analytische Chemie" ("Analytical Chemistry") of the DFG Commission for the Investigation of Health Hazards of Chemical Compounds in the Work Area has published in its collection "Analysen in biologischem Material" ("Analyses of Hazardous Substances in Biological Materials") a gas chromatographic method which fulfils the requirements of analytical reliability. After methylation of the free acids, the three isomeric toluric acids can be separated from one another and from hippuric acid by gas chromatography (42).

A high pressure liquid chromatographic method has also been published by the working group in its loose-leaf collection. It has the advantage that a derivatisation of the free acids can be dispensed with.

The gas chromatographic head-space technique is the preferred method for the determination of xylenes in blood. Such a procedure has been published in the loose-leaf collection "Analysen in biologischem Material" ("Analyses of Hazardous Substances in Biological Materials"). The working group "Analysen in biologischem Material" has also prepared a capillary gas chromatographic head-space method which allows the determination of most of the common organic solvents in blood in one analytical procedure. Using this procedure the isomeric xylenes can also be separated and determined.

6 Evaluation of the BAT Value

The results described in the literature (Tab. 1A) allow a relationship between the xylene concentration in the ambient air and the toluric acid concentration in the urine to be established. According to this, a metabolite excretion of

2 g toluric acids/l urine (2 g methylhippuric acids/l)

corresponds to an 8-hour xylene exposure at the level of the currently valid MAK value (100 ml/m^3).

This value is set as the BAT value.

At present there are no observations indicating the occurrence of disturbances in physical functions of toluric acid excretion at this level.

A relationship can also be calculated between the external exposure and the xylene concentration in the blood (Tab. 1B). According to this a concentration of

1.5 mg xylene/l blood

corresponds to a xylene exposure at the level of the MAK value. This value is also set as a BAT value.

Under laboratory experimental conditions Savolainen (37, 38) was able to demonstrate disturbances in the sense of balance at blood xylene concentrations of 1 mg/l. These cannot, however, be used for the setting of an occupational medical threshold limit value as even during the short term exposures to which the test persons were subjected habituation was seen.

Broadly based epidemiological investigations on the xylene exposure at the workplace are lacking. This is lamentable because these substances are of extraordinary importance for occupational and environmental medicine. The BAT value presented here must therefore be based above all on the effects of the xylenes which can be observed in laboratory experiments.

If under workplace conditions with concentrations below 100 ml/m^3 the changes in the blood count described from time to time and disturbances in the vegetative nervous system should be confirmed in future, a reduction of the BAT values might be necessary.

7 Interpretation of the Data

The urine samples for the determination of the toluric acid concentration should be collected at the end of exposure. Of course the metabolite concentration in the spontaneous urine samples is more likely to be subject to distorting influences (e.g. different amounts of fluid drunk and excreted etc.) than the 24-hour or 8-hour urinary excretion. Urine collection over these periods of time, however, cannot be carried out under workplace conditions. For practical reasons the collection of urine over a defined time is avoided due to the low probability that the collection is carried out reliably. This is also the reason against expressing the excreted amount in terms of time instead of volume. Furthermore, correction for specific weight and the creatinine content of the urine does not seem to be useful (40). However, the density of the urine should be used as an exclusion criterion in that samples with a density below 1.010 are not included in the evaluation. All these reasons lead to a wide fluctuation of the toluric acid concentrations in the spontaneous urine samples even under comparable conditions of exposure. For these reasons merely a single measurement which is numerically above or below the BAT value cannot be regarded as “adhering to” or “exceeding" it. This is only possible if the single measurement is not within the fluctuation range of the toluric acid concentration. According to the values described in the literature in all probability when the value measured is less than 0.5 or more than 4 g/l the BAT value is observed or exceeded, respectively.

Similar considerations also apply for fluctuation of the blood xylene concentration within wide limits. After a single measurement adherence to or exceeding of the BAT value can only be recognised if the xylene concentration in the blood is less than 0.4 or more than 3.0 mg/l, respectively. Due to the rapid decrease in the xylene concentration after the end of exposure blood sampling directly at the workplace at the end of exposure is recommended.

8 References

1. Šedivec, V., Flek, J.: Int. Arch. Occup. Environ. Health *37* (1976), 205–217
2. Šedivec, V., Flek, J.: Int. Arch. Occup. Environ. Health *37* (1976), 219–232
3. Åstrand, I., Engström, J., Övrum, P.: Scand. J. Work Environ. Health *4* (1978), 185–195
4. Senczuk, W., Orlowski, J.: Brit. J. Ind. Med. *35* (1978), 50–55
5. Riihimäki, V.: Scand. J. Work Environ. Health *5* (1979), 135–142
6. Engström, K., Husman, K., Riihimäki, V.: Int. Arch. Occup. Environ. Health *39* (1977), 181–189
7. Riihimäki, V., Pfäffli, P.: Scand. J. Work. Environ. Health *4* (1978), 73–85
8. Angerer, J.: Schriftenreihe Arbeitsmed. Sozialmed. Präventivmed. Bd. 71. Gentner Verlag, Stuttgart 1983
9. Riihimäki, V., Pfäffli, P., Savolainen, K., Pekari, K.: Scand. J. Work Environ. Health *5* (1979), 217–231
10. Hagemann, J., Angerer, J.: Verhandlungen der Deutschen Gesellschaft für Arbeitsmedizin e.V., 18. Jahrestagung in Frankfurt/M.-Hoechst vom 24.–27. 5. 1978. Loskant, H. (ed.). Gentner Verlag, Stuttgart 1978, pp. 365–371
11. National Institute for Occupational Safety and Health (NIOSH): Criteria for a recommended standard occupational exposure to xylene. H. E. W. Publication; No. 75/168 (1975)
12. World Health Oraganization (WHO): Study group on internationally recommended health based occupational exposure limits to selected organic solvents. Geneva 17.–23. 6. 1979
13. Henschler, D. (ed.): Xylol (alle Isomeren). Gesundheitsschädliche Arbeitsstoffe. Toxikologisch-arbeitsmedizinische Begründungen von MAK-Werten. 9th issue. VCH Verlagsgesellschaft, Weinheim 1983
14. Deutsche Gesellschaft für Mineralölwissenschaft und Kohlechemie: Wirkung von Xylol auf Mensch und Tier. Forschungsbericht, (1984), 174-8
15. Koelsch, F.: Handbuch der Berufskrankheiten, 2nd ed. Fischer Verlag, Jena 1959
16. Browning, E.: Toxicity and metabolism of industrial solvents. Elsevier, Amsterdam 1965, pp. 77-79
17. Sandmeyer, E. E. in: Patty's Industrial Hygiene and Toxicology, Vol. II B. Wiley & Sons, New York 1981
18. Valentin, H.: ASP *5* (1979), 105–110
19. Carpenter, C. P., Kinkead, E. R., Geary, D. L., Sullivan, I. J., King, J. M.: Toxicol. Appl. Pharmacol. *33* (1975), 543–558
20. Nelson, K. W., Ege, F. J., Ross. U., Woodman, L. E., Silverman, L.: J. Ind. Hyg. Toxicol. *25* (1943), 282
21. Sukhanova, V. A., Makar'eva, L. M., Boiko, V. I.: Gig. Sanit. *34* (1969), 130–132
22. Boiko, V. I.: Gig. Tr. Prof. Zabol. *6* (1970), 23–25
23. Stolbova, A. I.: Sborn. Trud. Kuybishevskoyo NII Gigieny, M. *7* (1972), 200
24. Gamberale, F., Annwall, G., Hultengren, M.: Scand. J. Work Environ Health *4* (1978), 204–211
25. Moeschlin, S.: Klinik und Therapie der Vergiftungen, 1st ed., Thieme Verlag, Stuttgart 1952
26. Smolik, R., Lange, A., Zatonski, W., Juzwiak, I., Andreasik, Z.: Polski Tygodnik Lekarski *28* (1973), 769–771

27. Lange, A., Smolik, R., Zatonski, W., Szymanski, J.: Int. Arch. Arbeitsmed. *31* (1973), 37–44
28. Lange, A., Smolik, R., Zatonski, W., Glazmann, H.: Int. Arch. Arbeitsmed. *31* (1973), 45–50
29. Ungvary, G., Tatrai, E., Hudak, A., Barcza, G., Lorincz, M.: Toxicology *18* (1980), 61–74
30. Ungvary, G., Varga, B., Horvath, E., Tatrai, E., Folly, G.: Toxicology *19* (1981), 263–268
31. Krotov, I. A., Chebotar, N. A.: Gig. Tr. Prof. Zabol. *16* (1972), 40–43, cited acc. NIOSH (1975) (11)
32. Hudak, A., Ungvary, G.: Toxicology *11* (1978), 55–63
33. Hofmann, A., Norpoth, K., Bolt, H. M., Gelbke, H.-P.: ASP *18* (1983), 181–185
34. Angerer, J., Lehnert, G.: Berufliche Belastung durch Xylol und Ethylbenzol. In: Konietzko/Schuckmann (eds.), 24. Jahrestagung der DGAUM vom 2.–5. Mai 1984, Mainz, Gentner Verlag Stuttgart, S. 267–270 (1984)
35. Engström, K., Husman, K., Pfäffli, P., Riihimäki, V.: Scand. J. Work Environ. Health *4* (1978), 114–121
36. Ogata, M., Tomokuni, K., Takatsuka, Y.: Brit. J. Ind. Med. *27* (1970), 43–50
37. Savolainen, K., Riihimäki, V., Seppäläinen, A. M., Linnoila, M.: Int. Arch. Occup. Environ. Health *45* (1980), 105–121
38. Savolainen, K., Riihimäki, V., Linnoila, M.: Int. Arch. Occup. Environ. Health *44* (1979), 201–211
39. Ogata, M., Yamazaki, Y., Sugihara R., Shimada, Y., Meguro, T.: Int. Arch. Occup. Environ. Health *46* (1980), 127–139
40. Norpoth, K., Heger, M.: Kreatinin als Bezugsgröße bei der Angabe von Stoffkonzentrationen im Harn. In: Henschler, D., Lehnert, G. (eds.): Biologische Arbeitsstoff-Toleranz-Werte und Expositionsäquivalente für krebserzeugende Arbeitsstoffe (EKA). Arbeitsmedizinisch-toxikologische Begründungen, 2nd issue. Deutsche Forschungsgemeinschaft, VCH Verlagsgesellschaft, Weinheim 1984
41. Angerer, J., Lehnert, G.: Verhandlungen der Deutschen Gesellschaft für Arbeitsmedizin e.V., 24. Jahrestagung in Mainz vom 2. bis 5. Mai 1984. Konietzko, J. (ed.). Gentner Verlag, Stuttgart 1984
42. Angerer, J., Schaller, K. H., Wardenbach P.: *o-*, *m-*, *p*-Tolursäure, Hippursäure in Harn. In: Henschler, D. (ed.): Analytische Methoden zur Prüfung gesundheitsschädlicher Arbeitsstoffe. Bd. 2: Analysen in biologischem Material, 6th issue. Deutsche Forschungsgemeinschaft, VCH Verlagsgesellschaft, Weinheim 1982

Author: J. Angerer
Approved by the Working Group: 17th February 1984

Tab. 1A: Investigations on xylene exposure of humans – A: Toluric acid excretion in urine

Collective; Duration of exposure; Substance	Xylene concentration air [ml/m³]	Toluric acid	Sampling time	Comments	Literature
23 ♂ test persons; 7 h; *m*-xylene					
a)	100	3140 mg/l	during the last 4 h of exposure	Decrease in the systolic blood pressure	Ogata, Tomokuni, Takatsuka [1970] (36)
b)	200	5790 mg/l	during the last 4 h of exposure	Increase in the reaction time	
4 ♂ test persons; 8 h; *o*-xylene, *m*-xylene, *p*-xylene	50	929.5 mg/24 h	during and 20 h after exposure	Respiratory minute volume 9 l/min	Šedivec, Fleck [1976] (2)
		527.4–2259.1 mg/l	during the last two hours of exposure	Respiratory minute volume 9 l/min	
6 ♂ test persons; 8 h; *o*-, *m*-, *p*-xylene	75	approx. 1130 mg/ 24 h	during and 18 h after exposure	at rest	Šedivec, Fleck [1976] (2)
15 painters (14 ♂; 1 ♀) 8 h; *o*-xylene, *m*-xylene, *p*-xylene, ethyl benzene	50	665 mg/g creatinine	during the last 3 h of exposure	The concentration in the urine was probably measured 15 % too low	Engström, Husman, Pfäffli, Riihimäki [1978] (35)
10 test persons (♂; 5 ♀) 8 h; *m*-xylene				Respiratory minute volume 7.6 l/min ♀ 9.6 l/min ♂	Senczuk, Orlowski [1978] (4)
a)	22.7	♂ 532.5 mg/24 h ♀ 429.3 mg/24 h	during and 16 h after exposure		
b)	68.1	♂ 1489.3 mg/24 h ♀ 1137.3 mg/24 h			
c)	136.2	♂ 2838.4 mg/24 h ♀ 2111.9 mg/24 h			

Tab. 1A: Continued

Collective; Duration of exposure; Substance	Xylene concentration air [ml/m^3]	Toluric acid	Sampling time	Comments	Literature
18 ♂ test persons; 6 h/d; 5 d; *m*-xylene					Riihimäki, Pfäffli Savolainen [1979] (9)
a)	90; constant	1427 mg/24 h	during and 18 h after exposure	Periodic physical work	
b)	93; 70–200	1610 mg/24 h		Periodic physical work	
c)	94; constant	1152 mg/24 h		(at rest)	
4 ♂ test persons; 3 h; *m*-xylene	138	1639 mg/l 479 mg/24 h	end of exposure		Ogata, Yanazaki, Sugihara, Shimada, Meguro [1980] (39)
4 ♂ med. tech. assistants; 8 h; *o*-xylene, *m*-xylene, *p*-xylene, ethyl benzene					Angerer [1983] (8)
a) 3 ♀	81	337–1201 mg/l	during the last 1.5 h of exposure		
b) 1 ♀	66	517 mg/l			
35 ♂ painters; 8 h; *o*-xylene, *m*-xylene, *p*-xylene ethyl benzene;	4.6–19.4	286–588 mg/l	end of exposure	The concentrations stated are average values at the individual work-places	Angerer [1984] (34)
6 workplaces	11.9	383		Average of all workplaces	

Tab. 1B: Investigations on xylene exposure of humans – B: Level of the toxic substance in the blood

Collective; Duration of exposure; Substance	Xylene concentration air [ml/m^3]	Xylene concentration in the blood [mg/l]	Sampling time	Comments	Literature
15 painters (14 ♂ ; 1 ♀) 8 h; *o*-xylene, *m*-xylene, *p*-xylene			1 min after exposure	Authors register great fluctuations in the blood concentration	Engström, Husman, Pfäffli, Riihimäki [1978] (35)
	1–20	0.07–0.42			
	21–40	0.33–0.62			
	41–60	0.31–1.36			
12 ♂ test persons; 2 h; *o*-xylene, *m*-xylene, *p*-xylene, ethyl benzene			at the end of exposure	90 min physical work 30 min rest	Åstrand, Engström, Övrum [1978] (3)
a)	196	6.1			
b)	98	5.2			
6 ♂ test persons; 6 h/d; 8 d; *m*-xylene			at the end of exposure	at rest	Savolainen, Riihimäki, Linnoila [1979] (38)
a)	100	1.05			
b)	200	2.11		Disturbances in the vestibular function	
c)	200 (130–400)	3.19		Severe disturbances in the sense of balance Feeling of drunkenness Reduced reaction time	
18 ♂ test persons; 6 h/d; 5 d; *m*-xylene			at the end of exposure		Riihimäki, Pfäffli, Savolainen [1979] (9)
a)	90	up to 2.01			
b)	93 (70–200)	up to 5.40		Periodic physical work	
c)	94	up to 1.06		at rest	

Tab. 1B: Continued

Collective; Duration of exposure; Substance	Xylene concentration air [ml/m^3]	Xylene concentration in the blood [mg/l]	Sampling time	Comments	Literature
8 ♂ test persons; 6 h/d; 6 d; *m*-xylene			continuously during exposure	Physical work: 100 W; 4 times a day 10 mins	Savolainen, Riihimäki, Seppäläinen, Linnoila [1980] (37)
a)	90	x = 1.7		Disturbances in the sense of balance, increase in the reaction time, disturbance in manual co-ordination	
b)	93 (64–200)	x = 2.3		Disturbance in the vestibular function, increase in the reaction time	
		as from 1.0		Disturbance in the vestibular function	Savolainen quoted in Savolainen et al. [1980] (37)
35 ♂ painters; 8 h/d; *o*-xylene, *m*-xylene, *p*-xylene, ethyl benzene; 6 workplaces			at the end of exposure		Angerer [1984] (34)
	4.6–19.4	0.058–0.226		Single values evaluated at the individual workplaces	
	11.9	0.164		Average of all persons and workplaces	

Index for Volumes 1–4

Acetic acid 2-butoxyethyl ester **3** 93
Acetic acid-2-ethoxyethyl ester **1** 71
Acetone **3** 65–77
Acetylcholinesterase inhibitors **2** 15–24
Acrylamide **3** 243–248
Acrylic acid amide **3** 243–248
Acrylonitrile **2** 183–192
Alkali chromates (Cr(VI) **1** 187–203
Alkyl phosphates **2** 15–24
Alkyl sulphates **2** 15–24
Aluminium **1** 3–16
Aluminium hydroxide **1** 3–16
Aluminium oxide **1** 3–16
Aminobenzene **2** 25–34
4-Aminodiphenyl **2** 193–201
p-Aminodiphenyl **2** 193–201
2-Aminonaphthalene **2** 213–221
2-Aniline **2** 25–34
Antimony and its inorganic compounds **4** 141-149
Arsenic and inorganic arsenic compounds **4** 171-178
Arsenic acid **4** 171-178
Arsenic pentoxide **4** 171-178
Arsenic trioxide **2** 124–136
Arsenic trioxide **4** 171-178
Arsenous acids **4** 171-178
Benzene **3** 217–231
Benzene-γ-hexachloride **2** 67–75
Beryllium and its inorganic compounds **4** 151-158
Blasting gelatin **3** 143–162
2-Bromo-2-chloro-1,1,1-trifluoroethane **2** 35-42
Bromomethane **3** 249–257
Bromomethane **4** 189-199
2-Butanone **2** 43–50
2-Butoxyethanol **3** 79–92
n-Butoxyethanol **3** 79–92
2-Butoxyethanol acetate **3** 93
2-Butoxyethyl acetate **3** 93
Butyl Cellosolve® **3** 79–92
Butyl Cellosolve® acetate **3** 93
Butylene oxide **2** 99–105
O-Butyl ethylene glycol **3** 79–92
Butyl glycol **3** 79–92
Butyl glycol acetate **3** 93
***p-tert*-Butyl phenol** **1** 17–21
Calcium arsenate **4** 171-178
Carbamates **2** 15–24
Carbinol **1** 99–114
Carbon disulphide **1** 23–29
Carbon monoxide **1** 31–35
Carbon tetrachloride **1** 153–161
Carbon tetrachloride **4** 117-118
Cellosolve® **1** 57–70
Cellosolve acetate® **1** 71
Chlorobenzene **1** 37–44
Chloroethylene **2** 173–179
Cinnamene **3** 163–184
Cinnamol **3** 163–184
Cobalt **1** 205–216
Cresols (all isomers) **4** 179-188
m-Cresol **4** 179-188
o-Cresol **4** 179-188
p-Cresol **4** 179-188
m-Cresylic acid **4** 179-188
o-Cresylic acid **4** 179-188
p-Cresylic acid **4** 179-188
Cyclohexane **4** 13-22
1,4-DCB **3** 95–104
p-DCB **3** 95–104
Diamide **2** 153–159
p,p'-Diaminodiphenylmethane **2** 203–212
4,4'-Diaminodiphenylmethane **2** 203–212
1,4-Dichlorobenzene **3** 95–104
1,4-Dichlorobenzene **4** 159
p-Dichlorobenzene **3** 95–104
Dichloromethane **1** 45–55
Dichloromethane **4** 123-126
Diethylene oxide **2** 99–105
Dimethylbenzene **2** 107–119
***N,N*-Dimethylformamide** **2** 51–57
Dimethylketone **3** 65–77
Dimethyl sulfate **3** 233–239
DMF **2** 51–57
DMS **3** 233–239
E 605 **2** 83–88
EGDN **3** 105–121
Ethene **2** 137–143
Ethenylbenzene **3** 163–184
2-Ethoxyethanol **1** 57–70
2-Ethoxyethyl acetate **1** 71

Essential BAT Value Documentations. DFG, Deutsche Forschungsgemeinschaft

ISBN 3-527-31477-6

Ethylene **2** 137–143
Ethylene glycol dinitrate **3** 105–121
Ethylene glycol monobutyl ether **3** 79–92
Ethylene glycol monobutyl ether acetate **3** 93
Ethylene glycol monoethyl ether **1** 57–70
Ethylene glycol monoethyl ether acetate **1** 71
Ethylene glycol *n*-butyl ether **3** 79–92
Ethylene oxide **2** 145–151
Ethyl glycol **1** 57–70
Ethyl glycol acetate **1** 71
Ethyl methyl ketone **2** 43–50
Formic acid methyl ester **4** 23-29
N-Formyldimethylamine **2** 51–57
Glycerol nitric acid triester **3** 143–162
Glyceryl trinitrate **3** 143–162
Glycide nitrate **3** 105–121
Glycol butyl ether **3** 79–92
Glycol dinitrate **3** 105–121
Glycol monobutyl ether acetate **3** 93
Glycol monoethyl acetate **1** 71
Halothane **2** 35–42
γ-HCH **2** 67–75
Hexachlorobenzene **2** 59–65
Hexachlorobenzene **4** 31-37
γ-1,2,3,4,5,6-Hexachlorocyclohexane **2** 67-75
Hexahydrobenzene **4** 13-22
Hexamethylene **4** 13-22
Hexanaphthene **4** 13-22
***n*-Hexane** **1** 73–85
2-Hexanone **1** 87
Hexone **1** 115–122
Hydrazine **2** 153–159
Hydrogen fluoride and inorganic fluorine compounds (fluorides) **1** 89–97
1-Hydroxy-2-methylbenzene **4** 179-188
1-Hydroxy-3-methylbenzene **4** 179-188
1-Hydroxy-4-methylbenzenel **4** 179-188
1-Hydroxy-4-*tert*-butylbenzene **1** 17–21
Hydroxytoluene **4** 179-188
2-Hydroxytoluene **4** 179-188
3-Hydroxytoluene **4** 179-188
4-Hydroxytoluene **4** 179-188
Isobutyl methyl ketone **1** 115–122
Isopropanol **1** 129–138
Isopropyl alcohol **1** 129–138
β-Ketopropane **3** 65–77
Lead and its compounds **4** 39-87
Lead arsenate **4** 171-188
Lead tetraethyl **2** 89–98
Lead tetramethyl **3** 185–187
Lindane **2** 67–75
Manganese and its inorganic compounds **4** 89-115
MBK **1** 87
MDA **2** 203–212
MEK **2** 43–50
Mercury, metallic mercury and inorganic mercury compounds **3** 123–142
Mercury, organic mercury compounds **4** 161-168
Methanol **1** 99–114
Methyl alcohol **1** 99–114
Methylbenzene 3 189-204
Methyl bromide **3** 249–257
Methyl bromide **4** 189-199
Methyl-*n*-butyl-ketone **1** 87
Methyl chloroform **1** 163–170
Methylene chloride **1** 45–55
Methylene chloride **4** 123-126
4,4-Methylenedianiline **2** 203–212
Methyl ethyl ketone **2** 43–50
Methyl formate **4** 23-29
Methyl isobutyl ketone **1** 155–122
Methyl methanoate **4** 23-29
4-Methylpentan-2-one **1** 155–122
Methylphenol **4** 179-188
2-Methylphenol **4** 179-188
3-Methylphenol **4** 179-188
4-Methylphenol **4** 179-188
Methyl sulfate **3** 233–239
MIBK **1** 155–122
Monobromethane **4** 189-199
Monobromomethane **3** 249–257
Monobutyl glycol ether **3** 79–92
Monochlorobenzene **1** 37–44
2-Naphthylamine **2** 213–221
β-Naphthylamine **2** 213–221
Nickel / sparingly soluble nickel compounds **2** 161-172
Nitrobenzene **2** 77–82
Nitroglycerin **3** 143–162
Nitroglycerol **3** 143–162
Nitroglycide **3** 105–121
Nitrostigmine **2** 83–88
Organic phosphates **2** 15–24
Organic sulphates **2** 15–24
3-Oxa-1-heptanol **3** 79–92
Oxolane **2** 99–105
Paraphos **2** 83–88
Parathion **2** 83–88
PCP **1** 217–235

Pentachlorophenol 1 217–235
Perchlorobenzene **2** 59–65
Perchloroethylene **1** 139–151
Perchloroethylene **4** 127-129
Phenol 1 123–128
Phenol 4 201-205
Phenylamine **2** 25–34
Phenylethylene **3** 163–184
Phenylmethane **3** 189–204
1,2,3-Propanetriol trinitrate **3** 143–162
2-Propanol 1 129–138
2-Propanone **3** 65–77
2-Propenamide **3** 243–248
Propenenitrile **2** 183–192
Sodium arsenite **4** 171-178
Stibium **4** 141-149
Styrene 3 163–184
Styrol **3** 163–184
Styrolene **3** 163–184
Sulfuric acid dimethyl ester **3** 233–239
Sulphonates **2** 15–24
Tetrachloroethene 1 139–151
Tetrachloroethene 4 127-129
Tetrachloromethane 1 153–161
Tetrachloromethane 4 117-118
Tetraethyllead 2 89–98
Tetraethylplumbane **2** 89–98
Tetrahydrofuran 2 99–105
Tetrahydrofuran 4 119-120
Tetramethylene oxide **2** 99–105
Tetramethyllead 3 185–187
Tetramethylplumbane **3** 185–187
Toluene 3 189–204
Toluol **3** 189–204
1,1,1-Trichloroethane 1 163–170
Trichloroethene 1 171–183
Trichloroethene 4 131-137
Trichloroethylene **1** 171–183
Trichloroethylene **4** 131-137
Trinitroglycerol **3** 143–162
Vanadic anhydride **3** 205–214
Vanadium(V) oxide **3** 205–214
Vanadium pentoxide 3 205–214
VCM **2** 173–179
Vinylbenzene **3** 163–184
Vinyl chloride 2 173–179
Vinyl cyanide **2** 183–192
Xylenes 2 107–119